Urinary Tract Health and Care

Urinary Tract Health and Care

Guest Editors

Matteo Frigerio
Stefano Manodoro

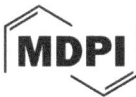

Basel • Beijing • Wuhan • Barcelona • Belgrade • Novi Sad • Cluj • Manchester

Guest Editors

Matteo Frigerio
Fondazione IRCCS San
Gerardo dei Tintori
Milano-Bicocca University
Monza
Italy

Stefano Manodoro
ASST Santi Paolo e Carlo
San Paolo Hospital
University of Milan
Milano
Italy

Editorial Office
MDPI AG
Grosspeteranlage 5
4052 Basel, Switzerland

This is a reprint of the Special Issue, published open access by the journal *Healthcare* (ISSN 2227-9032), freely accessible at: https://www.mdpi.com/journal/healthcare/special_issues/urinary_tract_health.

For citation purposes, cite each article independently as indicated on the article page online and as indicated below:

Lastname, A.A.; Lastname, B.B. Article Title. *Journal Name* **Year**, *Volume Number*, Page Range.

ISBN 978-3-7258-3750-2 (Hbk)
ISBN 978-3-7258-3749-6 (PDF)
https://doi.org/10.3390/books978-3-7258-3749-6

© 2025 by the authors. Articles in this book are Open Access and distributed under the Creative Commons Attribution (CC BY) license. The book as a whole is distributed by MDPI under the terms and conditions of the Creative Commons Attribution-NonCommercial-NoDerivs (CC BY-NC-ND) license (https://creativecommons.org/licenses/by-nc-nd/4.0/).

Contents

Preface vii

Ayman Qatawneh, Fatemah N. Lari, Wedad A. Sawas, Fatemah A. Alsabree, Mariam Kh. Alowaisheer, Marah A. Aldarawsheh and Renad A. Alshareef
Management of Stress Urinary Incontinence by Obstetricians and Gynecologists in Jordan: A Nationwide Survey Study
Reprinted from: *Healthcare* **2024**, *12*, 1489, https://doi.org/10.3390/healthcare12151489 1

Svetlana Jankovic, Marija Rovcanin, Milena Zamurovic, Branka Jovanovic, Tatjana Raicevic and Ana Tomic
Multifaceted Impact of CO_2 Laser Therapy on Genitourinary Syndrome of Menopause, Vulvovaginal Atrophy and Sexual Function
Reprinted from: *Healthcare* **2024**, *12*, 1385, https://doi.org/10.3390/healthcare12141385 10

Lorenzo Campanella, Gianluca Gabrielli, Erika Chiodo, Vitaliana Stefanachi, Ermelinda Pennacchini, Debora Grilli, et al.
Minimally Invasive Treatment of Stress Urinary Incontinence in Women: A Prospective Comparative Analysis between Bulking Agent and Single-Incision Sling
Reprinted from: *Healthcare* **2024**, *12*, 751, https://doi.org/10.3390/healthcare12070751 20

Tehila Fisher-Yosef, Dina Lidsky Sachs, Shiri Sacha Edel, Hanan Nammouz, Abd Ellatif Zoabi and Limor Adler
Pelvic Floor Dysfunction among Reproductive-
Age Women in Israel: Prevalence and Attitudes—A Cross-Sectional Study
Reprinted from: *Healthcare* **2024**, *12*, 390, https://doi.org/10.3390/healthcare12030390 30

Alessandro Ferdinando Ruffolo, Maurizio Serati, Arianna Casiraghi, Vittoria Benini, Chiara Scancarello, Maria Carmela Di Dedda, et al.
The Impact of Systemic Sclerosis on Sexual Health: An Italian Survey
Reprinted from: *Healthcare* **2023**, *11*, 2346, https://doi.org/10.3390/healthcare11162346 42

Milka B. Popović, Deana D. Medić, Radmila S. Velicki and Aleksandra I. Jovanović Galović
Purple Urine Bag Syndrome in a Home-Dwelling Elderly Female with Lumbar Compression Fracture: A Case Report
Reprinted from: *Healthcare* **2023**, *11*, 2251, https://doi.org/10.3390/healthcare11162251 53

Marta Barba, Alice Cola, Giorgia Rezzan, Clarissa Costa, Tomaso Melocchi, Desirèe De Vicari, et al.
Flat Magnetic Stimulation for Stress Urinary Incontinence: A 3-Month Follow-Up Study
Reprinted from: *Healthcare* **2023**, *11*, 1730, https://doi.org/10.3390/healthcare11121730 62

Gaetano Maria Munno, Marco La Verde, Davide Lettieri, Roberta Nicoletti, Maria Nunziata, Diego Domenico Fasulo, et al.
Pelvic Organ Prolapse Syndrome and Lower Urinary Tract Symptom Update: What's New?
Reprinted from: *Healthcare* **2023**, *11*, 1513, https://doi.org/10.3390/healthcare11101513 72

Pier Luigi Palma, Pierluigi Marzuillo, Anna Di Sessa, Stefano Guarino, Daniela Capalbo, Maria Maddalena Marrapodi, et al.
From Clinical Scenarios to the Management of Lower Urinary Tract Symptoms in Children: A Focus for the General Pediatrician
Reprinted from: *Healthcare* **2023**, *11*, 1285, https://doi.org/10.3390/healthcare11091285 82

Yoav Baruch, Stefano Manodoro, Marta Barba, Alice Cola, Ilaria Re and Matteo Frigerio
Prevalence and Severity of Pelvic Floor Disorders during Pregnancy: Does the Trimester Make a Difference?
Reprinted from: *Healthcare* **2023**, *11*, 1096, https://doi.org/10.3390/healthcare11081096 92

Esther Díaz-Mohedo, Itxaso Odriozola Aguirre, Elena Molina García, Miguel Angel Infantes-Rosales and Fidel Hita-Contreras
Functional Exercise Versus Specific Pelvic Floor Exercise: Observational Pilot Study in Female University Students
Reprinted from: *Healthcare* **2023**, *11*, 561, https://doi.org/10.3390/healthcare11040561 101

Mattia Dominoni, Annachiara Licia Scatigno, Marco La Verde, Stefano Bogliolo, Chiara Melito, Andrea Gritti, et al.
Microbiota Ecosystem in Recurrent Cystitis and the Immunological Microenvironment of Urothelium
Reprinted from: *Healthcare* **2023**, *11*, 525, https://doi.org/10.3390/healthcare11040525 111

María Paz López-Pérez, Diego Fernando Afanador-Restrepo, Yulieth Rivas-Campo, Fidel Hita-Contreras, María del Carmen Carcelén-Fraile, Yolanda Castellote-Caballero, et al.
Pelvic Floor Muscle Exercises as a Treatment for Urinary Incontinence in Postmenopausal Women: A Systematic Review of Randomized Controlled Trials
Reprinted from: *Healthcare* **2023**, *11*, 216, https://doi.org/10.3390/healthcare11020216 127

Matteo Frigerio, Marta Barba, Giuseppe Marino, Silvia Volontè, Tomaso Melocchi, Desirèe De Vicari, et al.
Coexistent Detrusor Overactivity-Underactivity in Patients with Pelvic Floor Disorders
Reprinted from: *Healthcare* **2022**, *10*, 1720, https://doi.org/10.3390/healthcare10091720 137

Chu-Ling Chang
Effect of Immersive Virtual Reality on Post-Baccalaureate Nursing Students' In-Dwelling Urinary Catheter Skill and Learning Satisfaction
Reprinted from: *Healthcare* **2022**, *10*, 1473, https://doi.org/10.3390/healthcare10081473 145

Preface

Dear Colleagues,

Lower urinary tract symptoms are common in women of all ages, with different causes and expressions according to patient age and condition. Most of the time, the symptoms are transitory and recover with no or simple therapy. Nevertheless, for some women, the symptoms are ongoing and interfere with normal routines, impacting the quality of life.

Urinary tract dysfunctions range from infective disorders to impaired continence physiology, with urinary incontinence and or urinary outlet obstruction, as well as chronic pelvic pain of unknown origin and dyspareunia. Frequently, these aspects combine with each other, leading to complex clinical presentations.

Many women never tell anyone about their symptoms and are reticent even with their gynecologist. Referral to a pelvic floor center is not usually required. On the other hand, the management of these conditions is never fulfilled by one single specialist but by a team of specialists who work together to ensure pelvic floor and urinary tract health.

This Special Issue of *Healthcare* is dedicated to offering an overview of female urinary tract health and care.

Matteo Frigerio and Stefano Manodoro
Guest Editors

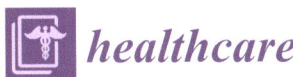

Article

Management of Stress Urinary Incontinence by Obstetricians and Gynecologists in Jordan: A Nationwide Survey Study

Ayman Qatawneh [1,*], Fatemah N. Lari [2], Wedad A. Sawas [2], Fatemah A. Alsabree [2], Mariam Kh. Alowaisheer [2], Marah A. Aldarawsheh [2] and Renad A. Alshareef [2]

1. Department of Obstetrics and Gynecology, The University of Jordan, Amman 11942, Jordan
2. Department of Medicine, The University of Jordan, Amman 11942, Jordan; fatimaa_lari@hotmail.com (F.N.L.); wedadsawas@gmail.com (W.A.S.); fatemah.alsabree@hotmail.com (F.A.A.); mkalowaisheer98@gmail.com (M.K.A.); m_aldarawsheh@yahoo.com (M.A.A.); renad.abdullah.alshareef@gmail.com (R.A.A.)
* Correspondence: a.qatawneh@ju.edu.jo

Abstract: Background: Stress urinary incontinence (SUI) is a common condition that can significantly impact a patient's quality of life. Although multiple diagnostic and treatment options exist, significant variability in SUI management exists between countries. Since women's SUI prevalence in Jordan is high, and Jordan is a lower-middle-income country, this study aimed to investigate how obstetricians and gynecologists (OBGYNs) across Jordan manage and treat women with SUI. Method: A Google Forms survey was prepared and sent out to Jordanian OBGYNs via WhatsApp. The results were collected and arranged in Microsoft Excel and then transferred to SPSS for statistical analysis. Results: Out of the 804 Jordanian registered OBGYNs, 497 could be reached, 240 conduct gynecological surgeries, and 94 completed the survey, providing a response rate of 39.2%. Most of the respondents were females between 41 and 55 years old. More than 70% of the OBGYNs worked in the private sector, and 88.3% operated in the capital of Jordan. Most of the respondents favored lifestyle and behavior therapy (43.6%) or pelvic floor physiotherapy (40.4%) as the first-line management for SUI. The transobturator mid-urethral sling (MUS) was the most common initial surgical treatment option. The physicians preferred two-staged procedures for the repair of pelvic organ prolapse alongside concomitant SUI. In the case of recurrent SUI following surgery, 77% of the respondents chose to refer to a urologist or urogynecologist. Conclusions: The Jordanian OBGYNs preferred using lifestyle/behavioral therapy and pelvic floor muscle physiotherapy as the first-line treatment to manage SUI. Secondly, the MUS would be the most frequently preferred surgical choice. To effectively manage SUI, adequate training in urogynecology and referral resources are essential in lower-middle-income countries.

Keywords: stress urinary incontinence; urogynecology; survey study; Jordan

1. Introduction

Urinary incontinence is a common global problem affecting around 423 million people over 20 years old [1], indicating a high incidence and prevalence. Furthermore, urinary incontinence is considered to be a major challenge for the health system. Urinary incontinence has different forms, including urge urinary incontinence and stress urinary incontinence (SUI) [2,3]. Urge urinary incontinence affects men, whereas SUI dominates in women [2,3]. According to the International Urogynecological Association (IUGA)/International Continence Society (ICS), SUI is defined as the involuntary leakage of urine upon effort, physical exertion, coughing, or sneezing [4,5]. The two main mechanisms behind SUI are urethral hypermobility, which occurs due to the loss of support from the pelvic floor muscles or vaginal connective tissue, and intrinsic sphincter deficiency, which occurs due to the loss of the mucosal and muscular tone in the urethra and tends to be more severe [6,7]. SUI affects the quality of life of millions of women worldwide, affecting their physical, social, and

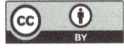

sexual health, thereby causing anxiety, depression, and the urge to withdraw from daily activities [8]. Therefore, it is paramount that viable treatment options with high curative rates and low complication rates are offered to women to improve their quality of life.

Conservative measures and surgical methods are recommended to patients to improve their quality of life [9–11]. The patient's assessment begins with a focused history and physical exam and can include different investigations, such as post-residual urine volume, urine testing, and urodynamic testing [10]. Similarly, the management can range from conservative options such as pelvic floor exercises with or without biofeedback that support dynamic lumbopelvic stabilization and lumbar muscle resistance training to various surgical procedures such as bladder neck injections, mid-urethral slings, and colposuspension [9–11].

Many scientific groups or institutions have already developed SUI diagnosis and management recommendations. Nevertheless, regional variations in practice patterns exist, especially in lower-middle-income countries (LMICs) [12]. With the different diagnostic and treatment modalities available, coupled with the bans on polypropylene mesh in certain countries, it is crucial to understand and analyze how physicians worldwide and from LMICs treat SUI [13]. In Jordan, which is an LMIC, several studies reported high SUI prevalence among women [14–16], with approximately 37% and 16% reporting moderate and severe symptoms, respectively [16]. Thus, the present study aimed to investigate how obstetricians and gynecologists (OBGYNs) in Jordan manage and treat women with SUI.

2. Methods

2.1. Study Design

This cross-sectional study was conducted from 20 December 2022 to 9 March 2023 using an online Google Forms-based survey questionnaire (see Supplementary Materials). The investigators used the Jordanian Medical Association to obtain the listed and registered OBGYNs in Jordan. It is understandable that not all registered OBGYNs perform gynecological surgeries; however, all were reached by the investigators using the study link via WhatsApp. Participants had to meet specific eligibility criteria; the most important criterion was having seen and treated women with SUI. The study's objectives and voluntary nature were explained on the first page of the questionnaire.

The survey, a collaborative effort with esteemed OBGYNs, comprised 19 questions divided into three main sections. The first part focused on collecting demographic and specialty data, where participants were asked to provide basic information such as age, gender, practice location, training level, and work experience. The second part delved into the management and diagnostic aspects of SUI, such as preferred diagnostic modalities preoperatively and first line of management. The final section consisted of questions about the surgical treatment option that the participant would choose in different scenarios. The full survey can be found in Supplementary Materials.

2.2. IRB Approval

The research study was approved by the Institutional Review Board RB at the Jordan University hospital (11/2023/9367). On the questionnaire's first page, it was written that "the data provided will only be used for research purposes and will be dealt with confidentially. None of the questions address your identity, which will be anonymous throughout. Proceeding in completing this questionnaire will be taken as consent to participate in this study, and you are always free to withdraw at any point".

2.3. Statistical Analysis

Data were collected and transferred to a Microsoft Excel (Version 2406) spreadsheet. After coding and through double-checking, the data were exported to SPSS version 26 for statistical analysis. The validity of the questionnaire was tested using the 2-tailed Pearson correlation. Frequencies, percentages, cross-tabulations, and chi-squared analyses were conducted on continuous variables. In addition, a univariate analysis was conducted to test for association between each dependent question and fixed parameter. A *p*-value of ≤0.05 was considered significant.

3. Results

Out of the 804 registered Jordanian OBGYNs, 497 could be reached, and 240 performed gynecological surgeries and therefore were eligible for the study. Out of the 240 OBGYNs, 94 completed the survey, providing a response rate of 39.2%. The majority of the OBGYNs were between 41 and 55 years old, and the female to male ratio was ~1.8 (Table 1). More than 70% of the respondents worked in the private sector, 88.3% worked in the capital of Jordan, Amman, and a few, 8.5%, had a urogynecology specialty. Over 58% had no subspeciality.

Table 1. The demography, practice, and experience of the OBGYN respondents.

Parameters	Characteristics	Number	Percentage (%)
Age	<30 years old	7	7.4
	30–40 years old	28	29.8
	41–55 years old	34	36.2
	>55 years old	25	26.6
Gender	Female	60	63.8
	Male	34	36.2
Specialty	Gynaecology	86	91.5
	Urogynecology	8	8.5
Practice setting	Private Practice	67	71.3
	Ministry of Health	10	10.6
	Academic	10	10.6
	Other	7	7.4
Location of Practice	Amman	83	88.3
	Alzarqa	4	4.3
	Irbid	3	3.2
	Albalqa	2	2.1
	Madaba	1	1.1
	Alkarak	1	1.1
Years Out of Fellowship/Subspecialty Training	<5 years	9	9.6
	5–10 years	9	9.6
	>10 years	21	22.3
	No fellowship/subspecialty training	55	58.5

Most of the physicians favored lifestyle and behavior therapy (43.6%) or pelvic floor physiotherapy (40.4%) as the first-line management for SUI (Figure 1). On the contrary, very few respondents (14.9%) would go for surgery, and only (1%) would start with medications to manage SUI. No significant association was evident between the first-line management and the physician's age group, gender, specialty, years out of fellowship, or practice setting.

The physicians were asked about their investigations of choice before the surgical management of SUI. In this question, three processes were preferred; 26.6% (n = 25) would only perform a physical exam, and an equal amount of other respondents (26.6%) would perform stress testing, uroflow, and measure the post-residual urine volumes, and 24.5% would conduct a multichannel urodynamics test (Figure 2). To a lesser extent, 9.6% would perform a stress test and post-void residual volume, 6.4% a stress test only, and 6.4% video urodynamics. Interestingly, all six respondents who chose video urodynamics as their initial presurgical diagnostic modality worked in private practice clinics.

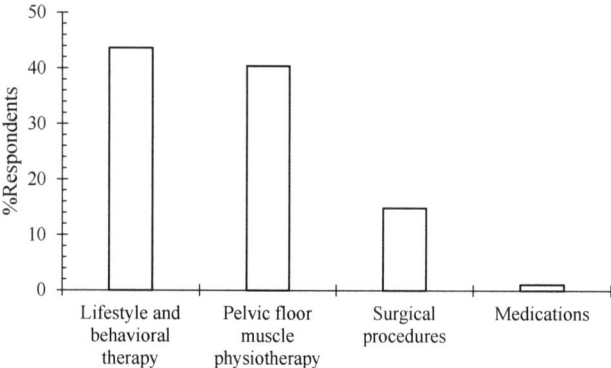

Figure 1. Breakdown of Jordanian OBJYNs' initial SUI management preferences.

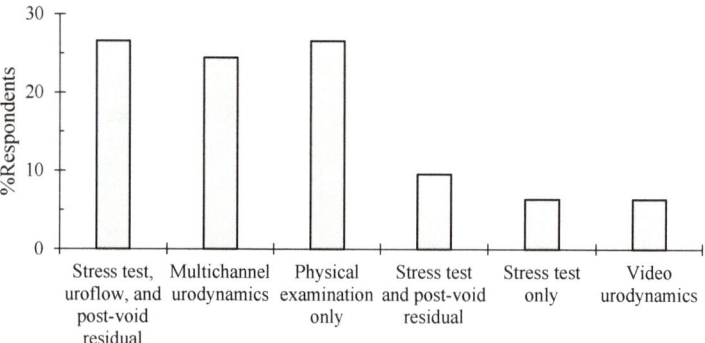

Figure 2. Breakdown of Jordanian OBJYNs' pre-surgical diagnostic modality preferences of SUI.

No significant association was established between the diagnostic modality preference and the physician's age group, gender, specialty, years out of fellowship, physician practice setting, or location.

When the OBGYNs were asked if they would repeat the urodynamics before a second operation, a significant association was found between repeating the urodynamics and the OBGYN's age group ($p < 0.01$). Seventy-one percent (71%) of the 30–40-year-old age group responded to repeat urodynamics testing all the time compared to 56%, 36%, and 14% for the 41–55, >50, and <30 age groups.

The primary surgical treatment option for the OBGYNs in Jordan was the transobturator mid-urethral sling (MUS-TO) procedure (46.8%), followed by the retropubic mid-urethral sling (MUS-RP) approach (17%), and Kelly plication (17%) was the next option in terms of frequency (Figure 3). On the other hand, bladder neck needle suspension and the Burch procedure were preferred by only 8.5% and 5.3%, respectively. Most of the physicians (79%) who had fellowship or subspecialty training favored the MUS-TO compared to 39% who did not have fellowship or OBGYN subspecialty training. These differences were significant ($p < 0.01$).

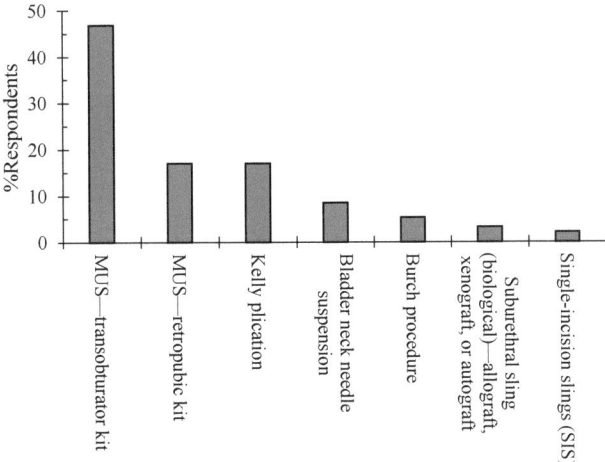

Figure 3. Jordanian OBJYNs' primary surgical treatment options for SUI.

The OBGYN's age group and gender were significantly associated with the choice regarding the primary surgical option ($p < 0.01$ and $p < 0.01$). The young OBGYNs were more prone to use the MUS-TO than older physicians. Interestingly, the percentages of using the MUS-TO were 71%, 64%, 44%, and 6% for the age groups <30, 30–40, 41–55, and >55. In addition, the male OBGYNs (62%) were more prone to use the MUS-TO compared to 38.2% of the female OBGYNs. No significant association was apparent between the primary surgical option and the specialty, years out of fellowship, or practice setting.

Next, the physicians were asked about urodynamic testing in the setting of repeat surgery. More than half (52.1%) indicated that they would always repeat the urodynamic testing, whereas 42.6% would repeat it some of the time, and 5.3% would never repeat it. Although many different treatment options were included in the questionnaire for the secondary surgical management of SUI after the failure of the primary procedure, most of the respondents (77%) stated that they would refer the patient to either a urologist or urogynecologist as a part of their management.

In the case of SUI with concomitant pelvic organ prolapse (POP), 34% of the Jordanian OBGYNs indicated that they would perform two-staged procedures, repairing the POP first, followed by SUI surgery at a later date, if indicated. Of the practitioners that would perform the surgery at the time of the POP repair, the MUS-TO was the most popular choice (21.3%), followed by Kelly plication (14.9%), the MUS-RP (9.6%), the Burch procedure (7.4%), bladder neck needle suspension (7.4%), single incision slings (4.3%), and lastly a urethral bulking agent (1.1%). No significant association was found between the preferred surgical treatment of the SUI option and the physician's age, gender, specialty, practice setting, fellowship, or years out of fellowship.

Furthermore, regarding the preferred surgical treatment to prevent de novo SUI when performing a simultaneous POP surgery in the absence of symptoms and objective evidence of SUI, the majority (66%) of the physicians indicated that they would not perform surgery. Out of the latter, most of them were female OBGYNs ($p < 0.05$) and those who did not have fellowship or subspecialty training ($p < 0.05$). On the other hand, some of the respondents (9.6%) chose Kelly plication, 8.5% selected the MUS-TO (8.5%), and 5.3% opted for the Burch procedure. The rest chose the MUS-RP (4.3%), single incision slings (3.2%), urethral bulking agents (2.1%), and bladder neck needle suspension (1.1%).

In the last two questions, the physicians were asked about the MUS material and the choice of the urethral bulking agent. Almost all the physicians (88.3%) chose synthetic material for the MUS, while only a small minority preferred autologous fascia (6.4%) and biologic materials (5.3%). As for the urethral bulking agents, the top three choices were polyacrylamide (Bulkamid) (26.6%), polytetrafluoroethylene (Teflon, PTFE) (23.4%), and bovine collagen (Contigen) (22.3%).

4. Discussion

The present study showed that the Jordanian OBGYNs preferred that the first-line treatment options follow the National Institute for Health and Care Excellence (NICE) 2023 guidelines [10], with 43.6% favoring lifestyle/behavioral therapy and 40.4% preferring pelvic floor muscle physiotherapy [9]. This preference is corroborated through research demonstrating improved quality of life and decreased urinary leakage measured by a 1 h pad test, Incontinence Quality of Life (IQOL), quality of life questionnaires, and King's health questionnaire using pelvic floor physiotherapy [17]. Furthermore, 14.9% of our target population preferred an initial surgical procedure instead of conservative measures. The latter preference is also evidenced by a multicenter, randomized study on 230 women with moderate to severe SUI whereby the initial MUS resulted in higher rates of subjective improvement and subjective and objective cure rates [18].

The Jordanian OBGYNs demonstrated that the MUS-TO is the method of choice for treating SUI at 46.8%, followed by the MUS-RP and Kelly plication at 17%. Our findings reinforce the research showing that the healthcare professionals in a tertiary-level hospital in the UK opted for the MUS as their preferred surgical approach for SUI patients [19]. On the other hand, a recent updated guideline study reported that there were conflicting studies on which one was more favorable between the MUS-TO and MUS-RP [9]. For instance, a slight advantage toward the MUS-RP was observed in a 5-year follow-up [20], whereas, in a systemic review study, no difference was found between the two treatments regarding patient satisfaction, QOL, and objective and subjective cure [21]. However, it is also essential to note that it is not only the preference of medical professionals but also patients demonstrated that a surgical curative approach was preferred when faced with severe SUI [22]. It was also observed that, when the patients were provided a scenario with a less invasive approach with similar curative rates, they opted for the less invasive option.

The less invasive advancements within the field include the use of urethral bulking agents (UBAs) [23]. Our data showed that 72.4% of the respondents have never used UBAs for SUI, and 27.6% opted for UBAs either initially or following the initial procedure failure. A systematic review and meta-analysis including 710 patients comparing the safety and effectiveness of UBAs and surgical methods demonstrated that the UBAs were less effective in terms of subjective improvement, and there was no significant difference in terms of complications following the intervention [24], thus demonstrating that the medical professional preference for surgery is validated through the merits of the procedure in terms of the balance between the outcome and complications.

Our findings showed that the diagnostic modality preference was associated with the fellowship experience. Furthermore, the primary selection of MUS-TO surgery and no need for SUI surgery when POP is present and with no symptoms of SUI were linked with or without fellowship/subspecialty training. Finally, the female OBGYNs were in favor of not performing SUI surgery when POP and SUI with no symptoms were present. This gender difference may be psychological. However, other socioeconomic factors did not affect the respondent preference when analyzing the practice settings. It is also worth noting that there was no difference in preference with respect to the geographic location or age of the respondent. It is also vital to demonstrate that our data are comparable to those in high-income countries (HICs), further demonstrating the lack of socioeconomic variables affecting the preference rather than substantiating the preference in terms of the merit of the procedure alone [19].

The European Association of Urology, NICE, and Cochrane guidelines posit that the initial surgical intervention offered to women with SUI should be an MUS [25]. Furthermore, the American Urological Association and Society of Urodynamics, Female Pelvic Medicine & Urogenital Reconstruction guidelines recommend that, if an MUS procedure is to be carried out, the surgeons should opt for a transobturator or retropubic approach [9,26].

Therefore, it is essential to substantiate the respondent's preference for the use of the MUS. However, post-operative mesh-related complications such as erosion into adjacent structures, pain during intercourse, and chronic pain were observed [19]. Although the US Food and Drug Administration and National Health Services England have banned the use of transvaginal mesh including the MUS, the incidence of these complications/symptoms to occur is low and the MUS is still the preferred surgical option for the healthcare professionals in the United Kingdom tertiary hospital [19]. Furthermore, several systematic review studies confirmed that the MUS-RP or MUS-TO are the preferred treatments for SUI [27,28].

It is vital to acknowledge the limitations of this study. Although we addressed all the OBGYNs in Jordan, most of our respondents were from one geographical region, Amman. Thus, one cannot generalize these data with certainty to the remainder of the country and other LMICs, especially when SUI is prevalent in the rural areas of Jordan and the incomes of the families are much less than in the capital, Amman [14,15]. More research would be essential comparing the medical professional preference in terms of SUI management between the LMICs and HICs. Secondly, the target population comprised OBGYNs only, posing another limitation; one could argue that the spread of preference might differ within other specialties, as demonstrated through other papers [19]. Therefore, it would be ideal if research was carried out using OBGYNs, urogynecologists, urologists, and actual patients to measure whether the medical specialty or lack thereof affects the preference. Interestingly, it is worth noting that the data gathered with regard to the management of SUI show a preference for treatment options that offer the highest symptomatic relief as well as ones with lower complication rates, which is in line with an MUS procedure [27–30].

5. Conclusions

The Jordanian OBGYNs preferred using lifestyle/behavioral therapy and pelvic floor muscle physiotherapy as the first-line treatment to manage SUI, which is according to the NICE guidelines. The MUS, mainly the MUS-TO, would be the most frequently preferred surgical choice. Furthermore, since 70% of OBGYNs refer recurrent SUI post-surgery to urogynecologists, this study supports the need for more specialization in urogynecology. Therefore, more efforts from Jordan's and LMICs' ministries of health are essential to acquire subspecialty training to tackle SUI, which is affecting millions of women's quality of life.

Supplementary Materials: The following supporting information can be downloaded at https://www.mdpi.com/article/10.3390/healthcare12151489/s1, Study questionnaire.

Author Contributions: A.Q.: Conceptualization, Project Administration, Visualization, Supervision, Writing—Review and Editing. F.N.L.: Questionnaire, Data Collection, Review of Literature, Data Analysis, Writing—original draft, Writing—review and editing. W.A.S.: Questionnaire, Data Collection, Review of Literature, Data Analysis, Writing—original draft, Writing—review and editing. F.A.A.: Data Collection, Writing—original draft. M.K.A.: Data Collection, Writing—original draft. M.A.A.: Data collection, Writing—original draft. R.A.A.: Data collection, writing—original draft. All authors have read and agreed to the published version of the manuscript.

Funding: This research received no external funding.

Institutional Review Board Statement: The research study was approved on 11 April 2023 by the Institutional Review Board IRB at the Jordan University hospital (11/2023/9367). All participants consented to participate in the study.

Informed Consent Statement: Informed consent was obtained from all subjects involved in the study.

Data Availability Statement: Data is contained within the article or Supplementary Material.

Conflicts of Interest: The authors declare no conflicts of interest.

References

1. Biswas, B.; Bhattacharyya, A.; Dasgupta, A.; Karmakar, A.; Mallick, N.; Sembiah, S. Urinary Incontinence, Its Risk Factors, and Quality of Life: A Study among Women Aged 50 Years and above in a Rural Health Facility of West Bengal. *J. Mid-Life Health* **2017**, *8*, 130–136. [CrossRef] [PubMed] [PubMed Central]
2. Broome, B.A. The impact of urinary incontinence on self-efficacy and quality of life. *Health Qual. Life Outcomes* **2003**, *1*, 35. [CrossRef] [PubMed] [PubMed Central]
3. Harland, N.; Walz, S.; Eberli, D.; Schmid, F.A.; Aicher, W.K.; Stenzl, A.; Amend, B. Stress Urinary Incontinence: An Unsolved Clinical Challenge. *Biomedicines* **2023**, *11*, 2486. [CrossRef]
4. Haylen, B.T.; de Ridder, D.; Freeman, R.M.; Swift, S.E.; Berghmans, B.; Lee, J.; Monga, A.; Petri, E.; Rizk, D.E.; Sand, P.K.; et al. An International Urogynecological Association (IUGA)/International Continence Society (ICS) joint report on the terminology for female pelvic floor dysfunction. *Int. Urogynecol. J.* **2010**, *21*, 5–26. [CrossRef] [PubMed]
5. Aoki, Y.; Brown, H.W.; Brubaker, L.; Cornu, J.N.; Daly, J.O.; Cartwright, R. Urinary incontinence in women. *Nat. Rev. Dis. Primers* **2017**, *3*, 17042, Erratum in *Nat. Rev. Dis. Primers* **2017**, *3*, 17097. [CrossRef] [PubMed] [PubMed Central]
6. Falah-Hassani, K.; Reeves, J.; Shiri, R.; Hickling, D.; McLean, L. The pathophysiology of stress urinary incontinence: A systematic review and meta-analysis. *Int. Urogynecol. J.* **2021**, *32*, 501–552. [CrossRef]
7. Wu, X.; Zheng, X.; Yi, X.; Lai, P.; Lan, Y. Electromyographic Biofeedback for Stress Urinary Incontinence or Pelvic Floor Dysfunction in Women: A Systematic Review and Meta-Analysis. *Adv. Ther.* **2021**, *38*, 4163–4177. [CrossRef] [PubMed] [PubMed Central]
8. AlQuaiz, A.M.; Kazi, A.; AlYousefi, N.; Alwatban, L.; AlHabib, Y.; Turkistani, I. Urinary incontinence affects the quality of life and increases psychological distress and low self-esteem. *Healthcare* **2023**, *11*, 1772. [CrossRef]
9. Kobashi, K.C.; Vasavada, S.; Bloschichak, A.; Hermanson, L.; Kaczmarek, J.; Kim, S.K.; Kirkby, E.; Malik, R. Updates to Surgical Treatment of Female Stress Urinary Incontinence (SUI): AUA/SUFU Guideline. *J. Urol.* **2023**, *209*, 1091–1098. [CrossRef] [PubMed]
10. NICE Guidance—Urinary incontinence and pelvic organ prolapse in women: Management: © NICE (2019) Urinary incontinence and pelvic organ prolapse in women: Management. *BJU Int.* **2019**, *123*, 777–803. [CrossRef] [PubMed]
11. Nightingale, G. Management of urinary incontinence. *Post Reprod. Health* **2020**, *26*, 63–70. [CrossRef]
12. Bazi, T.; Takahashi, S.; Ismail, S.; Bø, K.; Ruiz-Zapata, A.M.; Duckett, J.; Kammerer-Doak, D. Prevention of pelvic floor disorders: International urogynecological association research and development committee opinion. *Int. Urogynecol. J.* **2016**, *27*, 1785–1795. [CrossRef] [PubMed]
13. MacCraith, E.; Forde, J.C.; O'Brien, F.J.; Davis, N.F. Contemporary trends for urological training and management of stress urinary incontinence in Ireland. *Int. Urogynecol. J.* **2021**, *32*, 2841–2846. [CrossRef] [PubMed] [PubMed Central]
14. AlAzab, R.; Alomari, R.A.; Khader, Y.S.; Gharaibeh, M. Stress urinary incontinence among Jordanian women living in rural areas: Prevalence, associated factors and self-management behaviours. *Arab J. Urol.* **2021**, *19*, 469–472. [CrossRef] [PubMed] [PubMed Central]
15. Mahfouz, I.A.; Blanker, M.H.; Asali, F.; Al Mehaisen, L.; Al-Amoosh, H.; Mahfouz, S.A. Urinary incontinence among Jordanian women: Prevalence, types, and associated factors. *Asian J. Urol.* **2024**, in press. [CrossRef]
16. Sawaqed, F.; Al Kharabsheh, A.; Tout, M.; Zaidan, M.; Khashram, H.; AlShunaigat, N. Prevalence of stress urinary incontinence and its impact on quality of life among women in Jordan: A correlational study. *J. Int. Med. Res.* **2020**, *48*, 300060520925651. [CrossRef] [PubMed] [PubMed Central]
17. da Fonseca, L.C.; Giarreta, F.B.A.; Peterson, T.V.; Locali, P.K.M.; Baracat, E.C.; Ferreira, E.A.G.; Haddad, J.M. A randomized trial comparing vaginal laser therapy and pelvic floor physical therapy for treating women with stress urinary incontinence. *Neurourol. Urodyn.* **2023**, *42*, 1445–1454. [CrossRef] [PubMed]
18. Labrie, J.; Berghmans, B.L.; Fischer, K.; Milani, A.L.; van der Wijk, I.; Smalbraak, D.J.; Vollebregt, A.; Schellart, R.P.; Graziosi, G.C.; van der Ploeg, J.M.; et al. Surgery versus physiotherapy for stress urinary incontinence. *N. Engl. J. Med.* **2013**, *369*, 1124–1133. [CrossRef] [PubMed]
19. Araklitis, G.; Baines, G.; Da Silva, A.S.; Rantell, A.; Robinson, D.; Cardozo, L. Healthcare professional's choice for surgical management of stress urinary incontinence in a U.K. tertiary hospital. *Eur. J. Obstet. Gynecol. Reprod. Biol.* **2021**, *263*, 7–14. [CrossRef] [PubMed]
20. Kenton, K.; Stoddard, A.M.; Zyczynski, H.; Albo, M.; Rickey, L.; Norton, P.; Wai, C.; Kraus, S.R.; Sirls, L.T.; Kusek, J.W.; et al. 5-year longitudinal followup after retropubic and transobturator mid urethral slings. *J. Urol.* **2015**, *193*, 203–210. [CrossRef]
21. Juliato, C.; Santos, L., Jr.; Gomes, T.; Ranzani, F.; Castro, E.; Araujo, C. Long-term outcomes after mid-urethral slings for urinary incontinence: A systematic review and meta-analysis. *Int. Urogynecol. J.* **2018**, *29*, S138.
22. Shah, G.S.; Phillips, C. What women want now! *Eur. J. Obstet. Gynecol. Reprod. Biol.* **2023**, *286*, 118–120. [CrossRef] [PubMed]
23. Barba, M.; Frigerio, M.; Melocchi, T.; De Vicari, D.; Cola, A. Urethral Injury after Vaginal Birth and Stress Urinary Incontinence: Bulking Agents are Feasible Options. *Int. J. Women's Health* **2023**, *15*, 725–729. [CrossRef] [PubMed] [PubMed Central]
24. Pivazyan, L.; Kasyan, G.; Grigoryan, B.; Pushkar, D. Effectiveness and safety of bulking agents versus surgical methods in women with stress urinary incontinence: A systematic review and meta-analysis. *Int. Urogynecol. J.* **2022**, *33*, 777–787. [CrossRef] [PubMed]
25. Călinescu, B.C.; Neacșu, A.; Martiniuc, A.E.; Dumitrescu, D.; Stănică, C.D.; Roșu, G.-A.; Chivu, L.I.; Ioan, R.G. Surgical Treatments for Women with Stress Urinary Incontinence: A Systematic Review. *Life* **2023**, *13*, 1480. [CrossRef]

26. Kobashi, K.C.; Albo, M.E.; Dmochowski, R.R.; Ginsberg, D.A.; Goldman, H.B.; Gomelsky, A.; Kraus, S.R.; Sandhu, J.S.; Shepler, T.; Treadwell, J.R.; et al. Surgical Treatment of Female Stress Urinary Incontinence: AUA/SUFU Guideline. *J. Urol.* **2017**, *198*, 875–883. [CrossRef] [PubMed]
27. Ford, A.A.; Rogerson, L.; Cody, J.D.; Ogah, J. Mid-urethral sling operations for stress urinary incontinence in women. *Cochrane Database Syst. Rev.* **2015**, *7*, CD006375, Erratum in *Cochrane Database Syst. Rev.* **2017**, *7*, CD006375. [CrossRef] [PubMed]
28. Fusco, F.; Abdel-Fattah, M.; Chapple, C.R.; Creta, M.; La Falce, S.; Waltregny, D.; Novara, G. Updated Systematic Review and Meta-analysis of the Comparative Data on Colposuspensions, Pubovaginal Slings, and Midurethral Tapes in the Surgical Treatment of Female Stress Urinary Incontinence. *Eur. Urol.* **2017**, *72*, 567–591. [CrossRef] [PubMed]
29. Boyers, D.; Kilonzo, M.; Davidson, T.; Cooper, D.; Wardle, J.; Bhal, K.; N'Dow, J.; MacLennan, G.; Norrie, J.; Abdel-Fattah, M. Patient preferences for stress urinary incontinence treatments: A discrete choice experiment. *BMJ Open* **2023**, *13*, e066157. [CrossRef] [PubMed] [PubMed Central]
30. Sears, S.; Rhodes, S.; McBride, C.; Shoag, J.; Sheyn, D. Complications following retropubic versus transobturator midurethral synthetic sling placement. *Int. Urogynecol. J.* **2023**, *34*, 2389–2397. [CrossRef] [PubMed]

Disclaimer/Publisher's Note: The statements, opinions and data contained in all publications are solely those of the individual author(s) and contributor(s) and not of MDPI and/or the editor(s). MDPI and/or the editor(s) disclaim responsibility for any injury to people or property resulting from any ideas, methods, instructions or products referred to in the content.

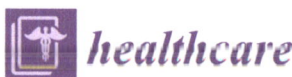

Article

Multifaceted Impact of CO_2 Laser Therapy on Genitourinary Syndrome of Menopause, Vulvovaginal Atrophy and Sexual Function

Svetlana Jankovic [1,2,*], Marija Rovcanin [1], Milena Zamurovic [1,2], Branka Jovanovic [1], Tatjana Raicevic [1] and Ana Tomic [3]

[1] Clinic for Gynecology and Obstetrics, Narodni Front, Kraljice Natalije 62, 11000 Belgrade, Serbia
[2] Faculty of Medicine, University of Belgrade, Dr Subotica Starijeg 8, 11000 Belgrade, Serbia
[3] Center for Radiology and Magnetic Resonance Imaging, University Clinical Center of Serbia, 11000 Belgrade, Serbia
* Correspondence: svetlanajankovic.r@gmail.com

Abstract: Genitourinary syndrome of menopause (GSM) encompasses a range of distressing symptoms in the vulvovaginal and/or bladder–urethral regions related to menopause changes, negatively influencing woman's quality of life and sexual activity. Fractional micro-ablative CO_2 laser therapy has shown the potential to reinstate the vaginal epithelium to a condition akin to the premenopausal state, thereby ameliorating the subjective symptoms associated with GSM. We conducted a prospective, pilot study in 73 sexually active postmenopausal women treated with CO_2 laser for their GSM symptoms, while assessing Vaginal Health Index Score (VHIS) and sexual function through the Female Sexual Function Index (FSFI) Questionnaire. The laser treatment resulted in a decrease in VHIS and patient-reported vulvovaginal atrophy (VVA) symptoms, with a significantly lower prevalence of vaginal itching, dryness, and burning ($p < 0.001$), as well as dyspareunia ($p = 0.002$). The occurrence of urinary incontinence, urgency, and vaginal heaviness significantly reduced, with an improvement in the staging of cystocele, either to Stage 1 or complete resolution ($p < 0.001$). FSFI total and domain scores were significantly higher after the treatment, indicating better sexual function, with a post-treatment score median of 25 ($p < 0.001$). Therefore, using a three-cycle fractional CO_2 laser was an effective choice for reducing urogenital discomfort related to GSM in postmenopausal women.

Keywords: genitourinary syndrome; menopause; female sexual health; fractional CO_2 laser

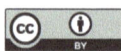

1. Introduction

Introduced a decade ago, genitourinary syndrome of menopause (GSM) encompasses a range of distressing symptoms in the vulvovaginal and/or bladder–urethral regions related to menopause changes [1]. Hence, GSM is not associated with any other medical conditions, as it is characterized by a menopause-induced decrease in sex steroids and entails alterations in the labia, clitoris, vestibule, vagina, urethra, and bladder [2]. GSM occurs in approximately 50% of menopausal women [3,4], characterized by its chronic and progressive nature [1]. The reluctance of both women and healthcare professionals to discuss issues related to vaginal health frequently results in underdiagnoses and undertreatment [1,4].

Women who are affected may experience symptoms that are associated with the vaginal tract, urinary tract, or both [4]. Genital symptoms are a manifestation of vulvovaginal atrophy (VVA), mostly consisting of vaginal dryness and pain during sexual intercourse, known as dyspareunia, arising due to a compromised response to sexual stimulation [4]. Prevalent urinary symptoms include frequency, urgency, dysuria and stress incontinence [2,4,5]. A number of surveys have provided comprehensive information regarding the adverse impacts of GSM on various aspects of menopausal women's lives, including their quality of life, emotional well-being, and sexual functioning [6,7]. Not less than roughly 50% of menopausal women experience symptoms of GSM in regard to sexual desire, intimacy, well-being, and self-worth [7].

The global significance of vaginal laser therapy in managing genitourinary syndrome of menopause is slowly increasing [8]. The utilization of laser therapy has been found to enhance the vascularization of the vaginal mucosa, promoting the production of newly derived collagen and matrix basic substance within the connective tissue, supporting the thickening of the epithelium that lines the vagina through the formation of new papillae, as it facilitates the restoration of mucosal equilibrium, consequently alleviating the aforementioned symptoms associated with GSM [9]. Hence, fractional micro-ablative CO_2 laser therapy has the potential to reinstate the vaginal epithelium to a condition akin to the premenopausal state, thereby ameliorating the subjective symptoms associated with GSM-associated VVA symptoms as well as lower urinary tract discomfort [10]. Moreover, it was observed that the CO_2 laser could be effective for treating urinary GSM symptoms because of the improvement in atrophy of the urethral and bladder mucosa. Additionally, it could ultimately result in enhanced genital health and increased satisfaction with sexual life among postmenopausal women [11–13].

Laser and radiofrequency techniques are currently being extensively researched in order to have a full understanding of their overall efficacy and safety [5], with a scarcity of research that has explored the impact of this intervention on sexual function, as well as GSM-associated urinary discomfort. Therefore, the objective of this study was to evaluate the impact of a micro-ablative fractional CO_2 laser on clinical symptoms of urinary and genital symptoms associated with GSM and concordant sexual function in postmenopausal women.

2. Materials and Methods

2.1. Study Design

This prospective, pilot study was conducted at our clinic between June and November of 2022 in order to evaluate GSM symptoms as well as concordant vaginal atrophy and sexual function after completing three cycles of laser treatment.

2.2. Participants

This study comprised a cohort of 73 postmenopausal women who were sexually active and experienced uncomfortable GSM symptoms resulting in sexual health complaints. The inclusion criteria included participants that had engaged in sexual activity within the past four weeks, with the absence of menstruation for at least one year, suffering at least one subjective GSM symptom (such as urinary incontinence, urgency, the presence of heaviness in vagina, vaginal itching, stinging, dyspareunia, dryness), and the presence of any severity of cystocele, diagnosed with VVA by a gynecologist. The exclusion criteria included the application/usage of any hormonal replacement therapy (HRT) (either systemic or local) within the past year, acute or recurrent urinary tract or genital infection, and suffering from hormonal imbalance or any serious disease, chronic condition, and or psychiatric disorders that could interfere with study compliance or which would prevent appropriate informed consent or study participation.

2.3. Data Collection and Intervention

The general questionnaire was administered to collect sociodemographic and anamnestic knowledge, including age, time since the last menstruation, past deliveries, and types of deliveries, prior to initiating the first laser application.

2.3.1. Urinary Symptoms and Cystocele Staging

Data pertaining to the presence of urinary GSM symptoms (incontinence, urgency, the presence of heaviness in vagina) were collected through respondents' answers to yes-or-no questions evaluated before starting the first laser application and 4 weeks after the third treatment. A cystocele, defined as a prolapse of the upper anterior vaginal wall involving the bladder was diagnosed and staged using the Pelvic Organ Prolapse Quantification System (POPQ), where stage 0 indicated no presence of prolapse, and stage 4 indicated complete vaginal eversion [14].

2.3.2. VVA Symptoms and Vaginal Health Index Score (VHIS)

Prior to treatment and 4 weeks after the third laser treatment, women were evaluated by using the Vaginal Health Index score (VHIS) that assesses 5 characteristics of the vaginal wall: elasticity, fluid volume, pH, epithelial integrity, and moisture. The severity of each characteristic was evaluated based on the 5-point Likert scale, ranging from 1 to 5. The total score of VHI varies from 5 to 25 with its cut-off point of 15, as a score less than 15 indicates atrophic vaginitis [15]. The severity of VVA symptoms (vaginal burning, vaginal itching, vaginal dryness, and dyspareunia) was self-evaluated by study participants using a 10 cm visual analogue scale (VAS), where the value of 1 represented the absence of symptoms, while values 2–10 indicated the presence of symptoms with varying degrees of severity, as the value of 10 represents the most severe form. Incidence of all noted VVA symptoms (positive clinical findings) were defined by all responses greater than 1.

2.3.3. Female Sexual Function Index (FSFI)

Prior to the initial laser treatment and four weeks after the third treatment, the assessment of sexual function was conducted using the Female Sexual Function Index Questionnaire [16]. The Female Sexual Function Index (FSFI) is an approved instrument assessing six domains of sexual function in women: desire, arousal, lubrication, orgasm, satisfaction, and pain as well as an overall score for sexual functioning (total FSFI). A cut-off score of 26.5 was used for the detection of Female Sexual Dysfunction [17].

2.3.4. Fractional CO_2 Laser Treatment

Postmenopausal women were treated intravaginally with the fractional micro-ablative CO_2 laser system (SmartXide2 V2 LR, Monalisa Touch; DEKA, Florence, Italy), using the following settings: dot power 35 W, dwell time 1000 µs, dot spacing 1000 µm, and the smart stack parameter from 1 to 3. The vaginal probe was inserted and rotated along the vaginal canal, applying laser energy to the full length of the vagina. A complete treatment cycle included three laser applications, spaced 6 to 8 weeks apart which all participants completed. The patients bore the expense of the procedure's treatment cost, which took place at the outpatient clinic without requiring any specific preparation or anesthesia.

2.4. Ethical Consideration

This study was implemented in accordance with the International Code of Medical Ethics of the World Medical Association (Declaration of Helsinki) and written informed consent was obtained from the participants after the nature and objectives of this study were fully explained to them. This study was approved by the institution's Ethical Committee (date of approval: 16 January 2022).

2.5. Data Analysis

Data presented in the text and tables are reported as means ± standard deviation or frequencies (n) and accordant percentages (%). A McNemar test and Wilcoxon signed ranks test were used to define statistical significance of continuous indicators before/after the treatment variables. The Chi-squared test was employed to assess disparities across various patient groups based on their prior delivery approach. Spearman's correlation analysis was employed to describe the relationships among two continuous variables. Statistical analysis was performed using IBM SPSS Statistics for Windows, version 23.0 (IBM Corp., Armonk, NY, USA). The significance level was set at $p < 0.05$. All 73 participants were included in this analysis.

3. Results

As presented in Table 1, our study involved 73 menopausal women, with mean deliveries of 55.6 ± 5.6 years old, with a menopause that averagely lasted for 6.6 ± 4.9 years. Our patients had a previous delivery in 63 (86.3%) cases, out of which 54 (74.0%) cases were vaginal deliveries, while 9 (12.3%) were deliveries by cesarean section.

Table 1. Patient characteristics.

Age (years)	55.6 ± 5.6
Menopause Duration (years)	6.6 ± 4.9
Previous Deliveries	63 (86.3%)
Previous Vaginal Delivery	54 (74.0%)
Previous Cesarean Section	9 (12.3%)

Values are presented as mean ± SD or frequencies and percentages (%).

3.1. Urinary GSM Symptms

We examined the extent to which urinary symptoms were completely alleviated following the laser therapy. As presented in Table 2, urinary incontinence, urgency, and heaviness in the vagina were significantly reduced ($p < 0.001$). After three cycles of laser treatment, the cystocele stage improved in a significant portion of our cohort ($p < 0.001$), to either stage 1 (37.0%) or was completely resolved. None of our patients exhibited a rectocele or a uterine prolapse.

Table 2. Urinary GSM symptoms at baseline level and after treatment with CO_2 laser.

Positive Clinical Finding	Baseline	After Completed Treatment	p Value *
Urinary Incontinence	48 (65.8%)	16 (21.9%)	<0.001
Urinary Urgency	45 (61.6%)	21 (28.8%)	<0.001
Vaginal Heaviness	34 (46.6%)	12 (16.4%)	<0.001
Cystocele (POPQ Staging)			
Stage 1	10 (13.7%)	27 (37.0%)	
Stage 2	24 (32.9%)	3 (4.1%)	<0.001
Stage 3	7 (9.6%)	0 (0%)	

POPQ—Pelvic Organ Prolapse Quantification System; data are expressed as n (%); * obtained with a McNemar test or Wilcoxon signed rank test when appropriate; significant at <0.05.

3.2. Vulvovagnal Atrophy Symptoms and Sexual Function

According to the data presented in Table 3, we examined the extent to which VVA symptoms were completely alleviated following the laser therapy. Any absence of observed pain was regarded as a positive clinical observation. VHIS and patient-reported VVA symptoms show a significant decrease following the administration of CO_2 laser treatment.

Table 3. Vulvovaginal atrophy symptoms presence at baseline level and after treatment.

Positive Clinical Finding	Baseline	After Completed Treatment	p-Value **
VVA (VHIS < 15)	54 (74.0%)	1 (1.4%)	<0.001
Vaginal Itching *	51 (69.9%)	30 (41.1%)	<0.001
Vaginal Burning *	55 (75.3%)	33 (45.2%)	<0.001
Vaginal Dryness *	71 (97.3%)	51 (69.9%)	<0.001
Dyspareunia *	64 (87.7%)	54 (74.0%)	0.002

VVA—vulvovaginal atrophy; VHIS—Vaginal Health Index Score; data are expressed as n (%); * VA Scale higher than 1 was equivalent to the presence of symptoms and positive clinical finding; ** obtained with McNemar test, significant at <0.05.

Upon examining the VHIS score, it was found that just 1 patient (1.4%) had a clinically relevant state of impaired vaginal health. Although the occurrence of VVA symptoms was diminished in a significant proportion of participants, a notable number of participants still reported experiencing a certain level of symptoms, particularly dyspareunia (74.0% of cases after the completed treatment) and vaginal dryness (69.9%).

As shown in Table 4, FSFI total and domain scores were significantly higher after the treatment, indicating better sexual function, with a total score median of 25.5, considered a clinically relevant level as compared to baseline median total score values (18.2).

Table 4. FSFI scores before and after treatment with CO_2 laser.

FSFI Scores	Before Treatment	After Treatment	p-Value *
Total	18.2 ± 6.5	25.5 ± 4.1	<0.001
Desire	3.0 ± 1.1	4.1 ± 0.8	<0.001
Arousal	3.0 ± 1.2	4.2 ± 0.8	<0.001
Lubrication	2.8 ± 1.3	4.2 ± 0.8	<0.001
Orgasm	3.2 ± 1.3	4.4 ± 0.9	<0.001
Satisfaction	3.3 ± 1.3	4.2 ± 1.0	<0.001
Pain	2.9 ± 1.5	4.3 ± 0.9	<0.001

FSFI—Female Sexual Function Index; * Values are presented as mean ± SD; * Wilcoxon signed rank test, significant at $p < 0.05$.

When correlating VHIS and VVA clinical findings to FSFI domain and total scores, all significant correlations were mostly weak to moderate strength (Table 5). VHIS correlated positively with all domain scores, as well as the total FSFI score, suggesting that higher VHS is associated with better sexual function. However, VVA symptoms intensity correlation coefficients were negative, indicating an inverse relationship, where lower FSFI scores were associated with more pronounced symptoms.

Table 5. Correlation coefficients.

	Desire	Arousal	Lubrication	Orgasm	Satisfaction	Pain	Total
VHIS	0.348 **	0.349 **	0.490 **	0.332 **	0.310 **	0.513 **	0.496 **
Vaginal Itching *	−0.145	0.081	−0.033	0.059	−0.028	−0.041	−0.044
Vaginal Burning *	−0.310 **	−0.008	−0.275 *	0.042	−0.010	−0.207	−0.209
Vaginal Dryness *	−0.043	−0.084	−0.206	0.028	−0.347 **	−0.220	−0.151
Dyspareunia *	−0.070	−0.196	−0.352 **	−0.059	−0.198	−0.427 **	−0.350 **

VHIS—Vaginal Health Index Score; Values are presented as spearman correlation coefficients; significant correlation coefficients are in bold; * $p < 0.05$; ** $p < 0.001$.

Vaginal burning showed significant correlation to FSFI desire and lubrication domain scores, while dryness intensity significantly correlated to satisfaction domain scores. Intensity of dyspareunia was correlated to lubrication and pain domain scores, while being the only symptom to exhibit significant correlation to FSFI total score. Surprisingly, vulvovaginal itching was not significantly correlated to any of the domains or total score.

Ultimately, no adverse reactions were recorded by the patients.

According to the data presented in Table 6, our analysis of urinary and VVA symptoms revealed that there were no statistically significant variations in the prevalence of most analyzed symptoms between women who had a vaginal delivery and those who had a cesarean section. Statistically significant changes were seen only in the prevalence of urinary incontinence ($p = 0.004$) and urinary urgency ($p = 0.014$).

Table 6. Urinary and vulvovaginal atrophy symptoms presence depending on the previous delivery type.

Positive Clinical Finding	Vaginal Deliveries (n = 54)	Cesarean Section (n = 9)	p-Value **
Urinary Incontinence	43 (79.6%)	3 (33.3%)	0.004 *
Urinary Urgency	31 (57.4%)	9 (100.0%)	0.014 *
Vaginal Heaviness	30 (55.6%)	3 (33.3%)	0.217
Cystocele Stage 1 Stage 2 Stage 3	8 (14.8%) 22 (40.7%) 6 (11.1%)	1 (11.1%) 2 (22.2%) 1 (11.1%)	0.292
VVA (VHIS < 15)	37 (68.5%)	2 (22.2%)	0.575
Vaginal Itching *	40 (74.1%)	6 (66.7%)	0.643
Vaginal Burning *	41 (75.9%)	8 (88.9%)	0.386
Vaginal Dryness *	52 (96.3%)	9 (100.0%)	0.557
Dyspareunia *	45 (83.3%)	9 (100.0%)	0.186

VVA—vulvovaginal atrophy; VHIS—Vaginal Health Index Score; data are expressed as n (%); * VA Scale higher than 1 was equivalent to the presence of symptoms and positive clinical finding; ** obtained with Chi-squared test, significant at <0.05.

4. Discussion

Our study has shown that both urinary and VVA symptoms that were registered in menopausal women were alleviated following the laser therapy in a majority of the participants. After three cycles of laser treatment, cystocele stage improved in a significant portion of our cohort to either Stage 1 or was completely resolved. VHIS correlated positively with all domain scores, as well as the total FSFI score, suggesting that higher VHS is associated with better sexual function, while VVA symptoms indicated an inverse relationship.

Similar to our results, previous studies showed that the intravaginal fractional CO_2 laser significantly improved urinary GSM symptoms such as nocturia and overall urinary frequency. Moreover, the mentioned authors reported a significant reduction in episodes of in women with urgency incontinence [18]. There are a small number of randomized control studies that tested the efficiency of CO_2 laser for GSM symptoms compared to sham-laser treated controls. A double-blind, randomized, sham-controlled trial by Salvatore et al. [19] showed that laser-induced changes were in favor of the CO_2-treated group, with a more pronounced effect for VVA symptoms like dryness, dyspareunia, and concomitant sexual dysfunction when compared to urinary symptoms such as dysuria. A study by Aguiar et al. [18] showed that only the intravaginal fractional CO_2 laser significantly improved urinary GSM symptoms such as nocturia, frequency, and episodes of urgency when compared to other, topical treatments such as estrogens and lubricants. A Brazilian study by Politano et al. [20] showed that the use of fractional CO_2 laser therapy to treat genitourinary syndrome resulted in better short-term effects than those of local estrogens or lubricant with respect to improving the VHIS score and overall vaginal health in postmenopausal women, with improvement in the desire and lubrication FSFI domains. Considering the regenerative impact of intravaginal fractional laser CO_2 therapy, which extends to the lower urinary tract and leads to an improvement of menopausal urogenital symptoms, it has been proposed as a potentially effective option for addressing GSM involving urinary symptoms [18].

Nevertheless, the literature presents varying outcomes about the efficacy of laser treatment in alleviating urinary symptoms. A study by Page et al. [21] reported that the laser treatment response was comparable to that of sham applications, as there were no obvious differences in observed outcomes, with no improvement when it came to both sexual and urinary functions. Similar results were reported when CO_2 was tested for GSM symptoms in breast cancer survivors [22]. Regrettably, a considerable amount of the existing literature does not provide sufficient evidence to support the superiority of laser treatment in alleviating GSM symptoms, as three-cycle laser treatment demonstrated comparable efficacy to other treatment options. Both fractionated CO_2 vaginal laser and vaginal estrogen treatment showed comparable efficacy in improving symptoms of genitourinary syndrome of menopause, as well as urine and sexual function, 6 months post-treatment [23]. Similarly, recognized GSM treatment modalities, such as laser, radiofrequency, and vaginal estrogen yielded similar and considerable enhancements in GSM symptoms for women with breast cancer, a highly vulnerable group who were undergoing adjuvant therapy for their disease. While laser therapy and topical estrogens have different mechanisms of action, data suggest that laser therapy is an equally effective approach for addressing the subjective discomfort caused by urogenital atrophy [24], with an improvement in sexual function and overall quality of life [25].

Nonetheless, while contemplating the assessment of treatments, it may be paramount to prioritize the assessment of lasers over hormone treatments due to health concerns associated with the latter [26]. When compared to vaginal estrogens or fractional radiofrequency, it was estimated that CO_2 laser was an adequate treatment alternative for noted treatment options, as hormonal treatment carries certain risk, while radiofrequency is rather often accompanied by pain [27]. Regarding hormone treatment, the lack of understanding of long-term follow-ups and limited data on the specific type, dosage, and method of administering hormones such as estrogens is particularly emphasized, as it has been observed that oral estrogens can exacerbate type-independent urinary incontinence in menopausal women [18]. What may set CO_2 laser treatment apart from other noted treatment modalities is patient satisfaction and adherence to the treatment cycles. Regarding the patient's overall impression, a study by Paraiso et al. [23] reported that 85.8% of participants rated their improvement as "better or much better" and 78.5% reported being either "satisfied or very satisfied" compared to 70% and 73.3% in the estrogen group. This is likely attributed to the enhanced laser treatment adherence, as the desired outcomes can be achieved in just three cycles with authors reporting that all patients who underwent the laser therapy successfully completed the whole treatment [28]. Furthermore, all the reported heterogenic results for the laser efficiency, we would like to emphasize that none of the above cited trials reported serious adverse effects, as it was the case in our study.

Prior research has observed that symptoms of VVA exhibit a roughly linear correlation with overall sexual functioning [29]. Accordingly, our analysis demonstrated a noteworthy enhancement in all FSFI domain scores following the treatment, consistent with the results previously reported by other authors [12,28,30]. Authors utilizing laser treatment showed significant improvement of total FSFI score and individual domains of desire and lubrication [20,31]. Moreover, literature-reported results showed that the improvement in the "Lubrication" domain of FSFI was only substantial when a laser with additional moisturizers was used [32]. However, some authors reported significant worsening of the pain FSFI domain [31]. It is imperative to carefully observe pain levels after laser procedures, as studies suggest that pain is the most influential element in predicting sexual functionality, compared to other domains whose effects contribute to overall sexual activity to a lesser extent [29]. According to our data, the pain domain exhibited greater scores in the presence of more pronounced dyspareunia, hence the highlighted post-treatment improvement of dyspareunia which may be imperative for optimal results for sexual function in menopause. Additionally, dyspareunia was the only subjective symptom that showed a significant correlation with the overall FSFI score, underscoring the significance of addressing and ameliorating this symptom of VVA.

Despite the compelling nature of our findings, some limitations should be considered. Compared to certain cited studies, our study lacks randomization and did not include a control group. However, it is important to mention that our study encompassed a wider range of investigated urinary GSM symptoms, such as urgency, frequency, heaviness in vagina, as well as the efficiency of laser treatment on the urinary organ prolapse-cystocele.

Nevertheless, available research is still limited, as more randomized controlled studies in particular are lacking. Most of available studies show a trend toward safe and effective treatment, but only in the short-term [8]. Therefore, a significant drawback of this study is that we did not examine the long-term results beyond the four-week period after treatment. This prevents us from comprehending the long-term efficiency and any delayed effects associated with CO_2 laser therapy. Although laser therapy for the treatment of the symptoms of GSM appears promising, there is currently a lack of high-level and long-term evidence regarding its safety and efficacy. Moreover, there is a lack of professional guidelines regarding this modality of treatment, specifically for GSM [10]. Opportunities exist for future research in this area, specifically to determine safety and long-term outcomes of therapy.

5. Conclusions

Our study found that using a three-cycle fractional CO_2 laser treatment is an effective choice for reducing genital discomfort related to vulvovaginal atrophy in postmenopausal women. Furthermore, it had a notable impact in reducing urinary symptoms. Subsequently, the improvements led to an increase in scores related to overall sexual functioning, as well as certain domains. Although these findings show promising possibilities for future therapeutic use, further research is required to evaluate its long-term efficacy, potential adverse effects, and safety considerations. Furthermore, a potential source of bias in our study is the relatively small number of participants, which could restrict the applicability of our findings and impact the strength of the statistical analysis.

Author Contributions: Conceptualization, S.J. and M.R.; methodology, S.J. and M.R.; formal analysis, A.T.; investigation, S.J., M.R., M.Z. and B.J.; data curation, S.J., M.Z., B.J. and T.R.; writing—original draft preparation, S.J., A.T. and M.R.; writing—review and editing, S.J., M.R., T.R. and A.T.; supervision, S.J. and M.R. All authors have read and agreed to the published version of the manuscript.

Funding: This research received no external funding.

Institutional Review Board Statement: This study was implemented in accordance with the International Code of Medical Ethics of the World Medical Association (Declaration of Helsinki). This study was approved by the ethical committee of the clinic (approval code 01/2022, approved on 16 January 2022).

Informed Consent Statement: Informed consent was obtained from all subjects involved in the study.

Data Availability Statement: The data presented in this study are available on request from the corresponding author.

Conflicts of Interest: The authors declare no conflicts of interest.

References

1. Cox, S.; Nasseri, R.; Rubin, R.S.; Santiago-Lastra, Y. Genitourinary Syndrome of Menopause. *Med. Clin. N. Am.* **2023**, *107*, 357–369. [CrossRef] [PubMed]
2. Kagan, R.; Kellogg-Spadt, S.; Parish, S.J. Practical Treatment Considerations in the Management of Genitourinary Syndrome of Menopause. *Drugs Aging* **2019**, *36*, 897–908. [CrossRef] [PubMed]
3. Marino, J.M. Genitourinary Syndrome of Menopause. *J. Midwifery Womens Health* **2021**, *66*, 729–739. [CrossRef] [PubMed]
4. Briggs, P. Genitourinary Syndrome of Menopause. *Post Reprod. Health* **2020**, *26*, 111–114. [CrossRef] [PubMed]
5. Phillips, N.A.; Bachmann, G.A. The Genitourinary Syndrome of Menopause. *Menopause* **2021**, *28*, 579–588. [CrossRef] [PubMed]
6. Moral, E.; Delgado, J.L.; Carmona, F.; Caballero, B.; Guillán, C.; González, P.M.; Suárez-Almarza, J.; Velasco-Ortega, S.; Nieto Magro, C. The Impact of Genitourinary Syndrome of Menopause on Well-Being, Functioning, and Quality of Life in Postmenopausal Women. *Menopause* **2018**, *25*, 1418–1423. [CrossRef] [PubMed]
7. Cumming, G.P.; Herald, J.; Moncur, R.; Currie, H.; Lee, A.J. Women's Attitudes to Hormone Replacement Therapy, Alternative Therapy and Sexual Health: A Web-Based Survey. *Menopause Int.* **2007**, *13*, 79–83. [CrossRef] [PubMed]
8. Ratz, C. Vaginal laser therapy for urinary incontinence and genitourinary syndrome of menopause: A review. *Urol. Ausg. A* **2019**, *58*, 284–290. [CrossRef] [PubMed]

9. Naumova, I.; Castelo-Branco, C. Current Treatment Options for Postmenopausal Vaginal Atrophy. *Int. J. Womens Health* **2018**, *10*, 387–395. [CrossRef]
10. Rabley, A.; O'Shea, T.; Terry, R.; Byun, S.; Louis Moy, M. Laser Therapy for Genitourinary Syndrome of Menopause. *Curr. Urol. Rep.* **2018**, *19*, 83. [CrossRef]
11. Salvatore, S.; Maggiore, U.L.R.; Origoni, M.; Parma, M.; Quaranta, L.; Sileo, F.; Cola, A.; Baini, I.; Ferrero, S.; Candiani, M.; et al. Microablative Fractional CO_2 Laser Improves Dyspareunia Related to Vulvovaginal Atrophy: A Pilot Study. *J. Endometr. Pelvic Pain Disord.* **2014**, *6*, 150–156. [CrossRef]
12. Salvatore, S.; Nappi, R.E.; Parma, M.; Chionna, R.; Lagona, F.; Zerbinati, N.; Ferrero, S.; Origoni, M.; Candiani, M.; Leone Roberti Maggiore, U. Sexual Function after Fractional Microablative CO_2 Laser in Women with Vulvovaginal Atrophy. *Climacteric J. Int. Menopause Soc.* **2015**, *18*, 219–225. [CrossRef]
13. Salvatore, S.; Athanasiou, S.; Candiani, M. The Use of Pulsed CO_2 Lasers for the Treatment of Vulvovaginal Atrophy. *Curr. Opin. Obstet. Gynecol.* **2015**, *27*, 504–508. [CrossRef] [PubMed]
14. Persu, C.; Chapple, C.; Cauni, V.; Gutue, S.; Geavlete, P. Pelvic Organ Prolapse Quantification System (POP–Q)—A New Era in Pelvic Prolapse Staging. *J. Med. Life* **2011**, *4*, 75–81. [PubMed]
15. Bachmann, G. Urogenital Ageing: An Old Problem Newly Recognized. *Maturitas* **1995**, *22*, S1–S5. [CrossRef] [PubMed]
16. Rosen, R.; Brown, C.; Heiman, J.; Leiblum, S.; Meston, C.; Shabsigh, R.; Ferguson, D.; D'Agostino, R. The Female Sexual Function Index (FSFI): A Multidimensional Self-Report Instrument for the Assessment of Female Sexual Function. *J. Sex Marital Ther.* **2000**, *26*, 191–208. [CrossRef] [PubMed]
17. Wiegel, M.; Meston, C.; Rosen, R. The Female Sexual Function Index (FSFI): Cross-Validation and Development of Clinical Cutoff Scores. *J. Sex Marital Ther.* **2005**, *31*, 1–20. [CrossRef] [PubMed]
18. Aguiar, L.B.; Politano, C.A.; Costa-Paiva, L.; Juliato, C.R.T. Efficacy of Fractional CO_2 Laser, Promestriene, and Vaginal Lubricant in the Treatment of Urinary Symptoms in Postmenopausal Women: A Randomized Clinical Trial. *Lasers Surg. Med.* **2020**, *52*, 713–720. [CrossRef] [PubMed]
19. Salvatore, S.; Pitsouni, E.; Grigoriadis, T.; Zacharakis, D.; Pantaleo, G.; Candiani, M.; Athanasiou, S. CO_2 Laser and the Genitourinary Syndrome of Menopause: A Randomized Sham-Controlled Trial. *Climacteric J. Int. Menopause Soc.* **2021**, *24*, 187–193. [CrossRef]
20. Politano, C.A.; Costa-Paiva, L.; Aguiar, L.B.; Machado, H.C.; Baccaro, L.F. Fractional CO_2 Laser versus Promestriene and Lubricant in Genitourinary Syndrome of Menopause: A Randomized Clinical Trial. *Menopause* **2019**, *26*, 833–840. [CrossRef]
21. Page, A.-S.; Verbakel, J.Y.; Verhaeghe, J.; Latul, Y.P.; Housmans, S.; Deprest, J. Laser versus Sham for Genitourinary Syndrome of Menopause: A Randomised Controlled Trial. *BJOG Int. J. Obstet. Gynaecol.* **2023**, *130*, 312–319. [CrossRef] [PubMed]
22. Mension, E.; Alonso, I.; Anglès-Acedo, S.; Ros, C.; Otero, J.; Villarino, Á.; Farré, R.; Saco, A.; Vega, N.; Castrejón, N.; et al. Effect of Fractional Carbon Dioxide vs Sham Laser on Sexual Function in Survivors of Breast Cancer Receiving Aromatase Inhibitors for Genitourinary Syndrome of Menopause: The LIGHT Randomized Clinical Trial. *JAMA Netw. Open* **2023**, *6*, e2255697. [CrossRef] [PubMed]
23. Paraiso, M.F.R.; Ferrando, C.A.; Sokol, E.R.; Rardin, C.R.; Matthews, C.A.; Karram, M.M.; Iglesia, C.B. A Randomized Clinical Trial Comparing Vaginal Laser Therapy to Vaginal Estrogen Therapy in Women with Genitourinary Syndrome of Menopause: The VeLVET Trial. *Menopause* **2020**, *27*, 50–56. [CrossRef]
24. Dutra, P.F.S.P.; Heinke, T.; Pinho, S.C.; Focchi, G.R.A.; Tso, F.K.; de Almeida, B.C.; Silva, I.; Speck, N.M.G. Comparison of Topical Fractional CO_2 Laser and Vaginal Estrogen for the Treatment of Genitourinary Syndrome in Postmenopausal Women: A Randomized Controlled Trial. *Menopause* **2021**, *28*, 756–763. [CrossRef] [PubMed]
25. Gold, D.; Nicolay, L.; Avian, A.; Greimel, E.; Balic, M.; Pristauz-Telsnigg, G.; Tamussino, K.; Trutnovsky, G. Vaginal Laser Therapy versus Hyaluronic Acid Suppositories for Women with Symptoms of Urogenital Atrophy after Treatment for Breast Cancer: A Randomized Controlled Trial. *Maturitas* **2023**, *167*, 1–7. [CrossRef] [PubMed]
26. Krause, M.; Wheeler, T.L.; Richter, H.E.; Snyder, T.E. Systemic Effects of Vaginally Administered Estrogen Therapy: A Review. *Female Pelvic Med. Reconstr. Surg.* **2010**, *16*, 188–195. [CrossRef]
27. de Oliveira, C.D.; de Mello Bianchi, A.M.H.; Campos, M.L.P.; Nogueira, M.C.C.; Sartori, M.G.F.; de Góis Speck, N.M. Women with Genitourinary Syndrome of Menopause Treated with Vaginal Estriol, Microablative Fractional CO_2 Laser and Microablative Fractional Radiofrequency: A Randomized Pilot Study. *Photobiomodul. Photomed. Laser Surg.* **2023**, *41*, 718–724. [CrossRef]
28. Pearson, A.; Booker, A.; Tio, M.; Marx, G. Vaginal CO_2 Laser for the Treatment of Vulvovaginal Atrophy in Women with Breast Cancer: LAAVA Pilot Study. *Breast Cancer Res. Treat.* **2019**, *178*, 135–140. [CrossRef] [PubMed]
29. Pinkerton, J.V.; Bushmakin, A.G.; Komm, B.S.; Abraham, L. Relationship between Changes in Vulvar-Vaginal Atrophy and Changes in Sexual Functioning. *Maturitas* **2017**, *100*, 57–63. [CrossRef]
30. Filippini, M.; Porcari, I.; Ruffolo, A.F.; Casiraghi, A.; Farinelli, M.; Uccella, S.; Franchi, M.; Candiani, M.; Salvatore, S. CO_2-Laser Therapy and Genitourinary Syndrome of Menopause: A Systematic Review and Meta-Analysis. *J. Sex. Med.* **2022**, *19*, 452–470. [CrossRef]

31. Cruz, V.L.; Steiner, M.L.; Pompei, L.M.; Strufaldi, R.; Fonseca, F.L.A.; Santiago, L.H.S.; Wajsfeld, T.; Fernandes, C.E. Randomized, Double-Blind, Placebo-Controlled Clinical Trial for Evaluating the Efficacy of Fractional CO_2 Laser Compared with Topical Estriol in the Treatment of Vaginal Atrophy in Postmenopausal Women. *Menopause* **2018**, *25*, 21–28. [CrossRef] [PubMed]
32. Alvisi, S.; Lami, A.; Baldassarre, M.; Lenzi, J.; Mancini, I.; Seracchioli, R.; Meriggiola, M.C. Short-Term Efficacy and Safety of Non-Ablative Laser Treatment Alone or with Estriol or Moisturizers in Postmenopausal Women with Vulvovaginal Atrophy. *J. Sex. Med.* **2022**, *19*, 761–770. [CrossRef] [PubMed]

Disclaimer/Publisher's Note: The statements, opinions and data contained in all publications are solely those of the individual author(s) and contributor(s) and not of MDPI and/or the editor(s). MDPI and/or the editor(s) disclaim responsibility for any injury to people or property resulting from any ideas, methods, instructions or products referred to in the content.

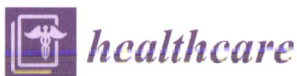

Article

Minimally Invasive Treatment of Stress Urinary Incontinence in Women: A Prospective Comparative Analysis between Bulking Agent and Single-Incision Sling

Lorenzo Campanella [1,2,*], Gianluca Gabrielli [1,2], Erika Chiodo [1,2], Vitaliana Stefanachi [1,2], Ermelinda Pennacchini [1,2], Debora Grilli [1,2], Giovanni Grossi [1], Pietro Cignini [1], Andrea Morciano [3,4], Marzio Angelo Zullo [4,5], Pierluigi Palazzetti [1], Carlo Rappa [4,6], Marco Calcagno [7], Vincenzo Spina [8], Mauro Cervigni [4,9] and Michele Carlo Schiavi [1,4]

1. Department of Obstetrics and Gynaecology, Ospedale Sandro Pertini, 00157 Rome, Italy; gianluca.gabrielli@aslroma2.it (G.G.); erika.chiodo@aslroma2.it (E.C.); vitaliana.stefanachi@aslroma2.it (V.S.); ermelinda.pennacchini@aslroma2.it (E.P.); debora.grilli@aslroma2.it (D.G.); giovanni.grossi@aslroma2.it (G.G.); pietro.cignini@aslroma2.it (P.C.); pierluigi.palazzetti@aslroma2.it (P.P.); michele.schiavi@aslroma2.it (M.C.S.)
2. Department of Obstetrics and Gynaecology, Università di Tor Vergata, 00133 Rome, Italy
3. Department of Obstetrics and Gynaecology, Pia Fondazione Cardinale G. Panico, 73039 Tricase, Italy; drmorciano@gmail.com
4. AIUG Research Groups, Associazione Italiana di UroGinecologia e del Pavimento Pelvico, 00168 Rome, Italy; m.zullo@unicampus.it (M.A.Z.); carlodok@gmail.com (C.R.); info@maurocervigni.it (M.C.)
5. Department of Week-Surgery, Policlinico Universitario Campus Bio Medico, 00128 Rome, Italy
6. Andrea Grimaldi Medical Care, 80122 Naples, Italy
7. Department of Obstetrics and Gynecology, Santo Spirito Hospital, 00193 Rome, Italy; marco.calcagno@aslroma1.it
8. Maternal and Child Department, S. Camillo de Lellis Hospital, 02100 Rieti, Italy; v.spina@asl.rieti.it
9. Department of Female Pelvic Medicine and Reconstructive Surgery, Istituto Marco Pasquali ICOT, 04100 Latina, Italy
* Correspondence: lorenzo.campanella@aslroma2.it; Tel.: +39-3277027221

Abstract: Introduction: The study aims to compare the efficacy and safety of bulking agents and single-incision slings in the treatment of urinary incontinence in 159 patients during a 29-month follow-up period. Material and methods: Of the 159 patients suffering from stress urinary incontinence, 64 were treated with bulking agents (PAHG Bulkamid®) and 75 with a single-incision sling (Altis®). The ICIQ-UI-SF (Incontinence Questionnaire-Urine Incontinence-Short Form), PISQ-12 (Pelvic Organ Prolapse/Urinary Incontinence Sexual Questionnaires short form), FSFI (Female Sexual Function Index), FSDS (Female Sexual Distress Scale), and PGI-I (Patient Global Improvement Index) were used to assess efficiency and quality of life. Results: The bulking agents showed high efficacy and safety during the 29-month follow-up. Post-operative complications were recorded in both groups, with only two significant differences. The Bulkamid group experienced no pain, while 10.8% of the ALTIS group experienced groin pain and 5% experienced de novo urgency. Furthermore, patients treated with bulking agents experienced reduced nicturia (0.78 vs. 0.92 in patients treated with single-incision slings.). In both groups, we noticed a significant improvement in QoL (quality of life), with a halved ICIQ-UI-SF (International Consultation on Incontinence Questionnaire-Urine Incontinence-Short Form) score which was completed to assess the impact of urine symptoms. After 24 months of therapy, the Bulkamid group saw a decrease from 14.58 ± 5.11 at baseline to 5.67 ± 1.90 ($p < 0.0001$), whereas the ALTIS group experience a decrease from 13.75 ± 5.89 to 5.83 ± 1.78. Similarly, we observed an improvement in sexual function, with the number of sexually active patients increasing from 29 to 44 (56.4%) in the Bulkamid group ($p = 0.041$) and from 31 to 51 (61.7%) in the ALTIS group ($p = 0.034$). According to the most recent statistics, the PISQ-12, FSFI, and FSDS scores all demonstrated an improvement in women's sexual function. Conclusions: In terms of efficacy and safety, bulking agents had notable results over the 29-month follow-up period. Furthermore, the patients treated with bulking agents reported a lower incidence of postoperative complications and no discernible difference in terms of quality of life and sexual activity compared to the ones treated

Citation: Campanella, L.; Gabrielli, G.; Chiodo, E.; Stefanachi, V.; Pennacchini, E.; Grilli, D.; Grossi, G.; Cignini, P.; Morciano, A.; Zullo, M.A.; et al. Minimally Invasive Treatment of Stress Urinary Incontinence in Women: A Prospective Comparative Analysis between Bulking Agent and Single-Incision Sling. *Healthcare* **2024**, *12*, 751. https://doi.org/10.3390/healthcare12070751

Academic Editors: Rainer W. G. Gruessner and Charat Thongprayoon

Received: 26 January 2024
Revised: 27 March 2024
Accepted: 28 March 2024
Published: 29 March 2024

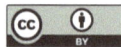

Copyright: © 2024 by the authors. Licensee MDPI, Basel, Switzerland. This article is an open access article distributed under the terms and conditions of the Creative Commons Attribution (CC BY) license (https://creativecommons.org/licenses/by/4.0/).

with single-incision slings. Bulking agents can be considered a very reliable therapeutic option based on accurate patient selection.

Keywords: stress urinary incontinence; single-incision sling; urethral bulking agents; Intrinsic Sphincteric Deficiency; midurethral sling

1. Introduction

The prevalence of urinary incontinence ranges from 10 to 60% of non-pregnant women above 20 years of age and from 50 to 70% of women older than 60 years of age [1–4].

In women with stress urinary incontinence (SUI), involuntary urine leakage occurs when intra-abdominal pressure increases (e.g., with exercise, sneezing, coughing, or laughing) in the absence of a bladder contraction. [5].

SUI is hypothesized to be caused by a lack of mechanical support of the urethra and/or poor coaptation of the urethral tissues, resulting in insufficient resistance to urine outflow with elevated abdominal pressures.

The two main mechanisms involved in the physiopathology of SUI are urethral hypermobility, which develops when pelvic-floor muscles and vaginal connective tissues provide insufficient urethral support, and Intrinsic Sphincteric Deficiency (ISD), which is caused by a loss of intrinsic urethral mucosal and muscle tone.

The usual argument for urethra support playing an important role in stress incontinence is the fact that urethral support operations are able to treat stress incontinence without changing urethral function [6].

However, contrary to the "pelvic-centric" theory, a new "urethro-centric" hypothesis is emerging, according to which urethral hypermobility is a characteristic that can be both associated and not with the condition of ISD but does not constitute the etiology of SUI.

This idea emphasizes how urethral hypermobility is not the primary cause of SUI and that ISD plays a critical part in the progression of this pathologic process [7,8].

The debate on the predominance of either of these two causes has dominated the urogynecological scene in terms of the interpretation of SUI physiopathology.

Worldwide, there is an ongoing search for increasingly minimally invasive urinary incontinence surgeries. In England, there was a 30% decrease in the use of urogynecological surgical mesh for SUI following the FDA warning [9] that prohibited the sale and use of these devices after recording a high number of postoperative complications and adverse effects.

Nowadays, international guidelines [10,11] recommend starting with conservative treatments such as rehabilitative therapy or lifestyle modifications before moving on to surgical options, with the midurethral sling (transobturatory or retropubic sling) being the most safe and effective surgical treatment available. Recently, single-incision slings, another form of midurethral sling, were developed as a novel technology capable of treating SUI while ensuring reduced invasiveness and postoperative complications for patients.

Evolving towards treatment requiring less invasiveness, next to single-incision slings, bulking agents represent, nowadays, an alternative option for patients with comorbidities and those who are less suitable for the usual surgical treatment due to the chance of having to repeat the procedure frequently and risk a higher tax of recurrences.

SIS (single-incision slings) and UBA (urethral bulking agents) are increasingly being used as first-line treatment options to try to reduce complications.

SISs are known to result in less post-operative groin pain, less bleeding, and shorter surgical times than traditional slings. On the other hand, UBAs are considered less effective in the long term but show fewer total complications.

UBA therapies were traditionally used to treat women with painful SUIs caused by ISD [12]. Currently, UBAs are rarely used as a first-line therapy for SUI; however, this procedure might be preferred by women who would rather have fewer postoperative problems, in lieu of performing this treatment several times to reduce the likelihood of a SUI recurrence.

In order to enhance the minimally invasive options available to patients who, in today's world, require effective and noninvasive treatments, this study compares UBAs and SISs in terms of efficacy, quality of life, and sexual function in women receiving first-line treatment for stress urinary incontinence. It also aims to demonstrate that UBA could be a viable first-line alternative to more invasive treatments.

2. Materials and Methods

From January 2016 to January 2021, 159 consecutive patients affected by SUI were included in the study. A prospective observational analysis was performed.

All data were prospectively evaluated from a urogynecological internal database. The Institutional Review Boards (IRB) approved the study (protocol number CD-27/2016). Informed written consent was obtained from all women. The research was conducted according to Good Clinical Practice Guidelines. Sixty-four patients underwent treatment with a UBA and 75 were treated with an SIS. As a multicentric prospective study, the clinical investigation was conducted at Sandro Pertini Hospital (Rome, Italy), Institute Marco Pasquali ICOT (Latina, Rome, Italy), Pia Fondazione G. Panico Hospital (Tricase, Italy), Policlinic Campus Biomedico Hospital (Rome), and Santo Spirito Hospital (Rome, Italy). Physical examinations, voiding diaries, and urodynamic tests were performed at our urogynecology outpatient clinic at the beginning and at the end of treatment.

The present study included only individuals who had symptoms for more than 1 year, had failed conservative treatment, and had incontinence episodes more than once every 24 h.

The following conditions were used as exclusion criteria: pelvic organ prolapse superior to grade 2(POP-Q system), neurogenic bladder, pure UUI (urgency urinary incontinence) and/or exclusive symptoms of OAB(overactive bladder), ongoing and/or suspected breast cancer, ongoing and/or suspected hormone-dependent tumors, urological tumors, endometrial hyperplasia and atypical uterine bleeding, ongoing or past venous thromboembolism, clinical evidence of chronic inflammation or urinary tract infection, and treatment history involving pelvic radiation.

Each patient conducted a supine and standing cough stress test at 300-mL bladder filling during the urogynecological examination. Urodynamic examinations were carried out in accordance with the International Continence Society (ICS) guidelines.

The maximum urethral closure pressure of 20 cm H_2O and the Valsalva leaking point pressure of 60 cm H_2O were regarded as indicators of intrinsic sphincter deficiency.

All patients in this investigation exhibited urodynamically verified urinary stress incontinence, with a median maximum cystometric capacity of 322 mL (ranging 245–498 mL) and a median Valsalva leaking pressure of 59 cm H_2O (ranging 40–100 cm H_2O), and no indication of outflow obstruction (Qmax 15 mL/s, Pvesmax > 50 cm H_2O). Patients with concurrent urinary tract infection, previous surgery for stress incontinence, functional bladder capacity of 200 mL, and stage 2 pelvic organ prolapse were excluded from the study.

Moreover, the patients completed a voiding diary before and after the treatment. Postoperatively, the International Consultation on Incontinence Questionnaire-Urine Incontinence-Short Form (ICIQ-UI-SF) was completed to assess the impact of urine symptoms. To assess sexual function, the standardized Female Sexual Function Index (FSFI), the Female Sexual Distress Scale (FSDS) and the Pelvic Organ Prolapse/Urinary Incontinence Sexual Questionnaires short form (PISQ-12) questionnaires were administered on the first visit and again after 3 months. Finally, after treatment, the Patient Global Index of Improvement (PGI-I) was calculated.

Cefazoline 2 g was administered to all patients as a preventative measure 30 min before surgery.

The patient was placed on the operation table with her hips slightly flexed.

In UBA group a local anesthetic-containing lubricant was applied within the urethra, followed by a gradual trans-urethral instillation of 2% lidocaine solution. The PAHG injection was performed under endoscopic control with a single-use PAHG Bulkamid® cystoscope (Contura International A/S, Sydmarken 23, 2860 Soeborg, Denmark) linked to a 0-degree optic to provide precise and accurate PAHG submucosal injection. The rotating sheath over the cystoscope allows the working channel to revolve 360-degrees, allowing for better access and visual control of the injection sites without having to move the entire cystoscope. Technique points include cautious needle advancement to avoid unintentional urethral mucosa injury and an angulation of fewer than 5-degrees to avoid too-deep injections. The best submucosal injection locations are at 2, 5, 7, 10 a.m., and 1 cm within of the bladder neck (proximal urethra). To ensure good urethral wall coaptation, 1–2 mL of Bulkamid® (Contura International A/S, Sydmarken 23, 2860 Soeborg, Denmark) are injected at four sites, with no more than 0.5 mL injected at each site.

In the SIS group, a spinal anesthesia was performed. The Altis® Single Incision Sling System is a transobturator MUS (midurethral sling) that is adjustable and authorized for the treatment of stress urine incontinence.

Approximately 1 cm proximal to the urethral meatus and extending downward towards the bladder neck, a 1.5 cm midurethral incision was made on the anterior vaginal wall. Then, the scissors are inserted into the vaginal incision and a "push spread" technique (at least 1.5 cm wide) is used to dissect back to the ipsilateral ischiopubic ramus. Secondly, the introducer and sling are inserted into the midline vaginal incision using an inside-out approach, with the tip of the introducer targeted via the previously dissected periurethral site towards the obturator membrane landmarks (a "10" and "2" o'clock locations). Finally, the sling is adjusted by dragging the suture loop across the patient's midline until the required support is attained, and it should be positioned tension-free beneath the urethra, allowing a right-angle tool to easily slip between the sling and the urethra. This sling employs one static and one dynamic anchor at either end of a pulley suture, allowing for simple intraoperative tension modulation.

Clinical evaluation and exam, uroflowmetry, urodynamic exam and questionnaires were performed at the first appointment and after at least 24 months after surgical intervention.

Using Fisher's exact test, we determined the statistical significance of each event based on its incidence. For each comparison, an odds ratio (OR) and 95% confidence interval (CI) were generated. To evaluate whether data were sampled from a Gaussian distribution, normality tests (D'Agostino and Pearson tests) were used. To compare continuous parametric and non-parametric variables (data that do not fall into a normal distribution), the t-test and Mann–Whitney U test were employed, respectively. The Spearman rank coefficient was used to calculate correlations between numerical parameters. A matched t-test was used to evaluate the change in questionnaire results (ICIQ-UI-SF, PISQ-12, FSFI, FSDS, PGI-I). All analyses were carried out with the Statistical Package for the Social Sciences (SPSS) 22.0 for Mac (SSPS, Chicago, IL, USA). A p-value of less than 0.05 was considered significant.

3. Results

The total number of patients was 211. Since 33 patients did not match the inclusion criteria and 39 were lost to follow-up, the sample consisted of 159 patients.

The 159 evaluated patients were divided into 2 groups: 64 patients who underwent UBA and 75 with SIS. Patients' characteristics as age, BMI, parity, menopausal status, use of HRT, previous hysterectomy and POPQ status are similar between the two groups and shown in Table 1.

Table 1. Patient characteristics.

Variable	Bulkamid Group (64 Patients)	ALTIS Group (75 Patients)	p
Age, year	55.8 ± 10.2	56.8 ± 8.9	0.06
Body mass index, kg/m^2	27.5 ± 3.4	26.8 ± 5.7	0.06
Parity, range	2 (1–3)	2 (1–3)	0.08
Menopausal status, n (%)	31 (48.4)	32 (42.7)	0.07
Hormone replacement therapy, n (%)	8/31 (25.8)	8/32 (25)	0.09
Previous hysterectomy, n (%)	9 (11.5)	7 (8.6)	0.08
POPQ system			
Stage 0 (%)	60 (76.9)	59 (72.8)	0.08
Stage 1 (%)	18 (23)	22 (27.1)	0.07

Values are given as mean ± standard deviation (SD).

Median follow-up was 29 months (24–37).

The two procedures had an almost overlapping intervention time (22.87 + 6.32 min. for the bulking-agents injection vs. 23.22 + 7.44 for ALTIS). We registered the post-operative complications in both groups (Table 2) but only two of them reached a statistical significance; no patients of the Bulkamid group complained about pain after the procedure, unlike the ALTIS group where 9 patients out of 75 (10.8%) experienced post-operative groin pain (p = 0.03). Five patients in the ALTIS group developed de novo urgency compared to none in the UBA group (0.04).

Table 2. Postoperative complications in 159 patients.

Variable	Bulkamid Group (64 Patients)	ALTIS Group (75 Patients)	p
Operative time, min	22.87 ± 6.32	23.22 ± 7.44	0.08
Fever, n (%)	1 (1.2)	0 (0)	0.09
Groin pain, n (%)	0 (0)	9 (10.8)	0.03
Urinary tract infection, n (%)	2 (2.6)	3 (3.6)	0.07
Deep vein thrombosis, n (%)	0 (0)	0 (0)	0.07
Urinary retention for up to 7 days, n (%)	1 (1.2)	1 (1.3)	0.08
Tape extrusion, n (%)	0 (0)	2 (2.5)	0.08
Severe pain, n (%)	0	0 (0)	0.09
Dyspareunia, n (%) †	0	2 (2.5)	0.06
De novo urgency (%)	0	5 (6.6)	0.04
Recurrent SUI (%)	4 (5.1)	4 (5)	0.09

SUI = Stress urinary incontinence. †: in patients who regularly practice sexual activity (>2 intercourses/month).

The comparison of the voiding diary before and 29 months after treatment also showed interesting results (Table 3).

Table 3. Comparison of Voiding Diary before and after treatment (29 months Follow-Up).

Variables	Bulkamid Group (64 Patients)			ALTIS Group (75 Patients)			
Follow Up	Baseline	Median FU	p	Baseline	Median FU	p	p
Positive Stress Test (%)	64 (100)	4 (5.1)	<0.0001	75 (100)	5 (6.2)	<0.0001	0.07
Q-Tip swab test (grade)	41.44 ± 12.10	23.15 ± 10.41	<0.0001	42.34 ± 11.11	21.87 ± 8.56	<0.0001	0.08
Mean number of voids (24 h)	7.72 ± 1.65	9.43 ± 2.22	0.04	7.34 ± 2.12	7.65 ± 1.98	0.08	0.03
Mean number of nocturia events	0.98 ± 0.43	0.78 ± 0.45	ns	1.12 ± 0.88	0.92 ± 0.95	0.06	0.09

Abbreviation: ns: not significant.

In the Bulkamid group, only 4 patients (5.1%) had a persistently positive Stress Test ($p < 0.0001$), as well as the ALTIS group in which 5 patients (6.2%) had a positive Stress Test ($p < 0.0001$).

The results of the urodynamic assessment conducted both before and after the therapy are shown in Table 4. In terms of first voiding desire (from 91 to 138 mL in the Bulkamid group and from 89 to 142 mL in the ALTIS group), maximal cystometric capacity (from 301 to 387 mL in the Bulkamid group and from 298 to 398 mL in the ALTIS group), detrusorial pressure at peak flow (from 18 to 14 cm H_2O in the Bulkamid group and from 19 to 13 cm H_2O in the ALTIS group), and peak flow (from 20 to 23 mL/s in the Bulkamid group and from 19 to 25 mL/s in the ALTIS group), the table demonstrates the significant outcomes achieved with these treatments and supports the efficacy of both methods without differences between the 2 groups.

Table 4. Pre- and post-urodynamic evaluation.

Urodynamic Data	Bulkamid Group (64 Patients)			ALTIS Group (75 Patients)			Bulkamid vs. Altis
	Baseline	12 Weeks	p	Baseline	12 Weeks	p	p
Peak flow (mL/s)	20.71 ± 3.60	23.23 ± 4.23	0.01	19.65 ± 4.23	24.81 ± 5.88	<0.0001	0.07
Flow time (mL/s)	26.22 ± 5.11	27.67 ± 5.18	0.11	25.68 ± 5.51	27.77 ± 5.11	0.09	0.81
Post-void residual (mL)	20.55 ± 6.28	19.54 ± 6.12	0.49	21.11 ± 7.09	20.13 ± 7.11	0.54	0.72
First voiding desire (mL)	91.76 ± 20.13	138.72 ± 19.24	0.004	89.23 ± 21.47	142.43 ± 19.98	<0.0001	0.32
Maximum cystometric capacity (mL)	301.31 ± 73.56	387.76 ± 82.44	0.002	298.65 ± 77.28	398.26 ± 91.21	0.0031	0.55
Detrusor pressure at peak flow (cm H_2O)	18.78 ± 5.63	14.45 ± 6.10	0.0012	19.11 ± 6.12	13.89 ± 4.89	<0.0001	0.21
Maximum Urethral Closure Pressure (cm H_2O)	69.87 ± 9.11	70.32 ± 8.34	0.69	68.91 ± 9.71	71.09 ± 7.91	0.51	0.72
Urethral Functional Length (mm)	28.10 ± 2.22	28.21 ± 2.33	0.41	28.43 ± 3.01	28.67 ± 2.93	0.65	0.81
Patients with detrusor overactive (%)	36 (60)	23 (38.3)	0.13	30 (57.7)	9 (17.3)	0.02	0.08

In both groups, we observed a notable improvement in the QoL (quality of life) with a halving score in ICIQ-UI-SF 29 months after treatment (Bulkamid group from 14.58 ± 5.11 at baseline to 5.67 ± 1.90 after 29 months; $p < 0.0001$ vs. ALTIS group from 13.75 ± 5.89 to 5.83 ± 1.78; $p < 0.0001$).

Likewise, we noted an improvement in sexual function, with the number of sexually active patients increasing from 29 to 44 (56.4%) in Bulkamid group ($p = 0.041$) and from 31 to 51 (61.7%) in ALTIS group ($p = 0.034$). In accordance with the last data, the scores derived from PISQ-12, FSFI and FSDS also showed an improvement in women's sexual function (Table 5).

Table 5. Quality of Life and Sexual Function at 29 months follow up.

Variables	Bulkamid Group (64 Patients)			ALTIS Group (75 Patients)		
	Preoperative	Median FU	p Value	Preoperative	Median FU	p Value
ICIQ-UI-SF	14.58 ± 5.11	5.67 ± 1.90	<0.001	13.75 ± 5.89	5.83 ± 1.78	<0.001
Sexual Activity † (%)	29 (37.2)	44 (56.4)	0.041	31 (38.2)	50 (61.7)	0.034
PISQ-12 ‡	30.44 ± 7.23	36.54 ± 6.98	<0.001	31.22 ± 5.65	38.33 ± 6.24	<0.001
FSFI ‡	20.43 ± 2.22	29.77 ± 1.89	<0.001	21.21 ± 1.43	29.34 ± 2.11	<0.001
FSDS ‡	21.65 ± 4.76	8.32 ± 3.56	<0.001	20.98 ± 5.43	7.86 ± 4.78	<0.001

Abbreviations: ICIQ-UI-SF: International Consultation on Incontinence Questionnaire–Urinary Incontinence Short Form; PISQ-12: Pelvic Organ Prolapse/Urinary Incontinence Sexual Questionnaire short form; FSFI: Female Sexual Function Index; FSDS: Female Sexual Distress Scale. †: Number of patients who regularly practice sexual activity (>2 intercourses/month). ‡: In patients who regularly practice sexual activity (>2 intercourses/month).

4. Discussion

Our analysis compares the two primary minimally invasive treatment choices for SUI above a wide range of additional possibilities for the first time in the literature: the contemporary SIS vs. UBAs. The comparison is based on the assessment of treatment effectiveness, safety, and enhancement of sexual function and quality of life.

SUI is a frequent condition among women and has a significant impact on quality of life (QoL). The first-line approach should include conservative therapies such as lifestyle advice, physical therapies (PFMT and pelvic-floor muscle training), scheduled voiding regimes, behavioral therapies, and medications [5]. When all of these therapies fail, patients with limited bladder-neck mobility may undergo the full range of surgical treatments, such as midurethral sling, gold standard treatment, or, when indicated, UBA injection.

Since retropubic and transobturator midurethral slings are associated with severe adverse effects (including bladder rupture, damage to blood vessels, and pelvic pain), today, single-incision midurethral slings (SISs) aim to reduce complications and be less invasive.

Nowadays, the literature acknowledges that SIS is an excellent and effective technique despite being minimally invasive, with significantly reduced operating times and pelvic inguinal pain compared to traditional approaches [13].

Contrary to UBAs, an SIS is also commonly used as a first-line treatment for SUI. UBAs are now largely indicated for IDS and/or urethral hypomobility. However, in both circumstances, they are considered a second-line alternative treatment.

Our initial goal was to compare UBAs and SISs in order to establish the efficacy of both these minimally invasive treatments.

Indeed, much has been published about women with SUI preferring less-successful interventions with fewer postoperative complications to more-effective procedures with significant side effects [14,15].

Regarding safety, only eight patients out of 64 from the UBA group showed complications. Only one patient experienced acute urinary retention, in contrast to Giammò et al. who described 8.2% of patients experiencing this self-limited side effect [16]. None of our patients reported de novo urgency, unlike Itkonen Freitas et al. [17] who described 9.3% of patients experiencing this complication. On the other hand, 26 patients out of 75 from SIS group showed side effects. The most frequent complication in this group was groin pain, in line with Moran et al. We also registered 6.6% of patients showing de novo urgency, which is comparable with the 5.3% of patients registered by Youxiang Han et al. [18], while Moran et al. reported a slightly higher rate of de novo urgency (8.1%) as well as a higher rate of urinary retention cases (7.2%) compared to our single case. Tape extrusion occurred in 2.5% of patients, in line with the literature [19,20].

SISs and UBAs were demonstrated to be highly effective. This is shown in the stress-test data. In fact, at the median follow-up (29 months), the number of patients with positive stress tests decreased drastically. Similarly, Q-Tip Swab Test grades were almost halved in both groups. These results appear to be better than the average "objective cure rate" drawn from the studies we analyzed [15,17,19,21].

We could justify this high cure rate because all procedures had been performed by the same expert (more than 100 procedures) surgeon, in the same center with a high volume of patients. Nevertheless, we believe in the need to standardize the parameters that define the "objective cure rate", to align outcomes of these two procedures.

Another fundamental parameter to assess the effectiveness of treatments is the "subjective cure rate", which could be defined as the personal perception of clinical improvement by the patients.

We obtained this data by submitting, to patients, questionnaires to evaluate their QoL, such as the ICIQ-UI-SF and the PGI-I scale. According to Kamarkar et al. [22], the cut-off points in the ICIQ to evaluate patients' satisfaction should be <6/21. These results are supported by the data in the literature which show a notable improvement in the ISIQ-UI-SF score after treatment [17,22]. The other item we used to evaluate QoL was the PGI-I scale. In our study, patients reported to feel "very much better" or "much better", so the "subjective cure rate" of both groups after treatment was approximately in line with the literature [15,17,19,21,23]. Hence, SISs and UBAs appeared to be totally comparable in effectiveness and safety at a 24-month follow-up. The only significant difference was the absence of groin pain after UBA treatment.

Another goal of our study was to investigate the changes in sexual function and sexual satisfaction of women treated with bulking agents vs. SIS. The number of sexually active patients (>2 intercourses/month) increased from 29 (37.2%) to 44 (56.4%) in the UBA group and from 31 (38.2%) to 50 (61.7%) in the SIS group. Similarly, the scores from the PISQ-12, FSFI, and FSDS showed an improvement in women's sexual function. There is limited literature available on the evaluation of sexual life after surgical SUI treatment. The two studies we found assess sexual function by using only one questionnaire out of the three we used in our study [24,25].

The strength of our study lies in the mid-term follow-up, which enables the evaluation of patients over time, unlike studies with only a short-term follow-up. As mentioned above, all patients underwent treatment by a single surgeon in the same high-volume center, minimizing the inter-operator outcome variability. Evaluation of sexual function via more than one questionnaire allows for the creation of a more precise score for sexual activity.

Some limitations include the small number of patients, the need of a longer follow-up (>60 months), the presence of selection bias, and the absence of randomization. In addition, we found, in Sekiguchi et al. [26], a cumulative cure rate of 91% after SIS treatment in a group of patients affected by mixed urinary incontinence, showing SUI together with ISD characteristics. According to these results, various research [27–29] showed high rates of success and enhanced quality of life following SIS therapy. This could widen the field of the application of SIS treatment, but further studies and investigations are needed, including a randomized double-blind-design study on a larger cohort of patients.

5. Conclusions

Overall, to the best of our knowledge, this is the first comparative evaluation of these therapies in two groups of patients with comparable features. Furthermore, using a variety of tools for evaluation, our study assesses both the objective and subjective success of the therapies.

Although further research and double-randomized trials are required, we have demonstrated that UBAs are highly successful when compared to minimally invasive surgical methods such as SISs, and they also have fewer side effects. Our study shows how a UBA can be used as a first-line therapy option since it helps reestablish the transient sphincteric mechanism of continence, which is the foundation of incontinence physiology. This gives women the option to choose the therapy that makes them feel more comfortable and gives them the possibility to choose a less invasive procedure.

Author Contributions: Conceptualization, M.C.S., A.M., M.C. (Mauro Cervigni), P.P., G.G. (Giovanni P.C.), V.S. (Vincenzo Spina), M.C. (Marco Calcagnoand), C.R., M.A.Z., D.G. and L.C.; methodology, M.C.S. and L.C.; software, M.C.S.; validation, M.C.S.; formal analysis, M.C.S.; investigation, M.C.S. and L.C.; resources, M.C.S. and L.C.; data curation, M.C.S. and L.C.; writing—original draft preparation, M.C.S., L.C., G.G. (Gianluca Gabrielliand), E.C. and V.S. (Vitaliana Stefanachiand); writing—review and editing, M.C.S., L.C., G.G. (Gianluca Gabrielliand), E.C., V.S. (Vitaliana Stefanachiand) and E.P.; visualization, M.C.S.; supervision, M.C.S.; project administration, M.C.S. All authors have read and agreed to the published version of the manuscript.

Funding: This research received no external funding.

Institutional Review Board Statement: This study was approved on 11 January 2016 by the Institutional Review Board (IRB) at Azienda Sanitaria Locale ASL Roma 2 (approval no. CD-27/2016).

Informed Consent Statement: Informed consent was obtained from all subjects involved in the study. Written informed consent has been obtained from the patients to publish this paper.

Data Availability Statement: Data are contained within the article.

Conflicts of Interest: The authors declare no conflicts of interest. The funders had no role in the design of the study; in the collection, analyses, or interpretation of data; in the writing of the manuscript; or in the decision to publish the results.

References

1. Abrams, P.; Cardozo, L.; Fall, M.; Griffiths, D.; Rosier, P.; Ulmsten, U.; van Kerrebroeck, P.; Victor, A.; Wein, A.; Standardisation Sub-committee of the International Continence Society. The standardisation of terminology of lower urinary tract function: Report from the Standardisation Sub-committee of the International Continence Society. *Neurourol. Urodyn.* **2002**, *21*, 167–178. [CrossRef]
2. Mardon, R.E.; Halim, S.; Pawlson, L.G.; Haffer, S.C. Management of urinary incontinence in Medicare managed care beneficiaries: Results from the 2004 Medicare Health Outcomes Survey. *Arch. Intern. Med.* **2006**, *166*, 1128–1133. [CrossRef]
3. Griffiths, A.N.; Makam, A.; Edwards, G.J. Should we actively screen for urinary and anal incontinence in the general gynaecology outpatients setting?--A prospective observational study. *J. Obstet. Gynaecol.* **2006**, *26*, 442–444. [CrossRef]
4. Minassian, V.A.; Yan, X.; Lichtenfeld, M.J.; Sun, H.; Stewart, W.F. The iceberg of health care utilization in women with urinary incontinence. *Int. Urogynecol. J.* **2012**, *23*, 1087–1093. [CrossRef]
5. Abrams, P.; Andersson, K.E.; Birder, L.; Brubaker, L.; Cardozo, L.; Chapple, C.; Cottenden, A.; Davila, W.; de Ridder, D.; Dmochowski, R.; et al. Fourth International Consultation on Incontinence Recommendations of the International Scientific Committee: Evaluation and treatment of urinary incontinence, pelvic organ prolapse, and fecal incontinence. *Neurourol. Urodyn.* **2010**, *29*, 213–240. [CrossRef]
6. Ashton-Miller, J.A.; Howard, D.; DeLancey, J.O. The functional anatomy of the female pelvic floor and stress continence control system. *Scand. J. Urol. Nephrol.* **2001**, *35*, 1–7; discussion 106–125.
7. Perucchini, D.; Fink, D. Stressinkontinenz der Frau: Theorien und moderne Operationstechniken in Vergleich [Urinary stress incontinence in the female: Comparison of incontinence theories and new tension-free surgical procedures]. *Gynäkologisch-Geburtshilfliche Rundsch.* **2002**, *42*, 133–140. (In German) [CrossRef]
8. Carone, R. *La Teoria Uretro-Centrica*, 1st ed.; Litografia Saba S.r.l.: Rome, Italy, 2011.
9. Obstetrics and Gynecology Devices Panel of the Medical Devices Advisory Committee Meeting Announcement. Available online: https://www.fda.gov/advisory-committees/advisory-committee-calendar/february-12-2019-obstetrics-and-gynecology-devices-panel-medical-devices-advisory-committee-meeting (accessed on 10 February 2024).
10. Kobashi, K.C.; Vasavada, S.; Bloschichak, A.; Hermanson, L.; Kaczmarek, J.; Kim, S.K.; Kirkby, E.; Malik, R. Updates to Surgical Treatment of Female Stress Urinary Incontinence (SUI): AUA/SUFU Guideline (2023). *J. Urol.* **2023**, *209*, 1091–1098. [CrossRef]
11. Nambiar, A.K.; Arlandis, S.; Bø, K.; Cobussen-Boekhorst, H.; Costantini, E.; de Heide, M.; Farag, F.; Groen, J.; Karavitakis, M.; Lapitan, M.C.; et al. European Association of Urology Guidelines on the Diagnosis and Management of Female Non-neurogenic Lower Urinary Tract Symptoms. Part 1: Diagnostics, Overactive Bladder, Stress Urinary Incontinence, and Mixed Urinary Incontinence. *Eur. Urol.* **2022**, *82*, 49–59. [CrossRef]
12. Abrams, P.; Cardozo, L.; Fall, M.; Griffiths, D.; Rosier, P.; Ulmsten, U.; Van Kerrebroeck, P.; Victor, A.; Wein, A.; Standardisation Sub-Committee of the International Continence Society. The standardisation of terminology in lower urinary tract function: Report from the standardisation sub-committee of the International Continence Society. *Urology* **2003**, *61*, 37–49. [CrossRef]
13. Kasi, A.D.; Pergialiotis, V.; Perrea, D.N.; Khunda, A.; Doumouchtsis, S.K. Polyacrylamide hydrogel (Bulkamid®) for stress urinary incontinence in women: A systematic review of the literature. *Int. Urogynecol. J.* **2016**, *27*, 367–375. [CrossRef]

14. Patel, T.; Sugandh, F.; Bai, S.; Varrassi, G.; Devi, A.; Khatri, M.; Kumar, S.; Dembra, D.; Dahri, S. Single Incision Mini-Sling Versus Mid-Urethral Sling (Transobturator/Retropubic) in Females With Stress Urinary Incontinence: A Systematic Review and Meta-Analysis. *Cureus* **2023**, *15*, e37773. [CrossRef]
15. Brosche, T.; Kuhn, A.; Lobodasch, K.; Sokol, E.R. Seven-year efficacy and safety outcomes of Bulkamid for the treatment of stress urinary incontinence. *Neurourol. Urodyn.* **2021**, *40*, 502–508. [CrossRef]
16. Giammò, A.; Geretto, P.; Ammirati, E.; Manassero, A.; Squintone, L.; Vercelli, D.; Carone, R. Urethral bulking with Bulkamid: An analysis of efficacy, safety profile, and predictors of functional outcomes in a single-center cohort. *Neurourol. Urodyn.* **2020**, *39*, 1523–1528. [CrossRef]
17. Anna-Maija, I.F.; Mentula, M.; Rahkola-Soisalo, P.; Tulokas, S.; Mikkola, T.S. Tension-Free Vaginal Tape Surgery versus Polyacrylamide Hydrogel Injection for Primary Stress Urinary Incontinence: A Randomized Clinical Trial. *J. Urol.* **2020**, *203*, 372–378.
18. Han, J.Y.; Huang, E.Y.; Liu, J.; Sultana, R.; Han, H.C. Short-medium term outcomes of Altis® single-incision sling for stress urinary incontinence in an Asian single-centre. *Continence* **2022**, *3*, 100498. [CrossRef]
19. Kocjancic, E.; Erickson, T.; Tu, L.M.; Gheiler, E.; Van Drie, D. Two-year outcomes for the Altis® adjustable single incision sling system for treatment of SUI. *Neurourol. Urodyn.* **2017**, *36*, 1582–1587. [CrossRef]
20. Dias, J.; Xambre, L.; Costa, L.; Costa, P.; Ferraz, L. Short-term outcomes of Altis single-incision sling procedure for SUI: A prospective single-center study. *Int. Urogynecol. J.* **2014**, *25*, 1089–1095. [CrossRef]
21. Morán, E.; Pérez-Ardavín, J.; Sánchez, J.V.; Bonillo, M.A.; Martínez-Cuenca, E.; Arlandis, S.; Broseta, E.; Boronat, F. Mid-term safety and efficacy of the ALTIS® single-incision sling for female stress urinary incontinence: Less mesh, same results. *BJU Int.* **2019**, *123*, E51–E56. [CrossRef]
22. Karmakar, D.; Mostafa, A.; Abdel-Fattah, M. A new validated score for detecting patient-reported success on postoperative ICIQ-SF: A novel two-stage analysis from two large RCT cohorts. *Int. Urogynecol. J.* **2017**, *28*, 95–100. [CrossRef]
23. Sokol, E.R.; Karram, M.M.; Dmochowski, R. Efficacy and safety of polyacrylamide hydrogel for the treatment of female stress incontinence: A randomized, prospective, multicenter North American study. *J. Urol.* **2014**, *192*, 843. [CrossRef] [PubMed]
24. Leone Roberti Maggiore, U.; Alessandri, F.; Medica, M.; Gabelli, M.; Venturini, P.L.; Ferrero, S. Periurethral injection of polyacrylamide hydrogel for the treatment of stress urinary incontinence: The impact on female sexual function. *J. Sex. Med.* **2012**, *9*, 3255–3263. [CrossRef] [PubMed]
25. Naumann, G.; Steetskamp, J.; Meyer, M.; Laterza, R.; Skala, C.; Albrich, S.; Koelbl, H. Sexual function and quality of life following retropubic TVT and single-incision sling in women with stress urinary incontinence: Results of a prospective study. *Arch. Gynecol. Obstet.* **2013**, *287*, 959–966. [CrossRef] [PubMed]
26. Sekiguchi, Y.; Kinjyo, M.; Inoue, H.; Sakata, H.; Kubota, Y. Outpatient mid urethral tissue fixation system sling for urodynamic SUI. *J. Urol.* **2009**, *182*, 2810–2813. [CrossRef] [PubMed]
27. Zullo, M.A.; Schiavi, M.C.; Luffarelli, P.; Bracco, G.; Iuliano, A.; Grilli, D.; Esperto, F.; Cervigni, M. Efficacy and safety of anterior vaginal prolapse treatment using single incision repair system: Multicentric study. *Taiwan. J. Obstet. Gynecol.* **2022**, *61*, 646–651. [CrossRef] [PubMed]
28. Schiavi, M.C.; Carletti, V.; Yacoub, V.; Cardella, G.; Luffarelli, P.; Valensise, H.C.C.; Palazzetti, P.; Spina, V.; Zullo, M.A. Evaluation of the efficacy and safety of single incision sling vs TVT-O in obese patients with stress urinary incontinence: Quality of life and sexual function analysis. *Taiwan. J. Obstet. Gynecol.* **2023**, *62*, 89–93. [CrossRef] [PubMed]
29. Zullo, M.A.; Schiavi, M.C.; Luffarelli, P.; Prata, G.; Di Pinto, A.; Oliva, C. TVT-O vs. TVT-Abbrevo for stress urinary incontinence treatment in women: A randomized trial. *Int. Urogynecol. J.* **2020**, *31*, 703–710. [CrossRef] [PubMed]

Disclaimer/Publisher's Note: The statements, opinions and data contained in all publications are solely those of the individual author(s) and contributor(s) and not of MDPI and/or the editor(s). MDPI and/or the editor(s) disclaim responsibility for any injury to people or property resulting from any ideas, methods, instructions or products referred to in the content.

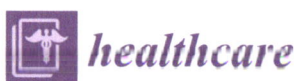

Article

Pelvic Floor Dysfunction among Reproductive-Age Women in Israel: Prevalence and Attitudes—A Cross-Sectional Study

Tehila Fisher-Yosef [1,2,*], Dina Lidsky Sachs [3], Shiri Sacha Edel [1], Hanan Nammouz [1], Abd Ellatif Zoabi [1] and Limor Adler [1,2]

1. Health Division, Maccabi Healthcare Services, Tel Aviv 6812509, Israel
2. Faculty of Medicine, Tel Aviv University, Tel Aviv 6997801, Israel
3. The Azrieli Faculty of Medicine, Bar Ilan University, Zefat 1311502, Israel
* Correspondence: fisher_t@mac.org.il

Abstract: Objectives: Our study aimed to investigate the prevalence of female pelvic floor dysfunction (PFD) in Israeli women who experienced vaginal delivery and are in their reproductive years (premenopausal), as well as to understand their attitudes and health-seeking behavior and barriers towards treating this problem. **Methods:** In this cross-sectional study, we conducted a questionnaire-based Internet survey. The surveys were sent to Israeli women in their fertile years (18–50 years old). We asked the women about their PFD symptoms, attitudes, and help-seeking behaviors. We used two validated questionnaires, including the USIQ and the PFDI-20. The combined questionnaire was submitted in both Hebrew and Arabic. We assessed the prevalence of PFD symptoms in the study population. Symptomatic women were asked about their help-seeking behaviors and their beliefs, desires, and barriers regarding the clinical management of symptoms. **Results:** Between July and September 2020, 524 women completed the questionnaire (response rate 44%). In total, 95% reported at least one symptom (mostly urinary-related) at any grade of severity in at least one category, and 66.8% suffered from at least one moderate to severe symptom in at least one category. Most women (93.7%) reported that they wanted to be asked and offered voluntary information about PFD from physicians and nurses; however, only 16.6% reported receiving such information. Barriers to seeking treatment were mainly related to low awareness. The study's main limitation was selection bias due to the questionnaire's design. **Conclusions:** These findings show the importance of raising awareness of the different therapeutic solutions to PFD symptoms and designing more available services for this common problem.

Keywords: pelvic floor dysfunction; women; parous; reproductive-age women; attitudes; prevalence

Citation: Fisher-Yosef, T.; Lidsky Sachs, D.; Edel, S.S.; Nammouz, H.; Zoabi, A.E.; Adler, L. Pelvic Floor Dysfunction among Reproductive-Age Women in Israel: Prevalence and Attitudes—A Cross-Sectional Study. Healthcare 2024, 12, 390. https://doi.org/10.3390/healthcare12030390

Academic Editors: Matteo Frigerio and Stefano Manodoro

Received: 14 December 2023
Revised: 30 January 2024
Accepted: 31 January 2024
Published: 2 February 2024

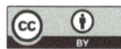

Copyright: © 2024 by the authors. Licensee MDPI, Basel, Switzerland. This article is an open access article distributed under the terms and conditions of the Creative Commons Attribution (CC BY) license (https://creativecommons.org/licenses/by/4.0/).

1. Introduction

Female pelvic floor dysfunction (PFD) is a term applied to a wide variety of clinical conditions, including urinary incontinence (stress, urge, and mixed), fecal and flatus incontinence, pelvic organ prolapse (POP), constipation, sexual dysfunction, and several chronic pelvic pain syndromes [1–3]. These conditions may cause significant suffering and impair the quality of life for many women, affecting their mental and sexual health as well as their social and physical activities [4–6]. The disorder is considered multifactorial, with vaginal parity being one of the leading risk factors for developing it [2,3,7,8], with a positive correlation to the number of vaginal births [4,7,8]. Assisted vaginal births (i.e., forceps and vacuum deliveries) were found to be contributing factors [2,5], as well as an extended second phase of labor (over 1 h), history of 3rd- or 4th-degree perineal tears, obesity, older age, positive family history of PFD, and smoking [2,6–9].

Estimating the prevalence of PFD is important for several reasons, including assessing the public health burden of these conditions as well as implementing healthcare strategies. Different studies have examined the prevalence of these conditions, usually using voluntary questionnaires [2,5,10–19]. Some studies have focused on urinary symptoms alone, some on the postpartum period, and some on the postmenopausal period. Correspondingly, there is a wide variation in the prevalence of PFD when comparing these studies and others, and any figure between 1.9 and 67% can be found. However, it is, without a doubt, not a rare condition. Nevertheless, the data on women in their reproductive years beyond the peripartum period are scarce.

PFD is a largely treatable problem. Pelvic floor muscle training (with or without biofeedback) has been shown to improve urinary incontinence, pain, and quality of life [20–23]; pessary surgery (implantation of sub-urethral tension-free slings, symmetric lateral levator myography colposuspension) is also an available treatment [23–25], as are botulinum toxin injections in selected cases [23]. Without early intervention, PFD may deteriorate and require more invasive and costly treatments. In a Cochrane meta-analysis by Dumoulin et al. involving a total of 165 patients, there was a cure rate of 56.1% in those who performed pelvic floor exercises and only 6% in those who did not (relative risk [RR] 8.38, 95% CI 3.68–19.07) [26]. The treated groups had significantly better outcomes concerning their quality of life, satisfaction with treatment, and need for further treatment compared with the control groups. Leaving PFD untreated could also be very costly: One study estimated the costs of ambulatory treatment for PFD in the United States to be as high as USD 300 million between 2005 and 2006 [27]. Left untreated, PFD has negative effects on women's health and quality of life, affecting their physical and mental health and sometimes even leading to social isolation, anxiety, and depression [28,29].

Despite the nature of PFD as a preventable and treatable condition affecting everyday life, most women avoid discussing this issue when encountering healthcare professionals [12,18,30,31]. The reasons for this are various: Some women have the perception that PFD is a normal part of aging, some expect it to wane eventually without intervention, some are too embarrassed to raise the issue, and some see it as an inevitable and untreatable adverse effect of parity, i.e., are unaware that treatment is available [18,32]. As a result, many women are left untreated or wait many years before seeking medical help [12,32].

Our study aimed to investigate the prevalence of PFD in Israeli parous women in their reproductive years and to investigate their needs, attitudes, barriers, and health-seeking behavior surrounding this problem. In addition, we wanted to evaluate which social-demographic and medical factors were associated with PFD and moderate-to-severe PFD. This would ideally assist us in understanding the key obstacles associated with addressing this medical condition and enhancing the quality of life for women.

2. Methods and Materials

2.1. Setting and Study Design

In this cross-sectional study, we conducted a questionnaire-based internet survey using PharmaQuest Ltd. (Ramat-Gan, Israel) company's platform. The company has an advanced, fully secured online system that enables questionnaire distribution and de-identified data collection that fully complies with EphMRA, ESOMAR, and ethical codes of conduct. It is a private independent research company and is not affiliated with any product.

The company distributes advertisements and invitations to join its databases on various websites such as Google and Facebook. Every internet-accessible citizen can be exposed to these invitations and links and can join the database, which is free and on a voluntary basis. Afterwards, a comparison is conducted between the demographic details of registered individuals and the overall demographic profile of Israeli citizens, as provided by the Central Bureau of Statistics in Israel, to generate a representative sample. The sample includes 100,000 people representing Israeli society. Registered individuals respond to population surveys and accumulate points with which they can purchase vouchers.

The company can activate filters when distributing questionnaires, such as selecting specific age groups or a particular gender.

The e-mail provided details about the study and invited the women to participate in an anonymous survey. Those who satisfied the age and parity inclusion criteria, determined by initial filtering questions, were allowed to proceed to the full questionnaire.

Within the survey, we inquired about the PFD symptoms, attitudes, and behaviors related to seeking help. The funding for these services was sourced from Marom, a research program catering to physicians and residents affiliated with Maccabi Healthcare Services.

2.2. Study Population

Inclusion criteria: women who experienced at least one vaginal delivery and are in their fertile years (18–50 years old).

2.3. The Questionnaire

We used two validated and well-established questionnaires for detecting PFD and assessing its effect on quality of life: the Pelvic Floor Distress Inventory (PFDI-20) [33–35] and the Urgency Severity and Impact Questionnaire (USIQ) [13,35]. The PFDI-20 questionnaire is a 20-item questionnaire divided into 6 items evaluating pelvic organ prolapse distress, eight items evaluating colorectal anal distress, and six items evaluating urinary distress. The USIQ focuses on urge urinary incontinence and has two parts: symptom severity and related quality of life. It includes 14 questions. Both questionnaires were previously validated in Hebrew [34,35]. After receiving permission from the original authors, we translated the questionnaires into Arabic using reverse translation and validation tools. Three native Arabic speaker doctors reviewed the questionnaire before distribution. Then, we designed a complete questionnaire that included four sections (see the full version in Supplementary Materials):

(a) Filtering questions for inclusion criteria (age, previous vaginal delivery)—2 questions;
(b) PFDI and USIQ questions for identifying symptomatic women—34 questions in total. These questions provided information on the prevalence of PFD in the study population;
(c) Beliefs, attitude, barriers, and treatment-seeking behaviors regarding PFD—9 questions. These questions explored symptomatic women's beliefs about their symptoms, willingness to seek and explore different medical solutions, and ability to adhere to recommended treatment methods;
(d) Medical, social, and demographic questions—18 questions. These included: age, number of births (both vaginal and cesarean), years since last delivery, types of vaginal deliveries (assisted or not), history of episiotomy, weight, height, smoking status, history of hormonal medication—both consumption and duration, ethnicity, education, marital status, and socio-economic status (based on income and residence).

The questionnaire was submitted in both Hebrew and Arabic. An English translation is available in the Supplementary Materials.

We divided the PFDI and USIQ answers into five categories: (1) bladder symptoms—mainly stress incontinence; (2) bladder symptoms—mainly overactive bladder/urge incontinence; (3) colorectal symptoms—mainly obstructive, i.e., constipation; (4) colorectal symptoms involving mainly incontinence—flatus and/or fecal; and (5) pelvic pain or discomfort and pelvic organ prolapse.

Each category was given a severity scale corresponding to the questionnaires we used (ranging from 0, as in never having these symptoms, to 5, as in having symptoms and finding them considerably bothersome). A score above 0 in each category was sufficient to define the patient as symptomatic, and a score of 3 and above (i.e., "yes, and it bothers me to a minor/moderate/great extent") defined a patient with moderate to severe symptoms.

2.4. Statistical Analysis

We used descriptive statistics to characterize the variables, including mean and standard deviation (SD) for continuous variables and counts and percentages for categorical variables. For the univariate comparison of continuous variables, we used the Student *t*-test for standard distribution variables and Mann–Whitney for non-normal distribution variables. For categorical variables, we used the chi-square test. We performed a multivariate analysis with logistic regression to test which factors were associated with PFD and moderate to severe PFD. In this regression, we inserted all sociodemographic and medical variables to test which affected the presentation of symptoms; these variables included age, number of vaginal deliveries, time since the last delivery, perineal stitching, assisted delivery (forceps/vacuum), socio-economic status, ethnic background (Arab, Orthodox Jewish, all others), BMI, and smoking. A p value < 0.05 was considered significant. All analyses were performed using SPSS Statistics version 27 (SPSS Inc., Chicago, IL, USA).

2.5. Ethical Considerations

The institutional review board of Assuta Health Care ASMC-0110-18 approved the study. Study participation was voluntary and anonymous. Consent to participate was granted by submission of a completed questionnaire.

3. Results

3.1. Participants

From July to September 2020, A total of 25,000 personal e-mail invitations were sent to all women under the age of 50 in the database. A total of 9907 women (4633 native Hebrew speakers and 5274 native Arabic speakers) accessed the questionnaire. This confirmed that they had seen the survey. Participants who answered the full survey were granted 20 NIS worth of vouchers.

The invitation to participate in the survey was emailed on six different occasions over these months (approximately once every two weeks). One thousand three hundred ninety-eight women answered the initial filtering questions. Out of the participants who fulfilled the inclusion criteria based on the initial filtering questions (i.e., being between the ages of 18–50 and having undergone at least one vaginal delivery), a total of 1178 women were identified. Among these, 524 completed the full questionnaire. They were considered responders, and 654 did not complete the rest of the questionnaire and were considered non-responders, resulting in a response rate of 44% for eligible participants (Figure 1).

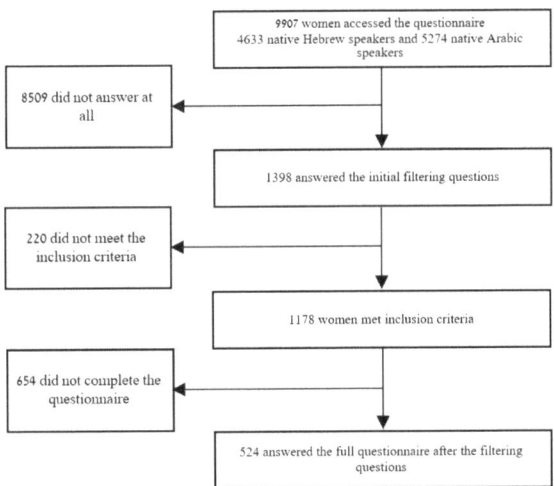

Figure 1. Flowchart.

3.2. Descriptive Data

Among the participants who completed the questionnaire, 80.5% (422) belonged to the Jewish sector, and 19.5% (102) represented the Arab sector. The average age was 35.9, with a standard deviation of 7.6 years. Most participants had an academic background, comprising 61.8% (324 individuals).

The average number of vaginal deliveries was 5.1, with a median of 3. In terms of delivery methods, 21.6% (113) had undergone both vaginal and cesarean deliveries, while 78.4% (411) had undergone exclusively vaginal deliveries. Furthermore, 17.6% of the women (92) had a history of at least one instrumental delivery (forceps or vacuum). Most women (72.1%, 378) required perineal stitches in at least one delivery. At the time of the questionnaire, 38.1% of the women (200) were at least five years postpartum, 39.7% (208) were between one and five years postpartum, and 22.2% (116) were less than a year postpartum. A positive smoking status was reported by 11.6% (61) of the respondents.

Stress urinary incontinence: A total of 370 participants (70.6%) reported having at least one symptom, and 193 (36.8%) reported moderate to severe symptoms.

Overactive bladder/urge urinary incontinence: A total of 394 participants (75.2%) reported having at least one symptom, and 215 (41%) reported moderate to severe symptoms.

Obstructive colorectal symptoms: A total of 331 participants (63.2%) reported having at least one symptom, and 150 (28.6%) reported moderate to severe symptoms.

Colorectal incontinence (gas and/or feces): A total of 325 participants (62%) reported having at least one symptom, and 123 (23.5%) reported moderate to severe symptoms.

Pelvic pain or discomfort and prolapse: A total of 433 participants (82.6%) reported having at least one symptom, and 242 (46.2%) reported moderate to severe symptoms.

Overall, 498 participants (95%) suffered from at least one symptom at any grade in at least one category, and 350 participants (66.8%) suffered from at least one moderate to severe symptom in at least one category (Figure 2). The differences in women with and without moderate to severe symptoms are outlined in Table 1.

The most common complaints were urinary-related (stress incontinence or overactive bladder). A total of 447 participants (85.3%) suffered from at least one urinary symptom in any grade, and 259 participants (49.4%) suffered from at least one moderate to severe symptom.

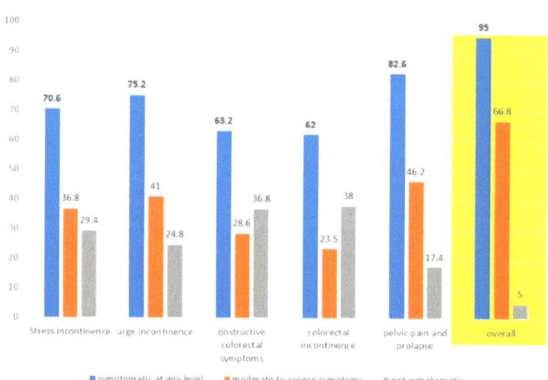

Figure 2. PFD prevalence in the study population.

Table 1. Characteristics of women with and without at least one moderate to severe pelvic floor complaint.

	Women without Any Moderate to Severe Pelvic Floor Complaints n = 174 (33.2%)	Women with at Least One Moderate to Severe Pelvic Floor Complaint n = 350 (66.8%)	p Value
	n (%)	n (%)	
Age			
18–24	11 (6.3)	29 (8.3)	
25–29	20 (11.5)	53 (15.1)	
30–34	50 (28.7)	83 (23.7)	0.173
35–39	36 (20.7)	48 (13.7)	
40–44	31 (17.8)	77 (22)	
45–50	26 (14.9)	60 (17.1)	
Age, mean ± SD	35.9 ± 7.1	35.9 ± 7.9	0.938
Only vaginal deliveries	138 (79.3)	273 (78)	0.737
Number of vaginal deliveries, mean ± SD	2.24 ± 1.5	2.24 ± 1.4	0.881
Duration since last delivery			
<2 months	11 (6.3)	16 (4.6)	
2–12 months	21 (12.1)	68 (19.4)	
1–5 years	74 (42.5)	134 (38.3)	0.231
5–10 years	39 (22.4)	68 (19.4)	
>10 years	29 (16.7)	64 (18.3)	
Duration since last delivery (years), mean ± SD	5 ± 5	5.2 ± 5.3	0.861
Assisted vaginal birth (forceps/vacuum)	21 (12.1)	71 (20.3)	0.021
Perineal tear/episiotomy stitching	127 (73)	251 (71.7)	0.330
Hormonal therapy			
OCP	37 (21.3)	69 (19.7)	0.767
IUD	26 (14.9)	63 (18)	
Ethnicity			
Jewish	143 (82.2)	279 (79.7)	0.559
Arab	31 (17.8)	71 (0.23)	
Smoker	16 (9.2)	45 (12.9)	0.249
Academic education	103 (59.2)	221 (63.1)	0.658
Married	161 (92.5)	297 (84.9)	0.077
BMI	24.4 ± 4.1	25.8 ± 5.5	0.015

3.3. Multivariate Analysis

In this study, there was no effect of age, number of vaginal deliveries, time since the last delivery, perineal stitching, assisted delivery (forceps/vacuum), or socio-economic status on the chance of suffering from PFD symptoms. Nevertheless, women in the Arab sector tended to suffer more from pelvic pain or pelvic organ prolapse (OR 2.046, CI [1.004–4.173], $p = 0.049$), obstructive colorectal symptoms (OR 2.017, CI [1.185–3.432], $p = 0.01$), and moderate to severe colorectal incontinence (OR 1.730, CI [1.035–2.892], $p = 0.036$). A BMI greater than 25 was found to be a risk factor for suffering from fecal incontinence (OR 1.043, CI [1.004–1.084], $p = 0.029$), pelvic pain, or organ prolapse (OR 1.045, CI [1.007–1.084], $p = 0.019$), as well as moderate to severe urinary stress incontinence (OR 1.085, CI [1.044–1.126], $p < 0.001$).

Smoking was found to increase the risk of colorectal obstruction symptoms by almost twofold (OR 1.995, CI [1.033–3.854], $p = 0.04$), an effect that was also found in stress urinary incontinence (OR 2.362, CI [1.137–4.907], $p = 0.021$), and moderate to severe overactive bladder symptoms (OR 2.062, CI [1.161–3.661], $p = 0.014$).

3.4. Quality of Life Assessment

In the questionnaire, women were asked to grade the influence of urinary urge incontinence on their daily lives on a scale of 0-4 according to the USIQ questionnaire ("How much does it affect your ability to..."), where zero corresponded to "Not at all", 1 to "Somewhat", 2 to "Moderately", 3 to "quite a bit", and 4 to "Very much". Urinary urge incontinence was found to influence many daily activities: working and studying (1.8 ± 1.2), social activities outside of the home (2.0 ± 1.3), ability to travel by car or bus for a duration greater than 30 min (2.1 ± 1.3), intimate relationships (2 ± 1.3), physical activities (2.2 ± 1.3), emotional health (1.8 ± 1.1), and frustration (2 ± 1.3).

3.5. Opinions and Health-Seeking Behaviors

Most women in our study (93.7%) believed they should receive voluntary information on PFD symptoms from medical personnel (Figure 3). These included gynecologists (91.2%), family physicians (57.6%), the caring staff at the time of discharge from maternity wards (64.7%), pregnancy care nurses or well-baby clinic nurses (56.5%), and antenatal visits for childbirth preparation courses (32.3%). However, only 16.6% of women reported that a gynecologist or a family physician had ever initiated a conversation on these issues.

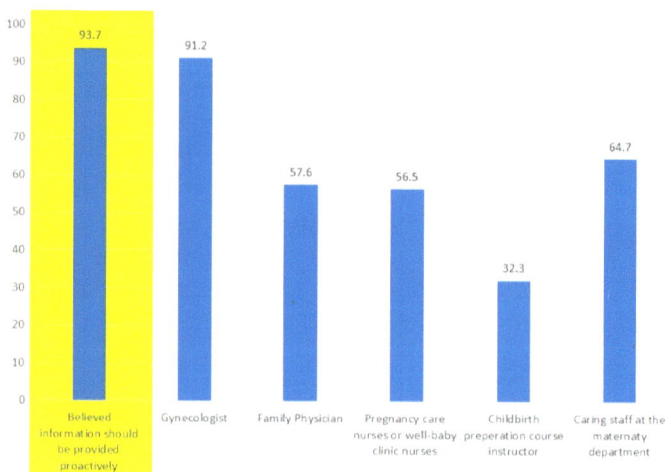

Figure 3. Participants answered that they wish to receive proactive information on PFD from healthcare personnel.

Women also showed a low level of initiative in seeking information and treatment for PFD symptoms. Among women who experienced PFD symptoms, 70.8% (n = 371) never sought professional help, 32.3% approached a gynecologist on their own initiative, 22.8% approached a family doctor, 18.3% approached a pelvic floor physiotherapist, 8.9% approached a urologist, and 12.7% approached a nurse. In addition, 19.7% approached a fitness trainer or Pilates instructor on their initiative, and 42% shared this with a friend or acquaintance.

Regarding the reasons why most symptomatic women did not seek professional help, 53.1% assumed that the symptoms would disappear over time, 44.7% thought that these were natural and normal symptoms that every woman experiences after vaginal birth, 28.3% did not seek help because they were busy with work or taking care of their children, 22.9% were not aware that such problems could be treated, 18.3% were embarrassed to raise the issue, and 12.4% felt they knew on their own how to treat the problem with pelvic floor exercises (Figure 4).

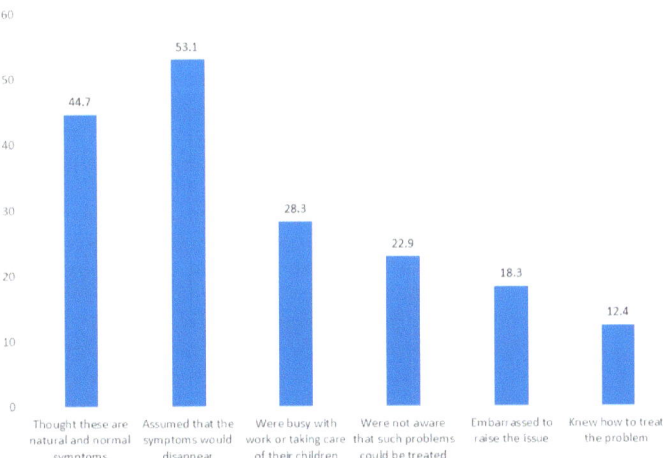

Figure 4. Reasons for avoiding healthcare in symptomatic women.

Women who did seek medical care were offered numerous treatments: Kegel exercises for activating the pelvic floor muscles (46%), referral to physiotherapy for pelvic floor rehabilitation (29%), lifestyle changes such as reducing caffeine consumption and timed urination (17%), breathing exercises (15%), pharmacological treatment such as stool softeners and alpha-blockers (7%), and the use of supportive devices such as a pessary (1%).

The degree of compliance with these treatments was inadequate, as only a small percentage of those who sought help followed through with all the recommended treatments (24.3%), while some completed only some of the treatments (20.3%) or planned to do so in the future (21.6%). Others did not complete the treatment and did not intend to (33.8%). The reasons for low compliance with recommended treatment were numerous and mainly stemmed from accessibility and awareness issues (Figure 5). Interestingly, 66% of those who reported no symptoms still sought treatment. This observation has several possible meanings, which will be discussed hereafter.

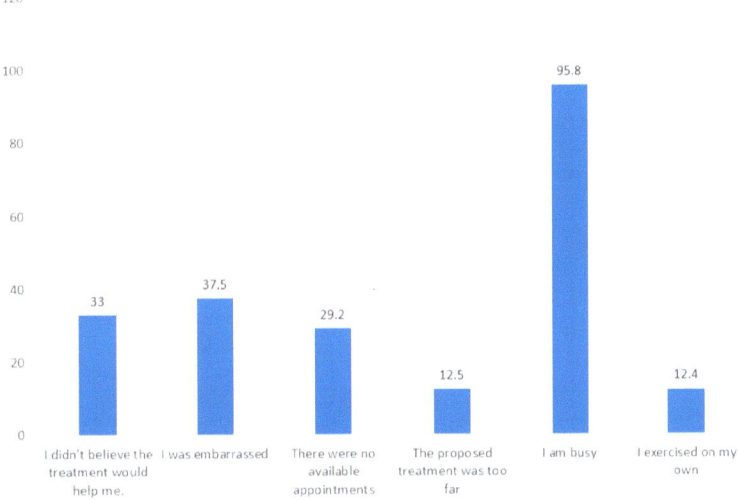

Figure 5. Reasons for low compliance with recommended treatment of PFD symptoms.

4. Discussion

4.1. Main Findings

In this study, we aimed to evaluate the prevalence of PFD among parous women in their fertile years using previously validated questionnaires and to characterize their approaches to treatment for these issues. To our knowledge, this study was the first in Israel to address women in their fertile years beyond the peripartum stage and to assess both symptoms and needs.

The study results suggest that up to 95% of women experienced PFD symptoms, with 85% experiencing urinary-related symptoms (stress incontinence and/or overactive bladder). Moderate to severe symptoms were observed in 66.8% of women. Arab women, smokers, and overweight women were at a higher risk of suffering from PFD.

Even though most symptomatic women (70.8%) did not proactively bring up their symptoms with any healthcare professional, almost all of them (93.7%) would have preferred to be approached and provided with information on the matter. Unfortunately, only 16.6% reported being actively approached by healthcare professionals.

4.2. Interpretation

The prevalence of the symptoms observed in this study exceeds what is known in most existing literature [2,4,5,10–14,16,17], in which most studies have estimated up to 60% prevalence. This difference may be attributed to volunteer bias in the women who chose to answer the questionnaire. This is a known problem in any questionnaire study and is more predominant when discussing a sensitive subject such as PFD. This is even more true when answering a long and thorough questionnaire, as was used in our study.

Another possible explanation is the gap between symptoms and bothersome symptoms. Some women were found to be symptomatic, but with no effect on their quality of life whatsoever and no wish for treatment, indicating that perhaps the USIQ and PFDI questionnaires were a little over-sensitive in our study. This might suggest that they were either experiencing mild levels of dysfunction, as evidenced by lower scores on the questionnaire, or they were adopting behaviors to cope with their symptoms. To diminish this effect, we chose to present women with moderate to severe symptoms separately—i.e., women with moderately to considerably bothersome symptoms. Even this restrictive analysis showed PFD to affect two-thirds of women in the study. Therefore, even if numerical accuracy has yet to be attained, it can be concluded that there is a considerable underestimation and underdiagnosis of these symptoms.

It should be noted that sources for comparison on this subject are even more limited than those for PFD in general, as the medical literature tends to focus on these issues mainly in the peripartum or menopausal periods.

Regarding risk factors, obesity and smoking are known risk factors and were found in this study as well. It was interesting to find that Arab Israeli women were at greater risk of PFD, regardless of the type of delivery (assisted or not), the age, and the number of children they had. This specific finding should be further researched.

One of the most important findings in our study was the discrepancy between women's desire to be asked and offered voluntary information about PFD from physicians and nurses (93.7%) and the low rate of it happening (16.6%). We may assume that physicians and nurses avoid the subject due to its sensitive nature or that they assume that women will raise the issue if they find it bothersome. This should be further studied. These findings clearly show that most women would like to be asked about it, and the reasons for them not seeking treatment are mainly lack of knowledge and inaccessibility, and are not due to embarrassment. These are all solvable problems.

A total of 66% of the women who reported no symptoms still stated that they sought treatment for PFD. This may be explained by the tendency to diminish symptom severity in self-reporting symptom scoring or by pursuing preventive treatments following parity.

Interestingly, when women did seek help for their symptoms, they tended to have low compliance with recommended methods. Only 24.3% of those seeking assistance completed all the recommended treatments. For the most part, the women were too busy to adhere, but other reasons included a lack of faith in the treatment, embarrassment, low availability, and self-management. These findings suggest that perhaps treating strategies in Israel may not correspond to a busy mother's life, and perhaps new and more available technologies, including remote treatment and self-care devices, should be implemented.

4.3. Limitations of the Study

This study has several limitations. First, a selection bias is probable. Women who chose to answer the questionnaire may suffer more or be more aware of PFD. Second, the response rate was only 44%, which may be improved using different approach models (telephone interviews, interviews in the clinic, etc.). Additional population biases stem from the research method and questionnaire distribution (via e-mail), including higher education and socioeconomic status, language, and technological literacy. This, again, can cause a selection bias.

This study only represents parous women. However, it is essential to explore nulliparous women in future studies to represent their PFD. To fully comprehend the scope of PFD in young women, it is necessary to conduct research that involves a control group consisting of women from the same age group who have never undergone vaginal delivery. This is another population that suffers from misrepresentation in the literature.

5. Conclusions

This study aimed to investigate the prevalence of female pelvic floor dysfunction in Israeli women who experienced vaginal delivery and are in their reproductive years, as well as to understand their attitudes and health-seeking behavior towards this problem. The topic is not novel. However, it is relevant in the field of pelvic floor dysfunction and addresses a specific gap in the field. Compared to the other published material, it adds further evidence to show the importance of raising awareness of the different therapeutic solutions to PFD symptoms and designing more available services for this common problem.

To date, unfortunately, there is still a cultural limit on addressing the problem of pelvic floor dysfunction with a gynecologist. In fact, to date, there is still the belief that these problems are inevitable and lack solutions. This leads women to accept this problem, with an enormous decline in their quality of life, without looking for possible solutions. It is the doctor's duty to educate women to be aware of these problems, which, although they appear, can be treated with medical and surgical rehabilitation therapy. The possibility of having various therapeutic opportunities based on the individual patient allows the woman to access an individualized therapeutic plan.

We anticipate that heightened awareness of this issue will eventually reach patients in diverse clinical settings, including doctor visits in various disciplines such as family medicine, gynecology, and urology, as well as during childbirth and parenting education courses, in nurses' clinics, and upon discharge from maternity departments. Beyond discussing the matter in medical appointments, other effective health interventions could involve addressing the problem through pregnancy tracking apps or children's developmental apps; distributing patient information leaflets, questionnaires, and signs; or providing specific pelvic floor examinations. Utilizing social media platforms or podcasts could also be effective in spreading awareness.

To tackle the accessibility challenges of care and treatment, it would be beneficial to establish standardized treatment plans, including remote pelvic floor physiotherapy and self-treatment solutions using readily available home devices. Subsidizing biofeedback tools for self-treatment could alleviate some of the significant accessibility barriers identified in this study.

This study highlights a significant yet often overlooked issue with a substantial public health burden. Various measures can be implemented to improve awareness, accessibility, and care in this regard. We believe that paying attention to patients' needs could contribute to designing better solutions and promoting a healthier life for them.

Supplementary Materials: The following supporting information can be downloaded at: https://www.mdpi.com/article/10.3390/healthcare12030390/s1, Women's Health Questionnaire.

Author Contributions: T.F.-Y.: conceptualization (lead); data curation (lead); funding acquisition (lead); writing—original draft (equal). D.L.S.: writing—original draft (equal). S.S.E.: writing—review and editing (supporting). H.N.: translating the questionnaire to Arabic (equal); writing—review and editing (supporting). A.E.Z.: translating the questionnaire to Arabic (equal); writing—review and editing (supporting). L.A.: formal analysis and methodology (lead); writing—original draft (equal). All authors have read and agreed to the published version of the manuscript.

Funding: This study was funded by Marom, a research program for physicians and residents in Maccabi Healthcare Services.

Institutional Review Board Statement: The institutional review board of Assuta Health Care 0110-18-ASMC approved the study. Date of approval: 28 November 2019.

Informed Consent Statement: The questionnaires were anonymous and voluntary. There was no identifying information in the process.

Data Availability Statement: The data supporting this study's findings are available upon request from the corresponding author, T.F.-Y. The data are not publicly available due to ethical restrictions.

Conflicts of Interest: The authors declare no conflict of interest.

Abbreviations

CI	Confidence interval
OR	Odds ratio
PFD	Pelvic floor dysfunction
PFDI20	Pelvic Floor Disability Index 20
POP	Pelvic floor organ prolapse
TVT	Tension-free vaginal tape
USIQ	Urgency, Severity, and Impact Questionnaire

References

1. Lawson, S.; Sacks, A. Pelvic floor physical therapy and women's health promotion. *J. Midwifery Women's Health* **2018**, *63*, 410–417. [CrossRef] [PubMed]
2. Peinado-Molina, R.A.; Hernández-Martínez, A.; Martínez-Vázquez, S.; Rodríguez-Almagro, J.; Martínez-Galiano, J.M. Pelvic floor dysfunction: Prevalence and associated factors. *BMC Public Health* **2023**, *23*, 2005. [CrossRef] [PubMed]
3. Li, M.; Shi, J.; Lü, Q.P.; Wei, F.H.; Gai, T.Z.; Feng, Q. Multiple factors analysis of early postpartum pelvic floor muscles injury in regenerated parturients. *Zhonghua Yi Xue Za Zhi* **2018**, *98*, 818–822. [CrossRef] [PubMed]
4. Handa, V.L.; Blomquist, J.L.; Knoepp, L.R.; Hoskey, K.A.; McDermott, K.C.B.; Muñoz, A. Pelvic floor disorders 5-10 years after vaginal or cesarean childbirth. *Obs. Gynecol.* **2011**, *118*, 777–784. [CrossRef] [PubMed]
5. Awwad, J.; Sayegh, R.; Yeretzian, J.; Deeb, M.E. Prevalence, risk factors, and predictors of pelvic organ prolapse: A community-based study. *Menopause* **2012**, *19*, 1235–1241. [CrossRef] [PubMed]
6. Bradley, C.S.; Kennedy, C.M.; Nygaard, I.E. Pelvic floor symptoms and lifestyle factors in older women. *J. Women's Health* **2005**, *14*, 128–136. [CrossRef] [PubMed]
7. NICE-National Institute for Health Care Excellence. *Pelvic Floor Dysfunction: Prevention And Nonsurgical Management—Risk Factors for Pelvic Floor Dysfunction*; NICE Guideline, NG210: London, UK, 2021.
8. Ge, J.; Wei, X.J.; Zhang, H.Z.; Fang, G.Y. Pelvic floor muscle training in the treatment of pelvic organ prolapse: A meta-analysis of randomized controlled trials. *Actas Urol. Esp.* **2021**, *45*, 73–82. [CrossRef] [PubMed]
9. Van Nieuwkoop, C.; Voorham-van der Zalm, P.J.; Van Laar, A.-M.; Elzevier, H.W.; Blom, J.W.; Dekkers, O.M.; Pelger, R.C.; Dalen, A.M.V.A.-V.; Van Tol, M.C.; Van Dissel, J.T. Pelvic floor dysfunction is not a risk factor for febrile urinary tract infection in adults. *BJU Int.* **2010**, *105*, 1689–1695. [CrossRef]
10. Olsen, A.L.; Smith, V.J.; Bergstrom, J.O.; Colling, J.C.; Clark, A.L. Epidemiology of surgically managed pelvic organ prolapse and urinary incontinence. *Obs. Gynecol.* **1997**, *89*, 501–506. [CrossRef]
11. Mardon, R.E.; Halim, S.; Pawlson, L.G.; Haffer, S.C. Management of urinary incontinence in Medicare managed care beneficiaries: Results from the 2004 Medicare Health Outcomes Survey. *Arch. Intern. Med.* **2006**, *166*, 1128–1133. [CrossRef]

12. Morrill, M.; Lukacz, E.S.; Lawrence, J.M.; Nager, C.W.; Contreras, R.; Luber, K.M. Seeking healthcare for pelvic floor disorders: A population-based study. *Am. J. Obs. Gynecol.* **2007**, *197*, 86.e1–86.e6. [CrossRef]
13. Lowenstein, L.; FitzGerald, M.P.; Kenton, K.; Hatchett, L.; Durazo-Arvizu, R.; Mueller, E.R.; Goldman, K.; Brubaker, L. Evaluation of urgency in women, with a validated Urgency, Severity and Impact Questionnaire (USIQ). *Int. Urogynecol. J. Pelvic Floor Dysfunct.* **2009**, *20*, 301–307. [CrossRef]
14. Kenne, K.A.; Wendt, L.; Brooks Jackson, J. Prevalence of pelvic floor disorders in adult women being seen in a primary care setting and associated risk factors. *Sci. Rep.* **2022**, *12*, 9878. [CrossRef] [PubMed]
15. Benti Terefe, A.; Gemeda Gudeta, T.; Teferi Mengistu, G.; Abebe Sori, S. Determinants of pelvic floor disorders among women visiting the gynecology outpatient department in wolkite university specialized center, wolkite. *Ethiop. Obs. Gynecol. Int.* **2022**, *2022*, 6949700. [CrossRef]
16. Malaekah, H.; al Medbel, H.S.; al Mowallad, S.; al Asiri, Z.; Albadrani, A.; Abdullah, H. Prevalence of pelvic floor dysfunction in women in Riyadh, Kingdom of Saudi Arabia: A cross-sectional study. *Women's Health* **2022**, *18*, 174550652110722. [CrossRef]
17. Dheresa, M.; Worku, A.; Oljira, L.; Mengiste, B.; Assefa, N.; Berhane, Y. One in five women suffer from pelvic floor disorders in Kersa district Eastern Ethiopia: A community-based study. *BMC Women's Health* **2018**, *18*, 95. [CrossRef]
18. Tinetti, A.; Weir, N.; Tangyotkajohn, U.; Jacques, A.; Thompson, J.; Briffa, K. Help-seeking behaviour for pelvic floor dysfunction in women over 55: Drivers and barriers. *Int. Urogynecol. J.* **2018**, *29*, 1645–1653. [CrossRef] [PubMed]
19. Mikuš, M.; Ćorić, M.; Matak, L.; Škegro, B.; Vujić, G.; Banović, V. Validation of the UDI-6 and the ICIQ-UI SF - Croatian version. *Int. Urogynecol. J.* **2020**, *31*, 2625–2630. [CrossRef] [PubMed]
20. Hagen, S.; Stark, D. Conservative prevention and management of pelvic organ prolapse in women. *Cochrane Database Syst. Rev.* **2011**, *12*, CD003882. [CrossRef]
21. Hagen, S.; Stark, D.; Glazener, C.; Dickson, S.; Barry, S.; Elders, A.; Frawley, H.; Galea, M.P.; Logan, J.; McDonald, A.; et al. Individualised pelvic floor muscle training in women with pelvic organ prolapse (POPPY): A multicentre randomised controlled trial. *Lancet* **2014**, *383*, 796–806. [CrossRef]
22. Braekken, I.H.; Majida, M.; Engh, M.E.; Bø, K. Can pelvic floor muscle training reverse pelvic organ prolapse and reduce prolapse symptoms? An assessor-blinded, randomized, controlled trial. *Am. J. Obs. Gynecol.* **2010**, *203*, 170.e1–170.e7. [CrossRef]
23. Jundt, K.; Peschers, U.; Kentenich, H. The investigation and treatment of female pelvic floor dysfunction. *Dtsch. Arztebl. Int.* **2015**, *112*, 564–574. [CrossRef] [PubMed]
24. Powers, S.A.; Burleson, L.K.; Hannan, J.L. Managing female pelvic floor disorders: A medical device review and appraisal. *Interface Focus* **2019**, *9*, 20190014. [CrossRef] [PubMed]
25. Scollo, P.; Pecorino, B.; Scibilia, G.; Guardalà, V.F.M.; Ferrara, M.; Mereu, L.; D'Agate, M.G. Scollo's symmetric lateral levator myorrhaphy (SLLM) for correction of rectocele in six steps. *Tech. Coloproctol.* **2023**, *27*, 497–498. [CrossRef] [PubMed]
26. Dumoulin, C.; Hay-Smith, E.J.; Mac Habée-Séguin, G. Pelvic floor muscle training versus no treatment, or inactive control treatments, for urinary incontinence in women. *Cochrane Database Syst. Rev.* **2014**, *5*, CD005654. [CrossRef] [PubMed]
27. Sung, V.W.; Washington, B.; Raker, C.A. Costs of ambulatory care related to female pelvic floor disorders in the United States. *Am. J. Obs. Gynecol.* **2010**, *202*, 483.e1–483.e4. [CrossRef] [PubMed]
28. Zhu, Q.; Shu, H.; Dai, Z. Effect of pelvic floor dysfunction on sexual function and quality of life in Chinese women of different ages: An observational study. *Geriatr. Gerontol. Int.* **2019**, *19*, 299–304. [CrossRef] [PubMed]
29. Reis, A.M.; Brito, L.G.O.; Lunardi, A.L.B.; Pinto e Silva, M.P.; Juliato, C.R.T. Depression, anxiety, and stress in women with urinary incontinence with or without myofascial dysfunction in the pelvic floor muscles: A cross-sectional study. *Neurourol. Urodyn.* **2021**, *40*, 334–339. [CrossRef] [PubMed]
30. Kinchen, K.S.; Burgio, K.; Diokno, A.C.; Fultz, N.H.; Bump, R.; Obenchain, R. Factors associated with women's decisions to seek treatment for urinary incontinence. *J. Women's Health* **2003**, *12*, 687–698. [CrossRef]
31. Dheresa, M.; Worku, A.; Oljira, L.; Mengistie, B.; Assefa, N.; Berhane, Y. Women's health seeking behavior for pelvic floor disorders and its associated factors in eastern Ethiopia. *Int. Urogynecol. J.* **2020**, *31*, 1263–1271. [CrossRef]
32. Wójtowicz, U.; Płaszewska-Zywko, L.; Stangel-Wójcikiewicz, K.; Basta, A. Barriers in entering treatment among women with urinary incontinence. *Ginekol. Pol.* **2014**, *85*, 342–347. [CrossRef] [PubMed]
33. Barber, M.D.; Walters, M.D.; Bump, R.C. Short forms of two condition-specific quality-of-life questionnaires for women with pelvic floor disorders (PFDI-20 and PFIQ-7). *Am. J. Obs. Gynecol.* **2005**, *193*, 103–113. [CrossRef]
34. Barber, M.D.; Chen, Z.; Lukacz, E.; Markland, A.; Wai, C.; Brubaker, L.; Nygaard, I.; Weidner, A.; Janz, N.K.; Spino, C. Further validation of the short form versions of the Pelvic Floor Distress Inventory (PFDI) and Pelvic Floor Impact Questionnaire (PFIQ). *Neurourol. Urodyn.* **2011**, *30*, 541–546. [CrossRef] [PubMed]
35. Lowenstein, L.; Levy, G.; Chen, K.O.; Ginath, S.; Condrea, A.; Padoa, A. Validation of hebrew versions of the pelvic floor distress inventory, pelvic organ prolapse/urinary incontinence sexual function questionnaire, and the urgency, severity and impact questionnaire. *Female Pelvic Med. Reconstr. Surg.* **2012**, *18*, 329–331. [CrossRef] [PubMed]

Disclaimer/Publisher's Note: The statements, opinions and data contained in all publications are solely those of the individual author(s) and contributor(s) and not of MDPI and/or the editor(s). MDPI and/or the editor(s) disclaim responsibility for any injury to people or property resulting from any ideas, methods, instructions or products referred to in the content.

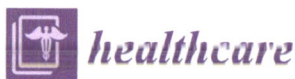

Article

The Impact of Systemic Sclerosis on Sexual Health: An Italian Survey

Alessandro Ferdinando Ruffolo [1,2], Maurizio Serati [3,*], Arianna Casiraghi [1], Vittoria Benini [1], Chiara Scancarello [3], Maria Carmela Di Dedda [4], Carla Garbagnati [5], Andrea Braga [6], Massimo Candiani [1] and Stefano Salvatore [1]

1. Obstetrics and Gynecology Unit, IRCCS San Raffaele Hospital, Vita-Salute University, 20132 Milan, Italy; alesruffolo@gmail.com (A.F.R.); casiraghi.arianna@hsr.it (A.C.); benini.vittoria@hsr.it (V.B.); candiani.massimo@hsr.it (M.C.); salvatore.stefano@hsr.it (S.S.)
2. Gynecological Department, Jeanne de Flandre Hospital, University Hospital of Lille, Avenue Eugène Avinée, 59037 Lille, France
3. Department of Obstetrics and Gynecology, Del Ponte Hospital, University of Insubria, 21100 Varese, Italy; chiarascanca@gmail.com
4. Department of Obstetrics and Gynecology, ASST FBF-SACCO Macedonio Melloni Hospital, 20129 Milan, Italy; maria.didedda@asst-fbf-sacco.it
5. Fondazione IRCCS Ca' Granda Ospedale Maggiore Policlinico, University of Milan, Via Commenda 12, 20122 Milan, Italy; carlagarbagnati@mac.com
6. Department of Obstetrics and Gynecology, EOC-Beata Vergine Hospital, 6850 Mendrisio, Switzerland; andrea.braga@eoc.ch
* Correspondence: maurizio.serati@uninsubria.it

Abstract: Objective: To evaluate the impact of systemic sclerosis (SSc) on vulvovaginal atrophy (VVA) and sexual health in an Italian population. Methods: An Italian survey about the prevalence and severity of VVA (on a 0 to 10 scale) and sexual dysfunction (using the Female Sexual Function Index—FSFI) through an anonymous online questionnaire. We investigated couple relationships and intimacy with partners, the predisposition of patients to talk about their sexual problems, physicians' receptivity, and treatment scenarios. Risk factors for VVA symptoms and sexual dysfunction were assessed. Results: A total of 107 women affected by SSc were enrolled. Of these, 83.2% of women (89/107) complained about VVA symptoms and 89.7% (among sexually active women; 87/97) about sexual dysfunction. Menopausal status did not affect VVA symptoms, while age was the only independent risk factor for sexual dysfunction. About 70% (74/107) of women reported a negative impact of disturbances on intimacy with their partner. A total of 63 women (58.9%) had never discussed their sexual problems and VVA condition with a physician. Lubricants were the only treatment prescribed, and 75% of women would welcome new therapies, even if experimental (62.9%). Conclusions: In women with SSc, VVA symptoms and sexual dysfunction are highly prevalent, independently from menopause. In more than half of the investigated women with SSc, we found reluctance to talk about their sexual problems, despite being symptomatic. This should encourage physicians to investigate vulvovaginal and sexual health. SSc patients would welcome the advent of new treatment possibilities for their VVA and sexual complaints.

Keywords: systemic sclerosis; sexual health; sexual dysfunction; genitourinary syndrome of menopause; vulvovaginal symptoms; quality of life

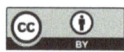

1. Introduction

Systemic sclerosis (SSc), also known as scleroderma, is an immune-mediated rheumatic disease that causes vasculopathy and fibrosis of the skin and internal organs [1]. SSc has been found to affect various aspects of life, including intimate health and sexuality [2]. Diminished intercourse frequency due to reduction in desire and satisfaction have been related to several SSc symptoms, such as mouth shrinking, skin tightening around vaginal introitus and breast, vaginal dryness, joint pain, muscle weakness, Raynaud phenomenon, reflux, vomiting, diarrhea, low self-esteem, as well as some drugs [3–6]. Indeed, decreased libido has been related to the use of prednisolone, vaginal ulceration to the use of colchicine, nausea and weakness to the use of nifedipine and prednisolone, and depression to the use of cimetidine [6]. Sexual function has been observed to be significantly impaired, and more sexual distress has been reported in women with SSc in comparison with healthy controls [7] or women affected by other chronic diseases [6]. Several issues, such as intimacy and their relationship with a partner, the spontaneous predisposition of patients to talk about their sexual problems, and physicians' awareness of or receptivity (meaning the ability to carefully listen to the woman and inquire with interest about possible intimate and relational disturbances) to women affected by SSc, remain largely under-reported [7]. The literature assessing sexuality impairment in women with SSc is growing [3–10]; however, these topics have never been previously explored.

We, therefore, designed this survey to evaluate the prevalence and severity of vulvo-vaginal atrophy (VVA) symptoms and sexual health, investigating patients' relationships with their partners, their physicians' receptivity, and patients' satisfaction with the available treatments for their genital and sexual disorders and expectations for alternative therapies in an Italian cohort of women affected by SSc.

2. Methods

2.1. Study Design

This is an Italian survey concerning the impact of SSc on VVA and sexual health. The questionnaire adopted in this study was designed in collaboration between the Italian National SSc Patient Association, named *Gruppo Italiano per la Lotta alla Sclerodermia* (GILS ODV), the Urogynecology Unit of IRCCS (Istituto di Ricovero e Cura a Carattere Scientifico) at the San Raffaele Hospital of Milan (where data were collected and analyzed), and the following national units: Scleroderma Unit of IRCCS Policlinico of Milan, Scleroderma Unit of ASST (Azienda Socio-Sanitaria Territoriale) Legnano, ASST Niguarda, IRCCS Humanitas Hospital of Milan. In addition to some demographic details and questions designed to investigate patients' subjective perception of their symptoms and the available solutions, the questionnaire also included the Female Sexual Function Index (FSFI), a validated questionnaire for sexual health assessment (Supplementary Materials). Approval for the study was obtained from the Institutional Review Board (number IRB 20/int/2020). All participants signed informed consent for the treatment of personal data. The study was conducted according to the Declaration of Helsinki [11].

2.2. Study Population

Women were enrolled between June 2019 and February 2020 by the previously mentioned Italian units.

Eligible patients were women with a diagnosis of SSc, according to the American College of Rheumatology [12], over 18 years of age, who signed an informed consent and were willing to fill out the questionnaire. Women who did not sign the informed consent for the treatment of personal data, did not complete the questionnaire, or did not fill in the questionnaire were not included in the study.

2.3. Study Procedures

During a routine rheumatologic examination, patients were informed about the possibility of answering anonymously to an online questionnaire based on vulvovaginal atrophy symptoms and sexual health related to systemic sclerosis.

The questionnaire included questions on general characteristics and medical and surgical history (gynecological surgery, presence or history of malignant neoplasia, frequency of gynecological medical examinations). Menopausal status was defined as "the absence of menstruation for at least 12 months". Vulvovaginal atrophy symptoms were then assessed through subjective parameters. Vaginal dryness and dyspareunia (defined in the questionnaire as "pain at intercourses") were investigated using a Visual Analogue

Scale (VAS) from 0 to 10 for intensity, where "0" indicated the absence of symptoms and "10" as the maximum intensity. To assess sexual function, we incorporated the Female Sexual Function Index (FSFI), a questionnaire composed of 19 questions to investigate 7 different domains (desire, arousal, lubrification, satisfaction, orgasm, pain, and a total FSFI score). Each domain of the FSFI includes a 0–6 scale where the lower score indicates the worst condition. In order to classify a woman as "sexually dysfunctioned", the overall FSFI score should be <26.55. Desire is the only item that may be considered separately, with a clinically significant cut-off score for dysfunction <5 [13,14]. FSFI analysis was carried out only for sexually active women, defined as women who had intercourse in the previous 4 weeks.

Couple relationships and intimacy with partners were then assessed. For this section of the questionnaire, the following questions were proposed to participants: "How much did these symptoms negatively influence your couple relationship and intimacy with partner?", "Do you think that these symptoms and their influence on sexual life are negatively perceived by your partner?". We also investigated the spontaneous predisposition of patients to talk about their sexual problems and physicians' receptivity: "Have you ever discussed about your symptoms (vulvovaginal and sexual) with your doctor?", "If the answer is yes, which physician did you discussed with?", "Was the doctor interested and receptive enough on the argument?", "Who started the conversation about the problem?".

Previous treatments for VVA complaints and their efficacy were recorded. Finally, we asked each participant if they would consider being submitted to a new or experimental therapy for their VVA symptoms or sexual dysfunction.

2.4. Statistical Analysis

IBM SPSS Statistics for Windows, version 21 (IBM Corp., Armonk, NY, USA) version 21.0 was used to perform data analysis.

Continuous variables were expressed as mean and standard deviation (SD). Categorical variables were expressed as n (%). Exploratory univariate was applied to test the association between risk factors for VVA-related symptoms and sexual dysfunction. Variables that had a significant association with the adopted scores at univariate analysis were eventually included in the multivariate analyses. A two-tailed p-value < 0.05 was considered statistically significant.

3. Results

3.1. General Characteristics

A total of 133 women were considered eligible for the study and signed the informed consent for the treatment of personal data. However, 19.54% (26/133) dropped out of the study: 53.84% (14/26) did not complete the whole questionnaire (missing data), while 46.16% (12/26) did not fill it at all.

A total of 107 women (80.46%; 107/133), with a mean age of 53.47 (SD ± 13.27) years, affected by SSc were recruited. The clinical and demographic characteristics of the study population are reported in Table 1. About half of the study population was in a menopausal status (58/107; 54.2%), with surgical menopause reported in 9.3% of women (10/107). Most of the included women were sexually active (97/107; 90.7%).

Table 1. Demographic and clinical characteristics of the study population. SD: Standard Deviation.

	N = 107
Age, mean (±SD), years	53.47 (±13.27)
Systemic sclerosis duration, mean (±SD), years	12.48 (±10.28)
Menopausal status, n (%)	58 (54.2)
Hysterectomy, n (%)	13 (12.1)

Table 1. *Cont.*

	N = 107
Bilateral salpingo-oophorectomy, n (%)	10 (9.3)
Malignant neoplasia, n (%)	3 (2.8)
Sexually active women, n (%)	97 (90.7)
Age of sexually active women, mean (±SD), years	53.28 (±13.70)
Systemic sclerosis duration of sexually active women, mean (±SD), years	12.76 (±10.34)

3.2. Vulvovaginal Atrophy (VVA) Symptoms

VVA symptoms are described in Table 2. Vaginal dryness was reported by 83.2% of women (89/107) with a mean severity score of 7.38 (SD ± 1.82), while dyspareunia by 82.2% of women (88/107) with a mean severity score of 7.72 (SD ± 1.44). Age, SSc duration, and menopause did not result related to VVA-related symptoms prevalence.

Table 2. Vulvovaginal atrophy symptoms of the study population. § Calculated among women complaining of vaginal dryness. * Calculated among women complaining of dyspareunia.

	N = 107
Vaginal dryness, n (%)	89 (83.2)
Vaginal dryness severity §, mean (±SD)	7.38 (±1.82)
Dyspareunia, n (%)	88 (82.2)
Dyspareunia severity *, mean (±SD)	7.72 (±1.44)

3.3. Sexual Function

In our population, 97/107 (90.70%) women were sexually active. The mean age of sexually active women was 53.28 (SD ± 13.70) years, with SSc duration of 12.76 (SD ± 10.34) years.

Table 3 shows in detail the FSFI results for a single domain and for the overall score. An FSFI total score < 26.55 was reported in 87/97 (89.7%) of sexually active women. Sexual desire, the only domain that can be considered separately from the FSFI final score, was 2.23 (SD ± 1.00), lower than the cut-off of 5.00 defining the impairment of this FSFI item. While the duration of the SSc and the menopausal status did not reach significance in uni- and multivariate analysis, age was the only condition that resulted as an independent risk factor for sexual dysfunction (Table 4).

Table 3. Sexual function evaluated by the Female Sexual Function Index of the study population. Calculated among sexually active women. SD: Standard Deviation.

	N = 97
Sexual dysfunction, n (%)	87 (89.7)
Desire, mean (±SD)	2.23 (±1.00)
Arousal, mean (±SD)	2.66 (±1.74)
Lubrification, mean (±SD)	2.56 (±1.91)
Orgasm, mean (±SD)	2.69 (±2.04)
Satisfaction, mean (±SD)	2.93 (±1.84)
Pain, mean (±SD)	2.57 (±2.05)
Total, mean (±SD)	15.66 (±9.36)

Table 4. Factors related to vulvovaginal atrophy-related symptoms and sexual dysfunction. * Calculated among sexually active women. HR: Hazard Ratio; CI: Confidence Interval.

	Univariate		Multivariate	
	HR (95%CI)	p-Value	HR (95%CI)	p-Value
	Vulvovaginal Atrophy Symptoms			
Age, years	1.05 (1.01–1.13)	**0.01**	1.04 (0.98–1.11)	0.17
Systemic sclerosis duration, years	1.06 (0.99–1.13)	0.09		
Menopause	3.43 (1.11–10.58)	**0.03**	1.44 (0.27–7.61)	0.66
	Sexual Dysfunction *			
	HR (95%CI)	p-Value	HR (95%CI)	p-Value
Age, years	1.08 (1.02–1.15)	**0.002**	1.08 (1.00–1.18)	**0.04**
Systemic sclerosis duration, years	1.01 (0.95–1.02)	0.61		
Menopause	5.16 (1.03–25.71)	**0.02**	0.90 (0.08–9.38)	0.93

Bold numbers evidence a statistical significance ($p < 0.05$).

3.4. Relationship with the Partner

This part of our questionnaire was designed to evaluate the impact of VVA symptoms on partner relationships and intimacy. Only 16/107 (15%) of women reported "no influence" on their intimate relationships, 17/107 (15.9%) reported "little", 32/107 (29.9%) "fairly", and 42/107 (39.2%) answered that they were "highly" influenced (Figure 1). Therefore, more than 2/3 of women in our population reported a negative impact on their intimacy because of VVA symptoms. Similarly, the partner's negative perception related to VVA condition on sexual life was reported by 67/107 (63.2%) women.

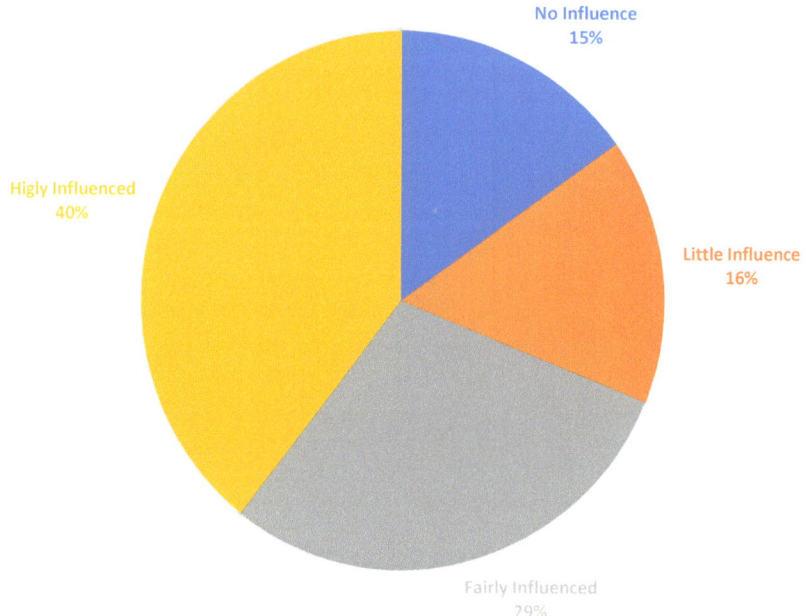

Figure 1. Influence of systemic sclerosis on intimacy with their partners reported by affected women.

3.5. Relationship with the Physician

In the study population, 68 (68/107; 63.6%) women had periodical annual gynecological evaluations. Of these, 63 women (63/107; 58.9%) had never discussed their VVA symptoms and the related sexual disorders with their doctor (Figure 2). Overall, 44/107 (41.1%) women revealed their bother to the following physicians: gynecologists in 75% (33/44) of cases, general practitioners in 13.6% (6/44), rheumatologists in 6.8% (3/44), and others in 4.5% (2/44). In the vast majority (40/44; 90.9%), the patient herself reported her symptoms to physicians who, according to the women's perception, manifested an interest in 84% (37/44) of cases.

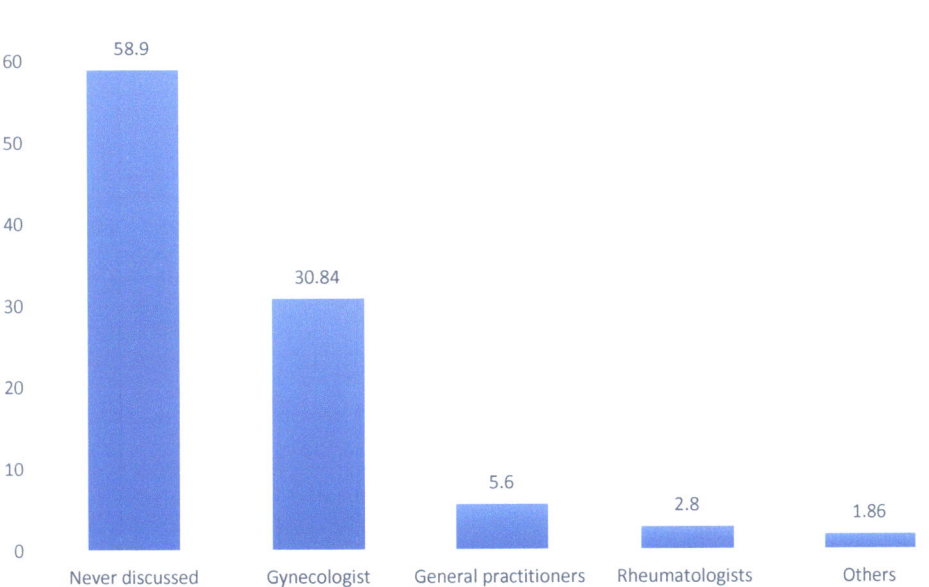

Figure 2. Kind of physicians involved in the assessment of women's vulvovaginal atrophy symptoms and sexual health.

3.6. Women's Considerations of Therapies

Only 15% (16/107) of women were on treatment for their VVA symptoms and, in all cases, with lubricants. Treatment satisfaction was reported as "fairly" in 56.3% (9/16) of cases, as "little" in 31.3% (5/16), and "not satisfied by the treatment" in 12.5% (2/16). The interest in an innovative medication or experimental treatment for their VVA symptoms and sexual dysfunction was expressed by 80/107 (75.5%) of women and 66/107 (62.9%) of cases, respectively.

4. Discussion

Chronic rheumatic diseases affect several aspects of women's life, including sexuality, intimate relationships with partners, and, therefore, their quality of life [15,16].

In women affected by SSc, skin tightening, muscle weakness, joint pain, deformity, and decreased physical function can have a negative impact on female sexuality and sexual functioning [8,17,18]. Common problems reported include vaginal dryness and discomfort, painful intercourse, and reduced frequency and intensity of orgasms [6,19], with a negative impact on intimate relationships and quality of life [20].

Our study, conducted on a cohort of 107 women with SSc, detected a VVA symptoms (vaginal dryness and/or dyspareunia) prevalence of 83.2% (89/107). The prevalence observed was greater than that reported in previous studies [6,21], with a severe perceived intensity of vaginal dryness and dyspareunia (7.38 and 7.72 on a 0 to 10 scale, respectively). As a consequence of VVA symptoms, sexual function was greatly impaired, too. Despite the high rate of sexually active women (90.7%; 97/107) in our population, 89.7% (87/97) of them were affected by sexual dysfunction, reporting low scores in all sexual domains, with a mean FSFI total score of 15.66. Moreover, even sexual desire, the only item that can be considered separate from the FSFI total score, was highly impacted with a mean of 2.23, far lower than the general cut-off of 5.00. In our analysis, the sexual dysfunction rate was higher than other rates reported in previous studies, while the intensity of sexual impairment evaluated with the FSFI total score was in line with the literature [20–22].

Levis et al. [9] led a study on 165 sexually active women affected by SSc and complaining of sexual impairment, reporting a 61.8% sexual dysfunction rate. The authors, however, adopted an FSFI total score cut-off of 22.5, lower than the cut-off of 26.55 commonly used, and included only a few women in menopause (less than 1/3 of the study population). Shouffer et al. [7] reported a sexual dysfunction rate of 70% in a population of 37 women affected by SSc, with only 27% of women in menopause. Menopause is known to be one of the main factors determining sexual dysfunction as a part of the genitourinary syndrome of menopause (GSM). Tissue changes in the external and internal female genitalia include retraction of the introitus, thinning and regression of the labia, and prominence of the urethral meatus [23], similar to changes reported in women affected by SSc [3–6], leading to VVA symptoms such as vaginal pain, dyspareunia, dryness, itching, and tissue friability. However, in our cohort of women affected by SSc, the disease itself seems to be a fundamental factor impacting VVA symptoms prevalence and sexuality, regardless of the menopausal status. Different authors have reported a worsening of sexual function impairment with age in women with SSc [6–10,18–22,24]. Our data demonstrated that SSc highly impacts VVA symptom prevalence and sexual dysfunction. In our study, when the risk factors for VVA symptoms and sexual dysfunction were assessed, patients' age resulted as the only risk factor related to sexual dysfunction. Indeed, while age, SSc duration, and menopause did not show to affect VVA symptom prevalence, older age was related to a higher sexual dysfunction prevalence. These findings led us to conclude that sexuality is affected independently by SSc but worsened by age.

Furthermore, the assessment of patients' relationships with their partners, communication with their physicians, and the desire for a novel outpatient treatment for genital symptoms was of primary importance in our survey.

Our data show that 70% of women affected by SSc felt a negative impact of VVA symptoms and impaired sexual function in intimacy with their partner and that in almost two-thirds of cases, these symptoms and their influence on sexual life are negatively perceived by the partner. Unfortunately, all these personal aspects still represent a taboo: sexual health is rarely investigated by physicians, and less than half of our patients (41.1%) search for a medical opinion. When a physician is involved by women in the assessment of VVA symptoms and sexual health, our survey reported gynecologists as the reference figure (30.84%). However, this study population, in which more than half of women have an annual gynecological examination, is only a part of a larger population in which the gynecologist could not be the reference figure. Therefore, it is possible that in other institutions, VVA symptoms and sexual problems are even less discussed by women to their own medical doctors. Indeed, while Schouffoer et al. recommended a routine interest of the physician about sexual problems in SSc women [16], Knafo et al. criticized this wide approach, finding that only a few patients desire to discuss sexual problems, with an infrequent involvement of rheumatologists [25], and suggesting, therefore, a routine assessment of sexual function only in the case of an effective intervention and patient benefit. In our opinion, educational activities on intimate aspects are needed for women with SSc in order to improve their awareness about this condition and the research of effective treatments. Educational activities about VVA symptoms and sexual disorders in women affected by SSc should be encouraged with two main targets: the patients and the medical caregivers. Firstly, women affected by SSc should be aware that VVA symptoms and sexual problems may be more frequent than in the healthy female population. Women affected by SSc should seek medical advice in case of vulvovaginal symptoms and sexual impairment, considering that appropriate treatments and strategies for this condition are available. Moreover, educational meetings should be encouraged through Patient Associations, with the aim of spreading awareness about this aspect of SSc among patients. On the other hand, educational activities should directly concern medical caregivers. Indeed, physicians assisting women with SSc should be systematically educated and trained in the screening and management of this important complication of SSc, which, even if it does not result in a decreased life expectancy, has a very high incidence with a huge impact on women's quality of life and health.

Concerning treatments, only a small part of the included women (16%) have adopted just lubricants for their symptoms without reaching satisfactory efficacy. Indeed, the majority of the study population would try a new (75.5%) or experimental (62.9%) treatment for vulvovaginal atrophy and sexual dysfunction treatment.

Several therapies are already available to treat VVA symptoms in menopausal women [26,27], including both systemic therapies such as ospemiphene [28], and local therapies such as vaginal estrogens and vaginal laser energies like the microablative fractional CO_2 laser or the erbium YAG laser [29,30], but none of these has been investigated in women affected by SSc. Further studies, however, are needed to evaluate the safety profile and the efficacy of these treatments on postmenopausal women affected by SSc complaining of VVA symptoms and sexual dysfunction.

The main strength of the current survey is the assessment of sexual health with a questionnaire carried out in collaboration with the National Italian Association of Scleroderma Patients named GILS ODV (*Gruppo Italiano Lotta alla Sclerosi Sistemica*) on the basis of the most frequent dilemma reported by SSc women, in association with a validated questionnaire (the FSFI). Moreover, the adoption of an anonymous questionnaire filled independently aimed to shield the result from the embarrassment provoked by the topic. Questionnaires, moreover, represent a feasible, non-invasive, and non-expensive method of investigation, making our study particularly acceptable to our patients.

Even if the sample size of 107 women with SSc can affect the statistical models, such as the multivariate analysis, we consider this population size as another strength of our investigation. SSc is, in fact, a rare medical condition with a prevalence that falls between 38 and 341 cases per million persons [31]. When assessing sexual function, our sample size of 107 women is one of the largest reported in the literature.

Furthermore, we deeply investigated new scenarios of SSc patients; we discovered an important negative influence on couple relationships due to sexual dysfunction, and we noticed communication difficulties with physicians. We highlighted the need for new effective therapies for this condition, as evidenced by the majority of SSc women. For vulvovaginal atrophy, therapeutic alternatives have increasingly been developed that result in improving symptoms and are also safe in terms of side effects and contraindications. Mechanical therapies, in particular, the vaginal CO_2 laser, are proving to be effective and safe in both clinical and histopathological terms [30]. The remodeling effect of the vaginal laser, which consists of the modification and regeneration of the vaginal mucosa through an increase in the content of collagen and elastic fibers, could be useful for women affected by SSc, considering the type of pathophysiology that sustains the tissue modification in affected women. In addition to that, in patients who are already using pharmacological therapies for their condition and have several comorbidities, offering a treatment that does not have severe side effects or pharmacological interactions may be of fundamental importance. Pilot studies and randomized control trials assessing the safety and efficacy of the different treatment strategies would be desirable in order to properly suggest adequate therapies for this condition.

However, this study presents several limitations, such as the impossibility of matching the results of the questionnaires to the clinical conditions related to SSc, because of the anonymous format of the questionnaire. Moreover, surveys may be affected by some typologies of bias intrinsic in such type of design. Indeed, considering the online design of the survey, participants may have answered questions inaccurately (response and recall bias). Moreover, wording differences can confuse the respondent or lead to incorrect interpretations of the question, especially for non-validated questions (question-wording). Furthermore, considering that 90.7% of the study population was sexually active, women who agreed to be enrolled in the study and completed the online questionnaire may be more interested in genital and sexual health than the general population of women affected by SSc (selection bias/sampling frame), making impossible an absolute generalizability to all patients with SSc.

5. Conclusions

Women with SSc present a high prevalence and severity of VVA symptoms and sexual dysfunction. These findings seem to be independent of the menopausal status and SSc duration. However, in a population of women affected by SSc, elderly patients are more frequently affected by sexual dysfunction. Relationships with their partners are highly impaired in this category of women. This increased awareness concerning the development of VVA and sexual dysfunction in women with SSc should help physicians investigate aspects that patients are partially reluctant to reveal spontaneously. Considering VVA management, not only lubricants should be considered as a possible treatment since patient satisfaction is not optimal. Research should be carried out in this field to explore new treatment strategies that would be welcome by women themselves.

Supplementary Materials: The following supporting information can be downloaded at: https://www.mdpi.com/article/10.3390/healthcare11162346/s1.

Author Contributions: Conceptualization, S.S. and C.G.; Methodology, S.S. and V.B.; software, A.F.R.; validation, M.S. and M.C.; investigation, C.S. and M.C.D.D.; data curation, V.B. and A.C.; writing—original draft preparation, A.F.R. and V.B.; writing—review and editing, M.S. and A.F.R.; visualization, A.B. and M.C.; supervision, S.S., A.B., M.C. and M.S.; project administration, C.G. and S.S. All authors have read and agreed to the published version of the manuscript.

Funding: This research received no external funding.

Institutional Review Board Statement: Obtained from the Institutional Review Boards.

Informed Consent Statement: Written informed consent has been obtained from the patient(s) to publish this paper.

Data Availability Statement: Data are available on request from the authors. The data that support the findings of this study are available from the corresponding author, AFR, upon reasonable request.

Acknowledgments: Gruppo Italiano per la Lotta alla Sclerodermia (GILS ODV) and ScleroNet, is a network of Hospitals and Universities in the Lombardia Region, Italy, specialized in the treatment of patients affected by SSc for the help in designing the questionnaire and data collection. ScleroNet affiliations are: 1. Beretta L, Carroni M, Bellocchi C. Scleroderma Unit, Fondazione IRCCS (Istituto di Ricovero e Cura a Carattere Scientifico) Ca' Granda Ospedale Maggiore Policlinico, Milano; 2. Epis O, Ughi N. Reumatologia ASST (Azienda Socio-Sanitaria Territoriale) Grande Ospedale Metropolitano Niguarda, Milano; 3. Mazzone A, Faggioli P. Scleroderma Unit, ASST Ovest Milanese, Legnano; 4. Selmi C, De Santis M. Reumatologia e Immunologia Clinica, IRCCS Istituto Clinico; 5. Humanitas, Milano.

Conflicts of Interest: The authors declare no conflict of interest.

References

1. Denton, C.P.; Khanna, D. Systemic sclerosis. *Lancet* **2017**, *390*, 1685–1699. [CrossRef] [PubMed]
2. Sampaio-Barros, P.D.; Samara, A.M.; Neto, J.F.M. Gynaecologic history in systemic sclerosis. *Clin. Rheumatol.* **2000**, *19*, 184–187. [CrossRef]
3. Saad, S.C.; Pietrzykowski, J.E.; Lewis, S.S.; Stepien, A.M.; Latham, V.A.; Messick, S.; Ensz, S.L.; Wetherell, C.; Behrendt, A.E. Vaginal Lubrication in Women with Scleroderma and Sjogren's Syndrome. *Sex. Disabil.* **1999**, *17*, 103–113. [CrossRef]

4. Schover, L.R.; Jensen, S.R. *Sexuality and Chronic Illness: A Comprehensive Approach*; Guilford: New York, NY, USA, 1988.
5. Trilpell, L.M.; Nietern, P.J.; Brown, A.N. (Eds.) Prevalence of female sexual dysfunction among women with systemic sclerosis. In Proceedings of the 9th International Workshop on Scleroderma Research, Boston, MA, USA, 5–9 August 2006.
6. Bhadauria, S.; Moser, D.K.; Clements, P.J.; Singh, R.R.; Lachenbruch, P.A.; Pitkin, R.M.; Weiner, S.R. Genital tract abnormalities and female sexual function impairment in systemic sclerosis. *Am. J. Obstet. Gynecol.* **1995**, *172*, 580–587. [CrossRef]
7. Schouffoer, A.A.; van der Marel, J.; Ter Kuile, M.M.; Weijenborg, P.T.M.; Voskuyl, A.; Vlieland, C.W.V.; van Laar, J.M.; Vlieland, T.P.M.V. Impaired sexual function in women with systemic sclerosis: A cross-sectional study. *Arthritis Rheum.* **2009**, *61*, 1601–1608. [CrossRef] [PubMed]
8. Knafo, R.; Thombs, B.D.; Jewett, L.; Hudson, M.; Wigley, F.; Haythornthwaite, J.A. (Not) talking about sex: A systematic comparison of sexual impairment in women with systemic sclerosis and other chronic disease samples. *Rheumatology* **2009**, *48*, 1300–1303. [CrossRef]
9. Levis, B.; Hudson, M.; Knafo, R.; Baron, M.; Nielson, W.R.; Hill, M.; Thombs, B.D.; Canadian Scleroderma Research Group (CSRG). Rates and correlates of sexual activity and impairment among women with systemic sclerosis. *Arthritis Care Res.* **2011**, *64*, 340–350. [CrossRef]
10. Tristano, A.G. The impact of rheumatic diseases on sexual function. *Rheumatol. Int.* **2009**, *29*, 853–860. [CrossRef]
11. World Medical Association. World Medical Association Declaration of Helsinki: Ethical principles for medical research involving human subjects. *JAMA* **2013**, *310*, 2191–2194. [CrossRef] [PubMed]
12. Subcommittee for scleroderma criteria of the American Rheumatism Association Diagnostic and Therapeutic Criteria Committee. Preliminary criteria for the classification of systemic sclerosis (scleroderma). *Arthritis Rheum.* **1980**, *23*, 581–590. [CrossRef]
13. Meston, M.; Freihart, B.; Handy, A.; Kilimnik, C.; Rosen, R. Scoring and Interpretation of the FSFI: What can be Learned From 20 Years of use? *J. Sex. Med.* **2020**, *17*, 17–25. [CrossRef] [PubMed]
14. Filocamo, M.T.; Serati, M.; Marzi, V.L.; Costantini, E.; Milanesi, M.; Pietropaolo, A.; Polledro, P.; Gentile, B.; Maruccia, S.; Fornia, S.; et al. The Female Sexual Function Index (FSFI): Linguistic Validation of the Italian Version. *J. Sex. Med.* **2014**, *11*, 447–453. [CrossRef]
15. Prady, J.; Vale, A.; Hill, J. Body image and sexuality. In *Rheumatology Nursing: A Creative Approach*; Hill, J., Ed.; Churchill Livingstone: Edinburgh, Scotland, 1998; pp. 109–124.
16. Wells, D. *Caring for Sexuality in Health and Illness*; Churchill Livingstone: Edinburgh, Scotland, 2000.
17. Impens, A.J.; Seibold, J.R. Vascular Alterations and Sexual Function in Systemic Sclerosis. *Int. J. Rheumatol.* **2010**, *2010*, 139020. [CrossRef]
18. Knafo, R.; Haythornthwaite, J.A.; Heinberg, L.; Wigley, F.M.; Thombs, B.D. The association of body image dissatisfaction and pain with reduced sexual function in women with systemic sclerosis. *Rheumatology* **2011**, *50*, 1125–1130. [CrossRef] [PubMed]
19. Impens, A.J.; Rothman, J.; Schiopu, E.; Cole, J.C.; Dang, J.; Gendrano, N.; Rosen, R.C.; Seibold, J.R. Sexual activity and functioning in female scleroderma patients. *Clin. Exp. Rheumatol.* **2009**, *27*, 38–43. [PubMed]
20. Jewett, L.R.; Hudson, M.; Haythornthwaite, J.A.; Heinberg, L.; Wigley, F.M.; Baron, M.; Thombs, B.D. Development and validation of the brief-satisfaction with appearance scale for systemic sclerosis. *Arthritis Care Res.* **2010**, *62*, 1779–1786. [CrossRef]
21. Bongi, S.M.; Del Rosso, A.; Mikhaylova, S.; Baccini, M.; Cerinic, M.M. Sexual Function in Italian Women with Systemic Sclerosis Is Affected by Disease-related and Psychological Concerns. *J. Rheumatol.* **2013**, *40*, 1697–1705. [CrossRef]
22. Frikha, F.; Masmoudi, J.; Saidi, N.; Bahloul, Z. Sexual dysfunction in married women with systemic sclerosis. *Pan Afr. Med. J.* **2014**, *17*, 82. [CrossRef]
23. Parish, S.J.; Nappi, R.; Krychman, M.L.; Spadt, K.; Simon, J.; Goldstein, J.; Kingsberg, S. Impact of vulvovaginal health on postmenopausal women: A review of surveys on symptoms of vulvovaginal atrophy. *Int. J. Women's Health* **2013**, *5*, 437–447. [CrossRef]
24. Sanchez, K.; Denys, P.; Giuliano, F.; Palazzo, C.; Bérezné, A.; Abid, H.; Rannou, F.; Poiraudeau, S.; Mouthon, L. Systemic sclerosis: Sexual dysfunction and lower urinary tract symptoms in 73 patients. *Presse Med.* **2016**, *45*, e79–e89. [CrossRef]
25. Knafo, R.; Jewett, L.R.; Ba, M.B.; Thombs, B.D. Sexual function in women with systemic sclerosis: Comment on the article by Schouffoer et al. *Arthritis Care Res.* **2010**, *62*, 1200–1202. [CrossRef] [PubMed]
26. North American Menopause Society. Management of symptomatic vulvovaginal atrophy: 2013 position statement of the North American Menopause Society. *Menopause* **2013**, *20*, 888–902. [CrossRef] [PubMed]
27. Salvatore, S.; Benini, V.; Ruffolo, A.F.; Degliuomini, R.S.; Redaelli, A.; Casiraghi, A.; Candiani, M. Current challenges in the pharmacological management of genitourinary syndrome of menopause. *Expert Opin. Pharmacother.* **2023**, *24*, 23–28. [CrossRef] [PubMed]
28. Portman, D.J.; Bachmann, G.A.; Simon, J.A. Ospemifene, a novel selective estrogen receptor modulator for treating dyspareunia associated with postmenopausal vulvar and vaginal atrophy. *Menopause* **2013**, *20*, 623–630. [CrossRef]
29. Filippini, M.; Porcari, I.; Ruffolo, A.F.; Casiraghi, A.; Farinelli, M.; Uccella, S.; Franchi, M.; Candiani, M.; Salvatore, S. CO_2-Laser therapy and Genitourinary Syndrome of Menopause: A Systematic Review and Meta-Analysis. *J. Sex. Med.* **2022**, *19*, 452–470. [CrossRef]

30. Benini, V.; Ruffolo, A.F.; Casiraghi, A.; Degliuomini, R.S.; Frigerio, M.; Braga, A.; Serati, M.; Torella, M.; Candiani, M.; Salvatore, S. New Innovations for the Treatment of Vulvovaginal Atrophy: An Up-to-Date Review. *Medicina* **2022**, *58*, 770. [CrossRef]
31. Ingegnoli, F.; Ughi, N.; Mihai, C. Update on the epidemiology, risk factors, and disease outcomes of systemic sclerosis. *Best Pract Res Clin Rheumatol.* **2018**, *32*, 223–240. [CrossRef]

Disclaimer/Publisher's Note: The statements, opinions and data contained in all publications are solely those of the individual author(s) and contributor(s) and not of MDPI and/or the editor(s). MDPI and/or the editor(s) disclaim responsibility for any injury to people or property resulting from any ideas, methods, instructions or products referred to in the content.

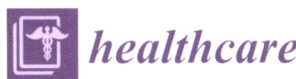

Case Report

Purple Urine Bag Syndrome in a Home-Dwelling Elderly Female with Lumbar Compression Fracture: A Case Report

Milka B. Popović [1,2,*], Deana D. Medić [3,4], Radmila S. Velicki [1,2] and Aleksandra I. Jovanović Galović [5,*]

1. Department of Hygiene, Faculty of Medicine, University of Novi Sad, Hajduk Veljkova 3, 21000 Novi Sad, Serbia; radmila.velicki@mf.uns.ac.rs
2. Center for Hygiene and Human Ecology, Institute of Public Health of Vojvodina, Futoška 121, 21000 Novi Sad, Serbia
3. Department of Microbiology, Faculty of Medicine, University of Novi Sad, Hajduk Veljkova 3, 21000 Novi Sad, Serbia; deana.medic@mf.uns.ac.rs
4. Center for Microbiology, Institute of Public Health of Vojvodina, Futoška 121, 21000 Novi Sad, Serbia
5. Faculty of Pharmacy Novi Sad, University of Business Academy, Trg Mladenaca 5, 21000 Novi Sad, Serbia
* Correspondence: milka.popovic@mf.uns.ac.rs (M.B.P.); aleksandra.jovanovic@faculty-pharmacy.com (A.I.J.G.)

Abstract: Purple urine bag syndrome (PUBS) is an uncommon, but usually benign, underrecognized clinical condition with the distressing presentation of purple, blue or reddish discoloration of a patient's catheter bag and tubing in the setting of catheter-associated urinary tract infections (UTIs). PUBS is the result of the complex metabolic pathway of the dietary essential amino acid tryptophan. Its urinary metabolite, indoxyl sulfate, is converted into red and blue byproducts (indirubin and indigo) in the presence of the bacterial enzymes indoxyl sulfatase and phosphatase. The typical predisposing factors are numerous and include the following: female gender, advanced age, long-term catheterization and immobilization, constipation, institutionalization, dementia, increased dietary intake of tryptophan, chronic kidney disease, alkaline urine, and spinal cord injury (SCI). Here, we present a case of PUBS in a home-dwelling elderly female patient with a history of long-term immobility after a pathological spinal fracture, long-term catheterization, constipation, and malignant disease in remission. Urine culture was positive for *Proteus mirabilis*. This state can be alarming to both patients and physicians, even if the patient is asymptomatic. Healthcare professionals and caregivers need to be aware of this unusual syndrome as an indicator of bacteriuria in order to initiate proper diagnostics and treatment.

Keywords: purple urine bag syndrome; purple urine discoloration; urinary tract infection; *Proteus mirabilis*; chronic indwelling urinary catheter; spinal cord injury; case report

1. Introduction

Purple urine bag syndrome (PUBS) is an uncommon, but usually benign, clinical condition with the purple discoloration of the patient's catheter bag and tubing [1]. The characteristic purple color is the result of the presence of predominantly Gram-negative bacteria in the urine. This urinary tract infection (UTI) may be completely asymptomatic or present with the classical bacteriuria symptoms. The mechanism of the characteristic discoloration of the Foley bag and the urine involves specific microbial enzymes. Bacteria-derived indoxyl sulfatase and phosphatase cause blue (indigo)- and red (indirubin)-pigmented breakdown products of dietary amino acid tryptophan metabolite (indoxyl sulfate). The different proportions of these two pigmented metabolites produce various shades of discoloration, ranging from purple and blue to a reddish color (Figure 1) [2,3]. The formed pigments predominantly bind to the synthetic materials, such as tubing and bags, whereas the fresh urine itself is not discolored.

Citation: Popović, M.B.; Medić, D.D.; Velicki, R.S.; Jovanović Galović, A.I. Purple Urine Bag Syndrome in a Home-Dwelling Elderly Female with Lumbar Compression Fracture: A Case Report. *Healthcare* **2023**, *11*, 2251. https://doi.org/10.3390/healthcare11162251

Academic Editors: Matteo Frigerio and Stefano Manodoro

Received: 29 June 2023
Revised: 4 August 2023
Accepted: 7 August 2023
Published: 10 August 2023

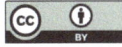

Copyright: © 2023 by the authors. Licensee MDPI, Basel, Switzerland. This article is an open access article distributed under the terms and conditions of the Creative Commons Attribution (CC BY) license (https://creativecommons.org/licenses/by/4.0/).

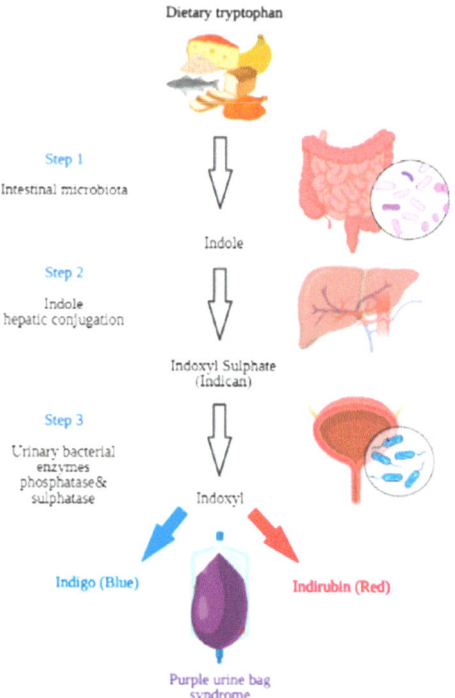

Figure 1. Metabolic pathway of dietary tryptophan leading to purple urine bag syndrome (PUBS) (created with BioRender.com).

According to systematic reviews, typical predisposing factors include female gender, advanced age, long-term immobilization and catheterization, constipation, institutionalization, dementia, increased dietary intake of tryptophan, chronic kidney disease, alkaline urine, and spinal cord injury (SCI).

In the study conducted by Sabanis et al., the mean age of 246 affected PUBS patients was 78.9 ± 12.3 years, of which 70.7% were female, with a high prevalence of alkaline urine (91.3%) and constipation (90.1%). More than 76% were bed-ridden, 45.1% were experiencing long-term catheterization, 42.8% had been diagnosed with dementia, 14.3% had recurrent urinary tract infections, and 14.1% were chronic kidney disease (CKD) patients [4].

The most common microbes identified as the causes of UTIs related to PUBS were as follows: *Escherichia coli, Proteus mirabilis, Klebsiella pneumoniae, Enterococcus, Pseudomonas aeruginosa, Providencia stuartii, Providencia rettgeri, Morganella morganii, Enterococcus faecalis*, etc. [4,5].

2. Case Presentation

Our case was a 79-year-old female with a history of long-term immobility after pathological spinal compression fracture, and urinary retention managed with a chronic indwelling Foley catheter, recurrent asymptomatic urinary tract infections, constipation, hypertension, prior malignant disease in remission, osteoporosis, and periodically altered mental status. The patient's routine medications included paracetamol, pantoprazol, diltiazem, ramipril, diazepam, vitamin D supplements, and melperon hydrochlorid.

The family reported that the patient lived at home with a professional home care service during the day. A compression fracture of the lumbar (lower) spine and a neurogenic bladder were diagnosed one year prior to the first urine discoloration. The first purple urine bag discoloration was misinterpreted as a dietary-related urine discoloration associated with beetroot or rosehip tea consumption, and did not receive an appropriate assessment or treatment. At the moment of the first PUBS onset, the catheter was 15 days "old". The family and caregiver noticed a recurrent light-purple discoloration of the patient's urine bag and a strong urine odor. The patient did not complain of any symptoms that could indicate urinary tract infection. In the following days, the family noticed a change in mental status indicated by mild signs of mental confusion.

The patient's overall clinical presentation was unremarkable. Apart from the elevated serum levels of lactic acid dehydrogenase (LDH), most biochemical parameters did not show any significant changes. Slightly elevated creatinine levels (reference interval: 49–97 µmol/L; the determined value was 115 µmol/L) and liver enzyme activity did not raise any concerns at the time. The physical examination recorded a slightly confused elderly female in no acute distress, with dry mucous membranes, active bowel sounds, without tenderness to deep low abdominal palpation, with both-sided lower extremity weakness and paresis, muscular atrophy, and a Foley bag with purple urine, as shown in Figure 2.

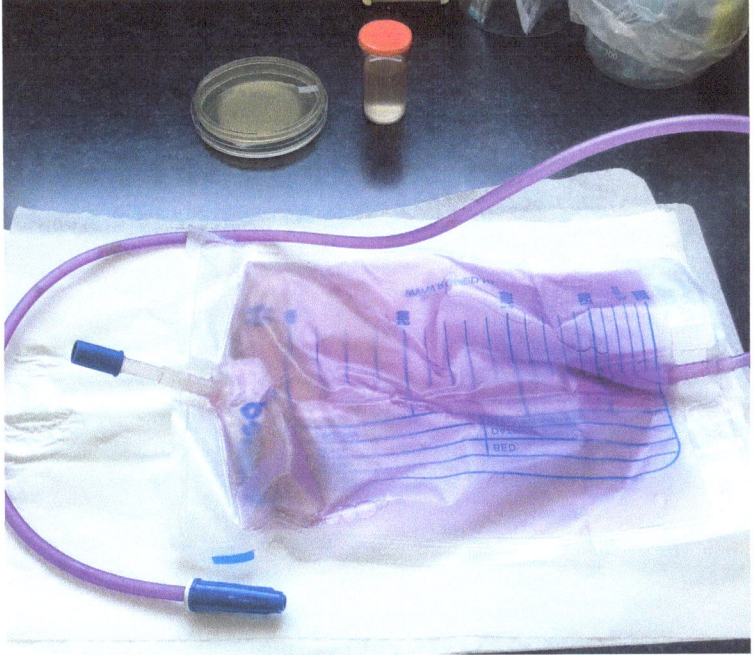

Figure 2. The purple urine bag and yellow-brown color of voided urine.

The purple color of the PE urine bag with the extended tubing was more intense than the color of the silicone catheter. A clear demarcation zone between the two grades of the same purple color was at the level of the urine drainage port of the Foley catheter. The more intense purple color of the urine tube implied that biofilm had formed.

Urinalysis revealed brownish, cloudy urine positive for nitrites, with more than 100 white blood cells per high-power microscopy field, without hematuria.

Immediately after the Foley catheter and urine bag change, the caregiver started with empiric antibiotics (fosfomycin), intensive per-oral rehydration, and bowel function normalization. Urine color and urine odor were normalized within 24 h. When the urine culture results became available, the patient started an antibiotic treatment course according to culture sensitivities. The urine color returned to clear yellow, without any sediment or purple shade. This case report was composed according to the CARE guidelines [6].

Microbiological Examination

A urine sample was collected from a urinary catheter and the complete urine bag was delivered to the laboratory. Urine samples were seeded with a sterile, calibrated, plastic 1 μL inoculation loop on the chromogenic medium CHROMID®CPS® Elite agar (bioMérieux, Marcy-l'Étoile, France). After incubation for 18–24 h at 35–37 °C, the plates were examined and a significant number of colonies of >10^5 CFU/mL of yellow-brown color with a characteristic smell of ammonia were established. MALDI-TOF/MS (Bruker, MA, USA) was used as an analytical tool for a further determination of the bacterial species in the urine samples.

The urine culture from both the sterile vial and Foley bag was positive for *Proteus mirabilis* (*P. mirabilis*) (Figure 3).

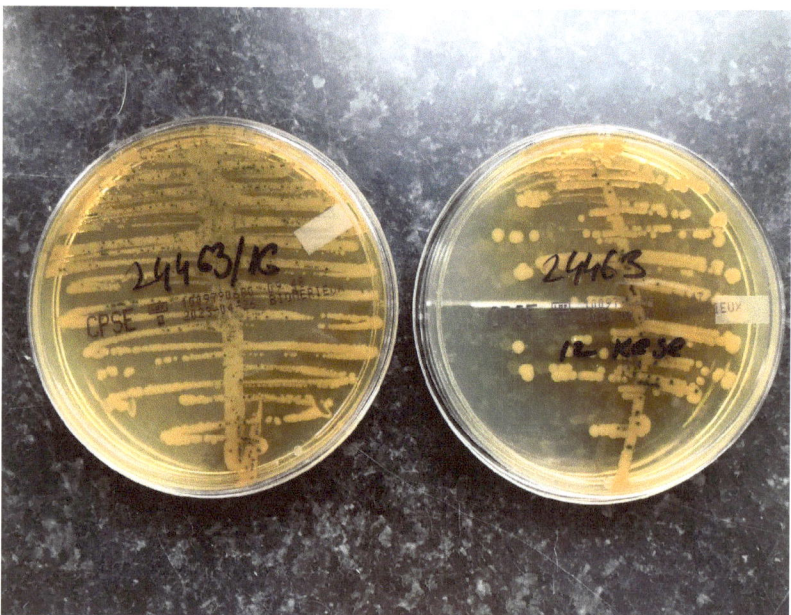

Figure 3. A positive urine culture on CHROMID®CPS® Elite agar (**left**—sample from the vial; **right**—sample from Foley bag).

After identification, an antibiotic sensitivity test was performed using the Kirby–Bauer disc diffusion method on Mueller–Hinton agar according to the recommendations of the European Committee on Antimicrobial Susceptibility Testing (EUCAST) standard [7]. The isolates showed sensitivity to aminopenicillins, aminopenicillins with beta-lactamase inhibitors, cephalosporins, aminoglycosides, quinolones, cotrimoxazole, and carbapenems (meropenem).

3. Discussion

The purple urine bag phenomenon was first described by Barlow and Dickson in 1978, who described the rare mechanism of purple color formation in urine bags in children with spina bifida in pediatric wards. The investigation elucidated the bacterial decomposition of dietary amino acid tryptophan in the gut lumen, producing indoxyl sulfate, which is consequently excreted in the urine, then oxidized to insoluble indigo upon contact with the air in a collecting bag [8,9]. A similar clinical manifestation in infants, known as "blue diaper syndrome" (Drummond syndrome), is also a consequence of abnormal tryptophan metabolism but is, however, genetically caused. In adults, a wide array of conditions may produce urinary discoloration: hematuria, myoglobinuria, porphyria, alkaptonuria, lipiduria, and the presence of certain microorganisms. In addition, numerous medications (amitriptyline, ibuprofen, propofol, L-dopa, phenytoin, flutamide, senna, and laxatives with a phenolphthalein component) as well as the consumption of intensively colored foods (beetroots, blackberries, fava beans, carrots, and rosehip tea) may produce changes in urine color, ranging from red or orange to blue-green [10,11].

Since it cannot be synthesized in the human body, tryptophan—an amino acid with an indole nucleus—is one of the essential amino acids and must be obtained through the diet. Tryptophan-rich foods include oats, bananas, dried prunes, milk, tuna fish, cheese, bread, chicken, turkey, peanuts, and chocolate [12]. In the gastrointestinal (GI) tract, due to the action of the GI microbiome, several metabolites of tryptophan can be produced. Most of these compounds arise from proteins which are not fully digested and, thus, are malabsorbed and, hence, remain in the colon (Figure 4). Bacteria may give rise to a number of tryptophan-derived, metabolically active molecules. It was experimentally proven that the amount of indole produced by bacteria is proportional to the amount of supplied tryptophan [13]. So, it is clear that tryptophan in the form of proteins incompletely digested from the human diet is a substrate for the intestinal microbiota. One of the enzymes responsible for indole production in the colon is tryptophanase [14,15].

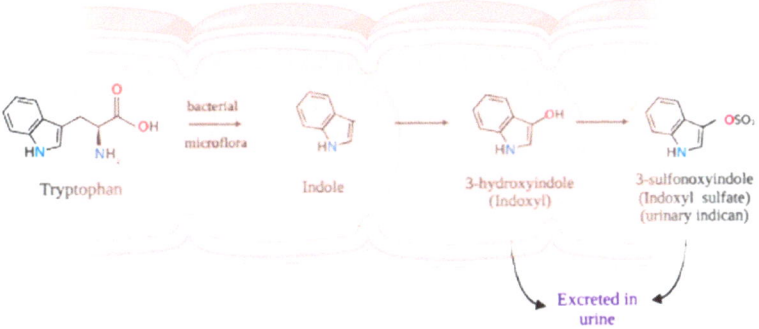

Figure 4. Pathway of bacterial transformation of tryptophan in the colon (created with BioRender.com).

In the case presented herein, the most probable dietary sources of tryptophan were bananas, meat, and chicken pâté, which were consumed in excessive amounts for a longer period before the onset of the urinary discoloration.

Indole is a precursor for several pivotal mediators including tryptamine, serotonin, melatonin, kynurenines, and nicotinic acid. Other indoles are considered waste products and are often conjugated prior to urinary excretion. The majority of indole is oxidized to indoxyl and conjugated with sulfate in the liver [16].

It has also been suggested that indoxyl sulfate is toxic to renal tubular cells, while increased indoxyl sulfate levels accelerate the progression of renal disease [17]. Thus, the produced physiologically active metabolites may be linked to the patient's altered mental state during bacteriuria.

The 3D structure of urinary sediments and urine bag walls of two cases of PUBS were observed using Low-Vacuum Scanning Electron Microscopy (LVSEM), which showed granular purple crystals around the bacilli, cocci, or mycelium that adhered to the walls of the bag [18].

As mentioned before, the discoloration in PUBS occurs when the two pigments come in contact with the synthetic materials of the catheter tubing and urinary bag, presumably already covered with biofilm. In some cases, the whole urine bag and the catheter are discolored. In other cases, the level of discoloration clearly indicates the area of prolonged contact between the urine and the synthetic material. A frequent misinterpretation is that the urine in PUBS itself is discolored [19,20].

P. mirabilis is a Gram-negative rod-shaped bacterium most noted for its swimming and swarming motility phenomenon and urease activity. It frequently causes catheter-associated urinary tract infections that are often polymicrobial, particularly in patients undergoing long-term catheterization. These infections may be accompanied by the development of bladder (urolithiasis) or kidney stones due to the alkalinization of urine from urease-catalyzed urea hydrolysis [21].

P. mirabilis is an opportunistic pathogen that uses a diverse set of virulence factors to access and colonize the host urinary tract and develop a crystalline biofilm [22]. Biofilm formation is a multistep process, which begins with migration by swarming motility along the catheter, followed by attachment to the surface through fimbriae adhesins. Once firmly attached, the number of *P. mirabilis* cells rises. They produce a substantial amount of urease enzyme which hydrolyses urea present in urine to ammonia and bicarbonate anion, inevitably raising the pH of the surrounding environment and leading to mineral precipitation in crystal form [22,23]. The increase in alkalinity leads to the deposition of struvite (ammonium magnesium phosphate) and hydroxyapatite (calcium phosphate) crystals on a developing biofilm. This process, named ureolytic biomineralization, is additionally aided by *P. mirabilis* capsular polysaccharide for biofilm matrix formulation and peptide efflux [23,24]. Fully developed crystalline biofilm formation by *P. mirabilis* unavoidably causes frequent catheter encrustation and blockage and, in most cases, is accompanied by urine retention and ascending UTIs, which may even lead to antibiotic treatment resistance [25,26].

P. mirabilis can be found in a wide variety of environments, including soil, water sources, and sewage, but it is predominantly a commensal of the gastrointestinal tracts of humans and animals. The majority of *P. mirabilis* UTIs are a consequence of the ascension of bacteria from the GI tract. There is literature evidence showing that patients with *P. mirabilis* infection have exactly the same bacterial strain present both in urine and the stool samples [22]. A certain percentage of cases are the result of person-to-person transmission, frequently in hospitals or nursing homes.

Several bacterial species that commonly infect the bladder after spinal cord injury can hydrolyze urea; apart from *Proteus*, these species are as follows: *Pseudomonas, Providencia, Klebsiella*, and *Morganella*. Interestingly, the *Proteus*' urease is one of the fastest-acting enzymes, so it is not surprising that this microbe is most commonly involved in catheter encrustation and blocking. Moreover, it may also lead to the formation of stones in the urinary tract, particularly in indwelling patients. Once stones are formed, antimicrobial therapy is usually not effective in eradicating *Proteus* and other organisms lodged in the of stones' crevices [27–29]. These infections are common in long-term catheterized patients, such as those who reside in nursing homes and chronic care facilities, and may be of particular danger to spinal cord injury patients. Recurrent UTIs are often seen in patients with spinal cord injuries (SCIs) and neurogenic bladders. It is well known that impaired bladder emptying, repeated catheterization, vesicoureteral reflux, and similar conditions that impair normal urine excretion are predisposing factors for infections of the urinary tract. Immobility is also one of the factors to be considered. In SCI patients, *Proteus* is more frequently found in individuals with a higher degree of damage to the spinal cord. In those patients, hospitalization, the onset of decubitus, and the use of indwelling catheter are highly probable. *Proteus* detection in urine is one of the predictive factors for urologic complications in persons with SCI [27,30]. Results from our laboratory for the previous period (2020–2023) show an average incidence of *P. mirabilis* presence in urine samples of 1.91% for both hospitalized patients and outpatients in the region of Vojvodina, Serbia (Table 1).

Table 1. Overall number of *P. mirabilis* positive urine analysis and the incidence (%) in the years 2020–2023 (until 30 June). Samples were obtained from both hospitalized patients and outpatients in the Vojvodina region (Serbia).

Year	Number of Microbiological Urine Analyses [1]	Number of P. mirabilis Detected	Incidence %
2023	21,558	410	1.90
2022	41,544	830	2.00
2021	34,730	658	1.89
2020	27,049	490	1.81
Total	124,881	2388	1.91 [2]

[1] All analyses were performed at the Center for Microbiology, Institute of Public Health of Vojvodina, Serbia; [2] average incidence.

Generally speaking, the incidence of PUBS in catheterized patients is fairly low, although the percentages vary depending on the geographical region and the population group enrolled in the study. According to the meta-analysis by Llenas-García [31], the prevalence of PUBS in observational studies was 11.7% in patients with long-term urinary catheterization. It is a widely accepted notion that PUBS may only reflect asymptomatic bacteriuria and, therefore, should not be treated with aggressive antibiotic therapy. However, taking into account data obtained in vitro [32] on the immunomodulatory capacity of *Proteus mirabilis* strains, it is worth considering the possibility of the scenario where *P. mirabilis* infection subdues the host immune response and that is the reason for the lack of symptoms in patients. If left untreated, such an infection may lead to a propagation of the possibility of biofilm formation on the catheter surface (possibly also on the bladder epithelium). Once formed, biofilm represents "a refuge" for microorganisms, protecting them from antibiotic action and the host immune cells. Well-established biofilm further leads to complications due to changes in the microenvironment (ammonia production, pH elevation, and crystal formation). While elevated ammonia concentrations are toxic on their own, crystals lead to catheter encrustation and blockage and are recorded as constituents of kidney stones in such patients [33,34].

Biofilm formation inhibition on catheters could become a promising alternative to conventional antimicrobial-based treatment, which may be associated with rapid resistance development [35]. Various modifications of materials and antimicrobial coatings on the catheter surface surely offer one of the possible solutions in order to prevent PUBS. The use of hydrogels, polytetrafluoroethylene (PTFE), polyethylene glycol (PEG), polyzwitterions, and specific enzymes as coatings all involve material modifications. As antimicrobial coatings, apart from various antibiotics (chosen for specific infecting agents), metallic ions, nanoparticles, nitric oxide bacteriophages, and antimicrobial peptides (AMPs) may be used in order to prevent biofilm formation [36]. Although there are numerous data from in vivo, in vitro, and clinical studies, a unanimous conclusion on which coating is the right choice for a specific pathogen has not been reached. Furthermore, with the possibilities offered by 3D printing, new options are available, like the coating of multiple drugs on catheters with different release profiles. Taking into account the fact that several phytochemicals—like curcumin, allicin, or proanthocyanidins—have shown in vitro effectiveness against *P. mirabilis* biofilm formation [23,24], it seems that there are a plethora of options available. According to some authors, a combination of various approaches will give the best results. However, more research efforts are needed in order to effectively translate scientific findings into clinical practice.

4. Conclusions

In this case report, we confirm that female gender, increased dietary tryptophan, long-term immobilization and catheterization, severe constipation, high urinary bacterial load, and renal failure are the risk factors for purple urine bag syndrome. Although this condition seems benign, it sometimes requires aggressive management.

In addition, we argue that purple urine bag syndrome should not be taken lightly, even if the patient is asymptomatic. In our opinion, it should be treated with the notion that it is a "warning signal". It indicates an ongoing urinary tract infection, which could develop into a serious health threat to the patient, usually heavily burdened with other chronic conditions in already-vulnerable patients [37].

Healthcare professionals—particularly urologists and geriatricians—need to be aware of this unusual syndrome so that an appropriate investigation and possible treatment can be initiated as soon as possible [38]. In spite of the fact that PUBS is a fairly rare condition today, with an aging population worldwide, its incidence is likely to increase in the future. In that respect, innovative solutions for biofilm prevention, combined with an effective antimicrobial therapy, may be of relevance.

Author Contributions: Conceptualization, M.B.P.; methodology, M.B.P.; investigation, M.B.P. and D.D.M.; resources, M.B.P.; writing—original draft preparation, M.B.P. and R.S.V.; writing—review and editing, A.I.J.G.; visualization, M.B.P. and R.S.V.; supervision, M.B.P.; funding acquisition, M.B.P. All authors have read and agreed to the published version of the manuscript.

Funding: This research received no external funding.

Institutional Review Board Statement: Ethical review and approval were waived for this study due to the fact that no intervention on the patient management was performed. This case study involved one patient only, from whom informed consent was obtained, both from the patient and a family member. Patient confidentiality was maintained at all times. The study involved observation only.

Informed Consent Statement: Informed consent was obtained from the person who was a subject involved in the case and a caregiver.

Data Availability Statement: The data presented in this study are available on request from the corresponding author. The data are not publicly available due to the patient's privacy protection.

Acknowledgments: The work was supported by the Institute of Public Health of Vojvodina, Novi Sad, Serbia, and we express our gratitude for the support.

Conflicts of Interest: The authors declare no conflict of interest.

References

1. Vallejo-Manzur, F.; Mireles-Cabodevila, E.; Varon, J. Purple urine bag syndrome. *Am. J. Emerg. Med.* **2005**, *23*, 521–524. [CrossRef]
2. Kumar, R.; Devi, K.; Kataria, D.; Kumar, J.; Ahmad, I. Purple Urine Bag Syndrome: An Unusual Presentation of Urinary Tract Infection. *Cureus* **2021**, *13*, e16319. [CrossRef] [PubMed]
3. DeRon, N., Jr.; Legan, C. Purple Urine Bag Syndrome: A Rare and Surprising Clinical Presentation. *Cureus* **2023**, *15*, e33354. [CrossRef] [PubMed]
4. Sabanis, N.; Paschou, E.; Papanikolaou, P.; Zagkotsis, G. Purple Urine Bag Syndrome: More Than Eyes Can See. *Curr. Urol.* **2019**, *13*, 125–132. [CrossRef] [PubMed]
5. Yang, H.W.; Su, Y.J. Trends in the epidemiology of purple urine bag syndrome: A systematic review. *Biomed. Rep.* **2018**, *8*, 249–256. [CrossRef]
6. Gagnier, J.J.; Kienle, G.; Altman, D.G.; Moher, D.; Sox, H.; Riley, D.; The CARE Group. The CARE guidelines: Consensus-based clinical case reporting guideline development. *J. Med. Case Rep.* **2013**, *7*, 223. [CrossRef] [PubMed]
7. The European Committee on Antimicrobial Susceptibility Testing. *Breakpoint Tables for Interpretation of MICs and Zone Diameters*; Version 13.0; EUCAST: Växjö, Sweden, 2023.
8. Barlow, G.B.; Dickson, J.A.S. Purple urine bags. *Lancet* **1978**, *311*, 220–221. [CrossRef]
9. Campagne, J.; Kurt, S.; Moulinet, T.; Mohamed, S.; Deibener-Kaminsky, J.; Jaussaud, R. Une couleur inhabituelle. *Rev. Med. Interne* **2021**, *42*, 61–62. [CrossRef]
10. Worku, D.A. Purple urine bag syndrome: An unusual but important manifestation of urinary tract infection. Case report and literature review. *SAGE Open Med. Case Rep.* **2019**, *7*, 2050313X18823105. [CrossRef]
11. Boo, W.H. An elderly man with purple urine. *Aust. J. Gen. Pract.* **2021**, *50*, 381–382. [CrossRef]
12. Richard, D.M.; Dawes, M.A.; Mathias, C.W.; Acheson, A.; Hill-Kapturczak, N.; Dougherty, D.M. L-Tryptophan: Basic Metabolic Functions, Behavioral Research and Therapeutic Indications. *Int. J. Tryptophan Res.* **2009**, *2*, 45–60. [CrossRef] [PubMed]
13. Li, G.; Young, K.D. Indole production by the tryptophanase TnaA in Escherichia coli is determined by the amount of exogenous tryptophan. *Microbiology* **2013**, *159*, 402–410. [CrossRef] [PubMed]
14. Banoglu, E.; Jha, G.G.; King, R.S. Hepatic microsomal metabolism of indole to indoxyl, a precursor of indoxyl sulfate. *Eur. J. Drug Metab. Pharmacokinet.* **2001**, *26*, 235–240. [CrossRef]

15. Michael, A.F.; Drummond, K.N.; Doeden, D.; Erson, J.A.; Good, R.A. Tryptophan metabolism in man. *J. Clin. Investig.* **1964**, *43*, 1730–1746. [CrossRef] [PubMed]
16. Huć, T.; Nowinski, A.; Drapala, A.; Konopelski, P.; Ufnal, M. Indole and indoxyl sulfate, gut bacteria metabolites of tryptophan, change arterial blood pressure via peripheral and central mechanisms in rats. *Pharmacol. Res.* **2018**, *130*, 172–179. [CrossRef] [PubMed]
17. Alan, S.L.; Yu, M.B.; Chir, B. The Pathophysiology of Uremia. In *Brenner and Rector's The Kidney*; Meyer, T.W., Hostetter, T.H., Eds.; Elsevier: Amsterdam, The Netherlands, 2020; Volume 52, pp. 1790–1804.e6.
18. Abe, M.; Furuichi, M.; Ishimitsu, T.; Tojo, A. Analysis of purple urine bag syndrome by low vacuum scanning electron microscopy. *Med. Mol. Morphol.* **2022**, *55*, 123–130. [CrossRef]
19. Chong, V.H. Misconception about purple urine bag syndrome. *QJM Int. J. Med.* **2020**, *113*, 445. [CrossRef]
20. Popoola, M.; Hillier, M. Purple Urine Bag Syndrome as the Primary Presenting Feature of a Urinary Tract Infection. *Cureus* **2022**, *14*, e23970. [CrossRef]
21. Armbruster, C.E.; Mobley, H.L.T.; Pearson, M.M. Pathogenesis of *Proteus mirabilis* Infection. *EcoSal Plus* **2018**, *8*, 10-1128. [CrossRef]
22. Schaffer, J.N.; Pearson, M.M. *Proteus mirabilis* and Urinary Tract Infections. *Microbiol. Spectr.* **2015**, *3*, 383–433. [CrossRef]
23. Wasfi, R.; Hamed, S.M.; Amer, M.A.; Fahmy, L.I. *Proteus mirabilis* Biofilm: Development and Therapeutic Strategies. *Front. Cell. Infect. Microbiol.* **2020**, *10*, 414. [CrossRef] [PubMed]
24. Ranjbar-Omid, M.; Arzanlou, M.; Amani, M.; Shokri Al-Hashem, S.K.; Amir Mozafari, N.; Peeri Doghaheh, H. Allicin from garlic inhibits the biofilm formation and urease activity of Proteus mirabilis in vitro. *FEMS Microbiol. Lett.* **2015**, *362*, fnv049. [CrossRef] [PubMed]
25. Yuan, F.; Huang, Z.; Yang, T.; Wang, G.; Li, P.; Yang, P.; Li, P.; Yang, B.; Li, J. Pathogenesis of Proteus mirabilis in Catheter-Associated Urinary Tract Infections. *Urol. Int.* **2021**, *105*, 354–361. [CrossRef] [PubMed]
26. Hung, E.W.; Darouiche, R.O.; Trautner, B.W. Proteus bacteriuria is associated with significant morbidity in spinal cord injury. *Spinal Cord.* **2007**, *45*, 616–620. [CrossRef]
27. Stover, S.L.; Lloyd, L.K.; Waites, K.B.; Jackson, A.B. Urinary tract infection in spinal cord injury. *Arch. Phys. Med. Rehabil.* **1989**, *70*, 47–54. [CrossRef]
28. DeVivo, M.J.; Fine, P.R.; Cutter, G.R.; Maetz, H.M. The risk of renal calculi in spinal cord injury patients. *J. Urol.* **1984**, *131*, 857–860. [CrossRef]
29. Tul Llah, S.; Khan, S.; Dave, A.; Morrison, A.J.; Jain, S.; Hermanns, D. A Case of Purple Urine Bag Syndrome in a Spastic Partial Quadriplegic Male. *Cureus* **2016**, *8*, e552. [CrossRef]
30. Kumar, U.; Singh, A.; Thami, G.; Agrawal, N. Purple urine bag syndrome: A simple and rare spot diagnosis in Uroscopic rainbow. *Urol. Case Rep.* **2020**, *35*, 101533. [CrossRef]
31. Llenas-García, J.; García-López, M.; Pérez-Bernabeu, A.; Cepeda, J.M.; Wikman-Jorgensen, P. Purple urine bag syndrome: A systematic review with meta-analysis. *Eur. Geriatr. Med.* **2017**, *8*, 221–227. [CrossRef]
32. Fusco, A.; Coretti, L.; Savio, V.; Buommino, E.; Lembo, F.; Donnarumma, G. Biofilm Formation and Immunomodulatory Activity of Proteus mirabilis Clinically Isolated Strains. *Int. J. Mol. Sci.* **2017**, *18*, 414. [CrossRef]
33. Rooney, H.; Mokool, L.; Ramsay, A.; Nalagatla, S. Purple urine bag syndrome: A truly harmless sign? *Scott. Med. J.* **2018**, *63*, 99–101. [CrossRef]
34. Ahmed, S.I.; Waheed, M.A.; Shah, S.; Muhammad Shah, S.Y.; Mumtaz, H. Purple urine bag syndrome: A case report. *Int. J. Surg. Case Rep.* **2022**, *99*, 107721. [CrossRef]
35. Amer, M.A.; Ramadan, M.A.; Attia, A.S.; Wasfi, R. Silicone Foley catheters impregnated with microbial indole derivatives inhibit crystalline biofilm formation by *Proteus mirabilis*. *Front. Cell. Infect. Microbiol.* **2022**, *12*, 1010625. [CrossRef]
36. Kanti, S.P.Y.; Csóka, I.; Jójárt-Laczkovich, O.; Adalbert, L. Recent Advances in Antimicrobial Coatings and Material Modification Strategies for Preventing Urinary Catheter-Associated Complications. *Biomedicines* **2022**, *10*, 2580. [CrossRef] [PubMed]
37. Yamamoto, S.; Mukai, T. Purple urine bags reflecting an aging society. *Clin. Case Rep.* **2021**, *9*, e04295. [CrossRef] [PubMed]
38. Alex, R.; Manjunath, K.; Srinivasan, R.; Basu, G. Purple urine bag syndrome: Time for awareness. *J. Fam. Med. Prim. Care* **2015**, *4*, 130–131. [CrossRef]

Disclaimer/Publisher's Note: The statements, opinions and data contained in all publications are solely those of the individual author(s) and contributor(s) and not of MDPI and/or the editor(s). MDPI and/or the editor(s) disclaim responsibility for any injury to people or property resulting from any ideas, methods, instructions or products referred to in the content.

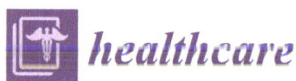

Article

Flat Magnetic Stimulation for Stress Urinary Incontinence: A 3-Month Follow-Up Study

Marta Barba [1,*], Alice Cola [1], Giorgia Rezzan [1], Clarissa Costa [1], Tomaso Melocchi [1], Desirèe De Vicari [1], Stefano Terzoni [2], Matteo Frigerio [1] and Serena Maruccia [2]

[1] Department of Gynecology, IRCCS San Gerardo dei Tintori, University of Milano-Bicocca, 20900 Monza, Italy; alice.cola1@gmail.com (A.C.); g.rezzan@campus.unimib.it (G.R.); c.costa14@campus.unimib.it (C.C.); t.melocchi@campus.unimib.it (T.M.); d.devicari@campus.unimib.it (D.D.V.); frigerio86@gmail.com (M.F.)
[2] Department of Urology, ASST Santi Paolo e Carlo, San Paolo Hospital, 20142 Milano, Italy; stefano.terzoni@asst-santipaolocarlo.it (S.T.); serena.maruccia@gmail.com (S.M.)
* Correspondence: m.barba8792@gmail.com; Tel.: +39-2339434

Abstract: Background: flat magnetic stimulation is based on a stimulation produced by electromagnetic fields with a homogenous profile. Patients with stress urinary incontinence (SUI) can take advantage of this treatment. We aimed to evaluate medium-term subjective, objective, and quality-of-life outcomes in patients with stress urinary incontinence to evaluate possible maintenance schedules. Methods: a prospective evaluation through the administration of the International Consultation on Incontinence Questionnaire-Short Form (ICIQ-SF), the Incontinence Impact Questionnaire (IIQ7), and the Female Sexual Function Index (FSFI) was performed at three different time points: at the baseline (T0), at the end of treatment (T1), and at 3-month follow-up (T2). The stress test and the Patient Global Impression of Improvement questionnaire (PGI-I) defined objective and subjective outcomes, respectively. Results: 25 consecutive patients were enrolled. A statistically significant reduction in the IIQ7 and ICIQ-SF scores was noticed at T1 returned to levels comparable to the baseline at T2. However, objective improvement remained significant even at a 3-month follow-up. Moreover, the PGI-I scores at T1 and T2 were comparable, demonstrating stable subjective satisfaction. Conclusion: despite a certain persistence of the objective and subjective continence improvement, the urinary-related quality of life decreases and returns to baseline values three months after the end of flat magnetic stimulation. These findings indicate that a further cycle of treatment is probably indicated after 3 months since benefits are only partially maintained after this timespan.

Keywords: quality of life; stress urinary incontinence; magnetic stimulation; pelvic floor disorders

Citation: Barba, M.; Cola, A.; Rezzan, G.; Costa, C.; Melocchi, T.; De Vicari, D.; Terzoni, S.; Frigerio, M.; Maruccia, S. Flat Magnetic Stimulation for Stress Urinary Incontinence: A 3-Month Follow-Up Study. *Healthcare* 2023, 11, 1730. https://doi.org/10.3390/healthcare11121730

Academic Editor: Edward J. Pavlik

Received: 4 May 2023
Revised: 5 June 2023
Accepted: 11 June 2023
Published: 13 June 2023

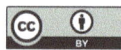

Copyright: © 2023 by the authors. Licensee MDPI, Basel, Switzerland. This article is an open access article distributed under the terms and conditions of the Creative Commons Attribution (CC BY) license (https://creativecommons.org/licenses/by/4.0/).

1. Introduction

Pelvic floor disorders include a series of diseases associated with pelvic floor weakening, which involve bowel, urinary, supports, and sexual dysfunctions [1]. Obstetric trauma is considered the primary damage to the pelvic floor giving the predisposition to develop pelvic floor disorders [2]. However, changes in the composition and enzymatic activity in the connective tissue play a role in the genesis of pelvic floor disorders [3]. Some of these changes in the collagenic patterns have been related to the menopausal decrease in estrogen [4]. Since pelvic floor disorders share risk factors, specific conditions may coexist, recur, or evolve into others as a consequence of treatment, such as surgery [5,6]. For instance, overactive bladder symptoms tend to improve after prolapse repair but may worsen if a suburethral tape is positioned at the time of surgery [7].

Stress urinary incontinence (SUI) represents one of the most common and bothersome pelvic floor disorders. Almost 50% of women in developed countries are estimated to be affected, and the lifetime risk of undergoing surgery is about 4% [8,9]. SUI is characterized by involuntary leakage of urine when the intra-abdominal pressure increases more than the urethral closure pressure such as during coughing, effort, or sneezing [10]. Pathogenetic mechanisms involve injuries to the connective tissue of the urethra, leading to urethral hypermobility and intrinsic urethral deficiency [11]. In addition, stress urinary incontinence may also occur (or persist) after pelvic floor surgery [12,13]. Stress urinary incontinence negatively affects women's quality of life in terms of social, domestic, and psychophysical well-being, with a negative effect on sexual function [14]. Urinary incontinence can reduce the opportunity to be part of intimate relationships, socialize, or the ability to perform daily activities [15]. SUI diagnosis and management need great expertise to approach the intimate sphere of patients who are unable to express themselves autonomously. During the visit, the gynecologist must be able to discuss any concerns and assess any problems related to the quality of life and sexual well-being [16].

Urodynamics may be useful to confirm the diagnosis since clinical and instrumental findings poorly agree in the evaluation of bladder dysfunction [17,18]. However, its diagnostic importance in the work-up of urinary incontinence is currently debated due to differences in performance and adopted definitions [19,20]. Stress urinary incontinence management involves both surgical and conservative treatments based on the patient's will, comorbidities, and quality-of-life impairment. According to the guidelines, conservative measures are considered the first-line choice, while surgical treatment is usually considered after the failure of conservative management. Different surgical options can be proposed for the treatment of SUI, such as anterior compartment repairs, bladder neck suspensions, midurethral slings, and injections [21–25]. To date, midurethral slings are considered the first option because of their high efficacy rates [26]. Retropubic tapes were introduced in 1995 and became the gold standard for SUI treatment [27]. To reduce the complications associated with the blind passage of needles in the retropubic space, the transobturator approach was developed in 2001 [28]. Finally, single-incision slings (SISs) were introduced in 2006. Their novelties were the shorter tape length and the limited intracorporeal dissection, avoiding the passage of tape and trocars through the obturator foramen, adductor tendons, and skin [24]. However, all surgical procedures have pitfalls, including visceral injuries, chronic pelvic pain, de novo bladder voiding dysfunctions, and overactive bladder symptoms [29,30]. As a consequence, conservative strategies should be preferred when possible. Options are represented by lifestyle modifications, pelvic floor exercises, electrical stimulations, biofeedback, and energy-based treatments [31].

An optional treatment for the treatment of stress urinary incontinence is represented by magnetic stimulation. Magnetic stimulators are extracorporeal devices that generate a specific electromagnetic field that interacts with pelvic floor neuromuscular tissue inducing intense muscular contractions and regulating neuromuscular control. Previous studies investigating magnetic stimulation for the treatment of female SUIs demonstrated a certain efficacy [32]. Specifically, systematic reviews and meta-analyses show significant improvements in quality-of-life questionnaires related to urinary incontinence [32,33]. In recent years, technological advancements have improved magnetic stimulator devices. One of them is represented by flat magnetic stimulation. This is characterized by homogeneous electromagnetic fields able to treat the entire pelvic area. In fact, this new magnetic field generates an equal distribution and intensity of stimulation. Consequently, flat magnetic stimulation allows for a large activation of muscle fibers without leaving areas of inconstant/suboptimal recruitment. This is thought to be associated with enhanced efficacy compared with standard magnetic stimulation treatment. The efficacy of this conservative treatment comes from the use of electromagnetic energy, the deep penetration of the waves, and the global stimulation of the pelvic floor. The magnetic field, through electrical tissue currents, induces changes in muscular contraction and allows neurons depolarization and blood supply enhancement. These modifications induce muscle fiber hypertrophy and hyperplasia due to more efficient stimulation. A previous experience has demonstrated the muscle hypertrophy of the urethral rhabdosphincter after flat magnetic stimulation, which has an established role in maintaining stress urinary continence. Similarly, preliminary reports of this new treatment option demonstrate exciting results in terms of quality-of-life improvements, but medium-term data, as well as optimal maintenance treatment schedules, are still unknown [34].

Consequently, the aim of our study is to analyze medium-term outcomes in patients with stress urinary incontinence undergoing flat magnetic stimulation in terms of objective and subjective cure rate and quality-of-life improvement and evaluate possible maintenance schedules.

2. Materials and Methods

This was a prospective interventional study. Recruitment occurred from August 2022 to September 2022 in the gynecologic outpatients at IRCCS San Gerardo dei Tintori Foundation in Monza, Italy. During the period of the study, a patient clinical interview to investigate the presence of lower urinary tract symptoms, such as urge urinary incontinence (UUI), stress urinary incontinence (SUI), overactive bladder (OAB), voiding symptoms (VS), or prolapse symptoms or anal incontinence was performed. All definitions conformed to IUGA/ICS terminology [10]. A gynecological examination was performed and, in case of prolapse, it was staged according to the POP-Q system.

Non-pregnant patients older than 18 years were included in the study if they had isolated SUI without surgical indication, confirmed with a standard 300 mL positive stress test. Exclusion criteria were a history of neoplasia, arrhythmia, congestive heart failure, recent deep venous thrombosis, fever, acute inflammatory diseases, or fractures in the area of treatment. Moreover, women with insufficient Italian language proficiency, a weight of more than 160 kg, neurostimulators, pacemakers, defibrillators, or ferromagnetic prostheses were excluded, as previously stated [J]. At the baseline (T0), the International Consultation on Incontinence Questionnaire-Short Form questionnaire (ICIQ-SF), the Female Sexual Function Index (FSFI-19) questionnaire, and the Incontinence Impact Questionnaire (IIQ-7) [35–37] were submitted and completed by all patients.

The ICIQ-SF questionnaire has been validated to measure the severity, frequency, and impact of urinary incontinence on quality of life [35]. The tool includes four questions, with the first three determining the total score: the leakage frequency, the perceived amount of leakage, and the level of impact on daily life [35]. The last item does not concur with the total score and is aimed to self-define the sub-type of incontinence [35]. This questionnaire showed high levels of validity, reliability, and sensitivity, and these parameters were evaluated through the use of standard psychometric tests [35]. The FSFI-19 questionnaire is a self-reported tool consisting of 19 items with a 5-point Likert scale addressing 6 domains of sexual function, including desire, lubrication, arousal, orgasm, pain, and satisfaction [36]. This instrument has consistently demonstrated satisfactory psychometric properties in evaluating the impact of several conditions on sexual well-being and the efficacy of different treatments [36]. Consequently, to investigate female sexual dysfunction at the baseline and after therapies, FSFI-19 represents one of the most valid, useful, popular, and powerful diagnostic tools [36]. For differentiating patients with and without sexual disorders, a cut-off of 26.5 points has been proposed to be the optimal [36]. The IIQ-7 questionnaire was introduced to investigate the impact of urinary incontinence on women's daily life [37]. The questionnaire consists of seven items with the aim to evaluate the perceived feelings and impact of urinary incontinence on daily life and relationships [37]. Each item has four answers that participants use to individually self-evaluate the impact of urine leakage on daily activities in four domains: physical activity (items #1 and #2), travel (items #3 and #4), social activities (item #5), and emotional health (items #6 and #7) [37]. Based on psychometric tests, across different countries and cultures, this tool was associated with an excellent level of validity, acceptability, and reliability [37].

After proper counseling, patients underwent flat magnetic stimulation with Dr. Arnold (DEKA, Calenzano, Italy) according to the following protocol: eight sessions (twice a week) of 25 min each, using the "Weakness 1" protocol from sessions 1 to 4 and the "Weakness 2" protocol from sessions 5 to 8. The "Weakness 1" protocol involves a primary warm-up phase and muscle activation and a second phase of muscle work based on recovering tropism and muscle tone (20–30 Hz) in a trapezoidal shape. The "Weakness 2" protocol involves a warm-up and muscle activation phase followed by muscle work with the aim of increasing tropism (volume), and a muscle strength phase (40–50 Hz) in a trapezoidal shape.

At the end of the treatment (T1), a 300 mL stress test was required to assess the objective cure rate, and patients compiled again the ICIQ-SF, IIQ-7, and FSFI-19 questionnaires. The subjective cure rate was evaluated through the results from the Patient Global Impression of Improvement (PGI-I) questionnaire [38]. The PGI-I questionnaire is a 7-point scale that ensures the clinician can assess how much the patient's disease has improved or worsened compared to a baseline state collected at the beginning of the treatment. This scale is described as follows: 1, very much improved; 2, much improved; 3, minimally improved; 4, no change; 5, minimally worse; 6, much worse; and 7, very much worse [38]. Subjective success was defined as an improvement in the PGI-I score ($\leq$3). Three months after the end of the treatment (T2), the ICIQ-SF, IIQ-7, FSFI-19, and PGI-I questionnaires were resubmitted to the patients, and the stress test was repeated.

The local Ethics Committee approval was obtained (protocol code PF-MAGCHAIR). The scores obtained from the questionnaires were described as the median and interquartile range (IQR) after the failure of the normality check and were performed by using the Shapiro–Wilk test. Friedman's non-parametric test [39] for repeated measures was then used to compare the IIQ-7, ICIQ-SF, and FSFI-19 questionnaire scores, as the small sample size did not allow obtaining normally distributed continuous variables, even after data transformation according to Blom's method [40]. Durbin–Conover pairwise comparisons were used to check for significant differences between the three moments of data collection; this method was preferred over the classic Durbin test to maximize statistical power [41]. Prior to comparing the scores obtained throughout the study, we used the Mann–Whitney U test to check if relevant covariates such as body mass index, number of deliveries, and age produced any statistically significant differences in baseline scores. Confidence intervals for binomial proportions were calculated according to the methods suggested by Ross [42]. Significant differences between proportions were checked by using McNemar's test, as the data came from repeated measures [43]. The significance threshold was established at 0.05 for all calculations; the analysis was conducted with R 4.1 (the R Core Team, Vienna, Austria, 2021) for MacOS®.

3. Results

Our study enrolled a total of 25 consecutive patients. Population characteristics are shown in Table 1. Baseline IIQ7 and ICIQ-SF scores were comparable by age, body mass index, and the number of deliveries ($p > 0.05$ for all calculations) as most women had normal weight (Me = 25.2, IQR = 3.10, eleven overweight and one obese with BMI = 31.8 kg/m^2), and there was only one nulliparous in the sample. Baseline FSFI-19 scores showed a significant, albeit weak, correlation with age (rho = -0.411, $p = 0.041$) and BMI (rho = -0.473, $p = 0.017$). These two variables were, therefore, considered as covariates in the analyses regarding sexual function scores, while all other analyses were unadjusted. No women reported adverse effects during the treatment. Outcome measures of objective, subjective, and quality-of-life questionnaires at the baseline (T0), end of treatment (T1), and 3-month follow-up (T2) are summarized in Table 2. After the treatment, the decrease in the IIQ7 scores (bothersome level of leakages) was statistically significant compared to the baseline ($p < 0.001$), thus supporting the clinical usefulness of this treatment. However, at the three-months follow-up evaluation, the IIQ7 scores showed a statistically significant increase ($p = 0.005$), thus returning to levels comparable to the baseline condition of the patients ($p = 0.135$). Similarly, at the end of the treatment, we observed a statistically significant decrease in the ICIQ-SF scores compared to the baseline ($p = 0.002$). However, the ICIQ-SF values also increased significantly after three months from the end of the sessions, becoming comparable to bothersome baseline levels. Regarding sexual function, the differences observed in the conditions reported by the patients through the FSFI-19 questionnaire did not reach statistical significance, neither between the scores before treatment and at the end of the sessions nor between the latter and those obtained three months after the end of the rehabilitation program. Regarding the overall perception of improvement reported by the women, the PGI-I scores reported no statistically significant differences ($p = 0.564$) three months after the end of treatment (T2) compared to those obtained at the end of the sessions (T1) even after adjusting the analysis for overweight or obesity and the number of deliveries. With respect to objective outcomes, at the end of the rehabilitation program (T1), the number of women with negative stress tests was 10 out of 25 (40.0%). After three months (T2) 5 out of 25 (20.0%) patients maintained this result (proportion difference = -0.200, 95%CI = $[-0.4225; 0.0533]$), as shown in Tables 2 and 3, and this decrease was statistically significant ($p = 0.025$).

Table 1. Population characteristics and baseline (T0) findings. Continuous data as mean ± standard deviation. ICIQ-SF: International Consultation on Incontinence Questionnaire-Short Form questionnaire; FSFI-19: Female Sexual Function Index questionnaire; IIQ-7: Incontinence Impact Questionnaire.

Age (years)	60.9 ± 12.7
Parity (n)	1.9 ± 0.7
BMI (kg/m^2)	25.4 ± 3.0
IIQ-7 score (T0)	33.7 ± 22.6
ICIQ-SF score (T0)	11.2 ± 3.6
FSFI-19 score (T0)	12.5 ± 11.2

Table 2. Outcome measures of objective, subjective, and quality-of-life questionnaires at the baseline (T0), end of treatment (T1), and 3-month follow-up (T2). Data are reported as median and interquartile range except for stress test proportion expressed as absolute (relative) frequencies. ICIQ-SF: International Consultation on Incontinence Questionnaire-Short Form questionnaire; FSFI-19: Female Sexual Function Index questionnaire; IIQ-7: Incontinence Impact Questionnaire; PGI-I: Patient Global Impression of Improvement questionnaire.

Questionnaire	Baseline	End of Treatment	3-Month Follow-Up
IIQ-7	33.00 (38.50)	16.50 (11.00)	22.00 (22.00)
ICIQ-SF	12.00 (4.00)	8.00 (6.00)	10.00 (5.00)
FSFI-19	7.80 (22.80)	6.70 (22.30)	6.00 (22.20)
PGI-I	N/a	3.00 (2.00)	3.00 (2.00)
Positive stress test	25 (100%)	15 (60%)	20 (80%)

Table 3. IIQ-7, ICIQ-SF, FSFI-19, and PGI-I scores and positive stress test rates comparisons among the endpoints of the study: the baseline (T0), end of treatment (T1), and 3-month follow-up (T2). P-values are provided. Durbin–Conover pairwise comparisons were performed to check for significant differences between the three moments of data collection. ICIQ-SF: International Consultation on Incontinence Questionnaire-Short Form questionnaire; FSFI-19: Female Sexual Function Index questionnaire; IIQ-7: Incontinence Impact Questionnaire; PGI-I: Patient Global Impression of Improvement questionnaire. N/A. not applicable. In bold statistically significant results.

	T0 vs. T1	T1 vs. T2	T0 vs. T2
IIQ-7	**<0.001**	**0.005**	0.135
ICIQ-SF	**0.002**	**0.034**	0.247

Table 3. Cont.

	T0 vs. T1	T1 vs. T2	T0 vs. T2
FSFI-19	0.394	0.495	0.864
PGI-I	N/A	0.564	N/A
Positive stress test	0.001	0.025	0.025

4. Discussion

International guidelines recommend, as the first-line treatment for SUI, conservative management. Among all conservative treatment options including PFMT, functional electrical stimulation, and biofeedback, MS offers some advantages. Concerning PFMT, patients may not be able to recruit, contract, and adequately train the pelvic floor muscle thus reducing its effectiveness and consistency over time [44]. As a consequence, patients who underwent PFMT may show reduced compliance and adherence rates and notice a slow progression of the improvements [45]. Due to the use of endocavitary devices, both functional electrical stimulation and biofeedback can be badly tolerated or even not possible due to impaired vaginal habitability, such as in the case of lichen sclerosis, previous surgery, or radiation. Moreover, mild local discomfort and side effects may cause treatment discontinuation in up to 12% of patients [46]. On the contrary, MS is a type of passive rehabilitation with no adverse effects described, which does not involve endocavitary probes, and patients stay dressed. Moreover, unlike the electrical current, tissue impedance does not affect the conduction of electromagnetic energy. With all these aspects, MS can be defined as a non-invasive, standardizable, and safe conservative treatment option for urinary incontinence management. In particular, the latest innovation in magnetic stimulation technology is represented by flat magnetic stimulation technology. Flat magnetic stimulation induces strong muscle contractions through the induction of electrical currents in the context of pelvic floor neuromuscular tissue. This, consequently, induces more efficient muscle fiber hypertrophy and hyperplasia, changing the muscle's structure. The hypertrophic effect of this technology on the skeletal muscles has been previously demonstrated. Leone et al. evaluated the impact of flat magnetic stimulation on the abdomens of 15 patients, demonstrating 1 month after the last treatment an increase in the abdominal muscle tissue thickness in the treated areas (lateral, upper, and lower abdomen) ranging from +14% to +23% [47]. Similarly, a significant (+15.4%) hypertrophy of the external urethral sphincter has been demonstrated in female patients with stress urinary incontinence [34]. However, the duration of this benefit and the optimal maintenance treatment schedule are still unknown.

For the first time, our study prospectively compared short- and medium-term outcomes of flat magnetic stimulation in patients with stress urinary incontinence. We found that, despite a certain persistence of the objective and subjective continence improvement, urinary-related quality-of-life tends to return to baseline values three months after treatment. Among the quality-of-life outcomes, a statistically significant reduction in the IIQ7 scores (a bothersome number of leakages) was observed after the treatment compared to the baseline but the IIQ7 scores significantly increased ($p = 0.005$), returning to levels comparable to the baseline condition at three months follow-up. Similarly, a statistically significant reduction in the ICIQ-SF scores at the end of the treatment compared to the baseline was followed by a significant increase in the ICIQ-SF values after three months from the end of the sessions, becoming comparable to the baseline. The subjective outcome evaluated by the PGI-I score showed no statistically significant differences ($p = 0.564$) three months after the end of treatment (T2) compared to the end of the sessions (T1), even after adjusting the analysis for overweight or obesity and the number of deliveries. In addition, after three months (T2), 5 out of 25 (20.0%) patients maintained a negative stress test compared to 10 out of 25 (40%) at the end of the rehabilitation program (T1). These findings indicate that a further eight-session cycle of treatment is probably indicated after 3 months since benefits are only partially still present at this time point.

To date, few pieces of evidence are available about the role of flat magnetic stimulation in the treatment of SUI, and there are none about the maintenance schedule. Lopopolo et al. evaluated improvement in the quality of life in 50 female patients with mixed urinary incontinence [48]. All patients underwent six sessions (twice a week) of 28 min each of Dr. ARNOLD magnetic stimulation. The first two minutes of warm-up were followed by the two protocols, Hypotonus/Weakness 1 and Hypotonus/Weakness 2. The ICIQ-UI-SF questionnaire, the Incontinence Questionnaire Overactive Bladder Module (ICIQ-OAB), and the IIQ-7 questionnaire were compiled at the baseline, during the treatment, and after three months. Quality of life improved from the second treatment session to the last one by 91%, 86%, and 98% according to the ICIQ-UI-SF, ICIQ-OAB, and IIQ-7 respectively. After three months, a small increase in scores was noticed, and the scores were better compared to the baseline; this can be probably explained by the return to a physiological hypotonus in the absence of long-term exercise.

Another study by Biondo et al. analyzed eighty-one female patients with urinary incontinence to evaluate the safety and the effectiveness of flat magnetic stimulation [49]. Women were divided into two groups: group A included 35 female patients who met the criteria for stress urinary incontinence, while group B enrolled 46 women with urge urinary incontinence. All patients underwent eight sessions of treatment for 28 min each twice a week for 4 straight weeks with the DR. ARNOLD system. Firstly, all patients started with a short warm-up phase followed by four sessions with the Hypotonus/Weakness 1 protocol and four sessions with the Hypotonus/Weakness 2 protocol for group A. There were eight sessions with the Overtone/Pain protocol (muscle work aimed at muscle inhibition) for group B.

Two questionnaires were completed before each treatment and at 3 months follow-up. The ICIQ-OAB questionnaire was compiled by the patients in group B, while the IIQ-7 questionnaire was assigned and filled out by the patients of group A. According to questionnaire results, there was an improvement in urge and stress urinary incontinence symptoms at the baseline and after treatment sessions at 3 months follow-up [49].

While specific data about the loss of hypertrophy on pelvic floor muscles due to detraining are not available, some studies have examined the effects of detraining on other muscles. In athletes' hearts, the regression of the physiological left ventricular hypertrophy seems to occur already during the first month of detraining, with no further reduction between 1 and 3 months [50]. Regarding skeletal muscles, Narici et al. found a decrease of 4% in the muscle cross-sectional area (CSA) after a period of 40 days of detraining in the quadriceps muscles [51]. Similarly, Psillander et al. aimed to determine if a previously strength-trained leg would respond better to a period of strength training than a previously untrained leg, hypothesizing that the trained leg would have an enhanced hypertrophic response and an increased number of myonuclei compared with the untrained leg. Using muscle biopsies and ultrasounds, they showed that the increase in muscle thickness seen during the training period was completely lost after a 20-week period of detraining, but a relatively large increase in muscle thickness was observed during retraining in both the trained leg and the untrained leg (~10%) [52]. These findings are consistent with our study, which enlightens the necessity of performing retraining after a few months from the first stimulation to maintain the benefits in the long term. From the point of view of physiology, as reported by Terzoni et al., in a previous study on magnetic innervation, the lack of persistence of the results obtained with this rehabilitation method can be explained by the fact that, if no maintenance exercises are performed after the end of the stimulation program, muscular performance can rapidly decrease due to lack of exercise [53].

To date, this is the first study on women with stress urinary incontinence comparing short- and medium-term data about flat magnetic stimulation treatment to try to define an optimal maintenance schedule. Other strengths involve the prospective design and the multimodal evaluation of benefits, including objective cure rate, subjective impression of improvements, and multiple validated quality-of-life questionnaires. A limitation is the small sample size analyzed. Future research can include the evaluation of flat magnetic stimulation benefits in a larger population study compared to a control group. Another reasonable purpose would be to collect data after a prolonged period of observation, maybe after further sessions of treatment.

5. Conclusions

Our analysis concluded that flat magnetic stimulation represents a safe and effective stress urinary incontinence's conservative treatment in terms of incontinence cure rate and quality-of-life improvement. However, despite a certain persistence of the objective and subjective continence improvement, the benefit in terms of quality of life tends to return to baseline values three months after the end of the treatment. These findings indicate that probably, after 3 months, a further cycle of treatment is indicated since benefits are only partially maintained after this timespan.

Author Contributions: Conceptualization, M.B., A.C., G.R., C.C., T.M., D.D.V., S.T., M.F. and S.M.; formal analysis, M.B., A.C., G.R., C.C., T.M., D.D.V., S.T., M.F. and S.M.; investigation, M.B., A.C., G.R., C.C., T.M., D.D.V., S.T., M.F. and S.M.; data curation, M.B., A.C., G.R., C.C., T.M., D.D.V., S.T., M.F. and S.M.; writing—original draft preparation, M.B., A.C., G.R., C.C., T.M., D.D.V., S.T., M.F. and S.M.; writing—review and editing, M.B., A.C., G.R., C.C., T.M., D.D.V., S.T., M.F. and S.M.; project administration, M.B., A.C., G.R., C.C., T.M., D.D.V., S.T., M.F. and S.M. All authors have read and agreed to the published version of the manuscript.

Funding: This research received no external funding.

Institutional Review Board Statement: The study was conducted in accordance with the Declaration of Helsinki and was approved by the Institutional Review Board of ASST Monza (protocol code PF-MAGCHAIR).

Informed Consent Statement: Informed consent was obtained from all subjects involved in the study.

Data Availability Statement: The data presented in this study are available upon request from the corresponding author.

Conflicts of Interest: The authors declare no conflict of interest.

References

1. Palmieri, S.; Cola, A.; Ceccherelli, A.; Manodoro, S.; Frigerio, M.; Vergani, P. Italian validation of the German Pelvic Floor Questionnaire for pregnant and postpartum women. *Eur. J. Obstet. Gynecol. Reprod. Biol.* **2020**, *248*, 133–136. [CrossRef] [PubMed]
2. Frigerio, M.; Mastrolia, S.A.; Spelzini, F.; Manodoro, S.; Yohay, D.; Weintraub, A.Y. Long-term effects of episiotomy on urinary incontinence and pelvic organ prolapse: A systematic review. *Arch. Gynecol. Obstet.* **2019**, *299*, 317–325. [CrossRef] [PubMed]
3. Manodoro, S.; Spelzini, F.; Cesana, M.C.; Frigerio, M.; Maggioni, D.; Ceresa, C.; Penati, C.; Sicuri, M.; Fruscio, R.; Nicolini, G.; et al. Histologic and metabolic assessment in a cohort of patients with genital prolapse: Preoperative stage and recurrence investigations. *Minerva Ginecol.* **2017**, *69*, 233–238. [CrossRef] [PubMed]
4. DeLancey, J.O.; Trowbridge, E.R.; Miller, J.M.; Morgan, D.M.; Guire, K.; Fenner, D.E.; Weadock, W.J.; Ashton-Miller, J.A. Stress urinary incontinence: Relative importance of urethral support and urethral closure pressure. *J. Urol.* **2008**, *179*, 2286–2290. [CrossRef] [PubMed]
5. Milani, R.; Frigerio, M.; Vellucci, F.L.; Palmieri, S.; Spelzini, F.; Manodoro, S. Transvaginal native-tissue repair of vaginal vault prolapse. *Minerva Ginecol.* **2018**, *70*, 371–377. [CrossRef]
6. Milani, R.; Frigerio, M.; Spelzini, F.; Manodoro, S. Transvaginal uterosacral ligament suspension for posthysterectomy vaginal vault prolapse repair. *Int. Urogynecol. J.* **2017**, *28*, 1421–1423. [CrossRef]
7. Frigerio, M.; Manodoro, S.; Cola, A.; Palmieri, S.; Spelzini, F.; Milani, R. Risk factors for persistent, de novo and overall overactive bladder syndrome after surgical prolapse repair. *Eur. J. Obstet. Gynecol. Reprod. Biol.* **2019**, *233*, 141–145. [CrossRef]
8. Ford, A.A.; Rogerson, L.; Cody, J.D.; Ogah, J. Midurethral sling operations for stress urinary incontinence in women. *Cochrane Database Syst. Rev.* **2015**, *7*, CD006375.
9. Iosif, C.S.; Batra, S.; Ek, A.; Åstedt, B. Oestrogen receptors in the human female lower urinarytract. *Am. J. Obstet. Gynecol.* **1981**, *141*, 817–820. [CrossRef]
10. Bo, K.; Frawley, H.C.; Haylen, B.T.; Abramov, Y.; Almeida, F.G.; Berghmans, B.; Bortolini, M.; Dumoulin, C.; Gomes, M.; McClurg, D.; et al. An International Urogynecological Association (IUGA)/International Continence Society (ICS) joint report on the terminology for the conservative and nonpharmacological management of female pelvic floor dysfunction. *Neurourol. Urodyn.* **2017**, *36*, 221–244. [CrossRef]

11. D'Alessandro, G.; Palmieri, S.; Cola, A.; Barba, M.; Manodoro, S.; Frigerio, M. Clinical and urodynamic predictors of Q-tip test urethral hypermobility. *Minerva Obstet. Gynecol.* **2022**, *74*, 155–160. [CrossRef] [PubMed]
12. Frigerio, M.; Manodoro, S.; Palmieri, S.; Spelzini, F.; Milani, R. Risk factors for stress urinary incontinence after native-tissue vaginal repair of pelvic organ prolapse. *Int. J. Gynaecol. Obstet.* **2018**, *141*, 349–353. [CrossRef] [PubMed]
13. Palmieri, S.; Frigerio, M.; Spelzini, F.; Manodoro, S.; Milani, R. Risk factors for stress urinary incontinence recurrence after single-incision sling. *Neurourol. Urodyn.* **2018**, *37*, 1711–1716. [CrossRef] [PubMed]
14. Frigerio, M.; Barba, M.; Cola, A.; Braga, A.; Celardo, A.; Munno, G.M.; Schettino, M.T.; Vagnetti, P.; De Simone, F.; Di Lucia, A.; et al. Quality of life, psychological wellbeing, and sexuality in women with urinary incontinence—Where are we now: A narrative review. *Medicina* **2022**, *58*, 525. [CrossRef]
15. Bientinesi, R.; Coluzzi, S.; Gavi, F.; Nociti, V.; Gandi, C.; Marino, F.; Moretto, S.; Mirabella, M.; Bassi, P.; Sacco, E. The Impact of Neurogenic Lower Urinary Tract Symptoms and Erectile Dysfunctions on Marital Relationship in Men with Multiple Sclerosis: A Single Cohort Study. *J. Clin. Med.* **2022**, *11*, 5639. [CrossRef]
16. Bientinesi, R.; Gavi, F.; Coluzzi, S.; Nociti, V.; Marturano, M.; Sacco, E. Neurologic Urinary Incontinence, Lower Urinary Tract Symptoms and Sexual Dysfunctions in Multiple Sclerosis: Expert Opinions Based on the Review of Current Evidences. *J. Clin. Med.* **2022**, *11*, 6572. [CrossRef]
17. D'Alessandro, G.; Palmieri, S.; Cola, A.; Barba, M.; Manodoro, S.; Frigerio, M. Correlation between urinary symptoms and urodynamic findings: Is the bladder an unreliable witness? *Eur. J. Obstet. Gynecol. Reprod. Biol.* **2022**, *272*, 130–133. [CrossRef]
18. Frigerio, M.; Barba, M.; Marino, G.; Volontè, S.; Melocchi, T.; De Vicari, D.; Torella, M.; Salvatore, S.; Braga, A.; Serati, M.; et al. Coexisting detrusor overactivity-underactivity in patients with pelvic floor disorders. *Healthcare* **2022**, *10*, 1720. [CrossRef]
19. D'Alessandro, G.; Palmieri, S.; Cola, A.; Barba, M.; Manodoro, S.; Frigerio, M. Detrusor underactivity prevalence and risk factors according to different definitions in women attending urogynecology clinic. *Int. Urogynecol. J.* **2022**, *33*, 835–840. [CrossRef]
20. Frigerio, M.; Barba, M.; Cola, A.; Volontè, S.; Marino, G.; Regusci, L.; Sorice, P.; Ruggeri, G.; Castronovo, F.; Serati, M.; et al. The learning curve of urodynamics for the evaluation of lower urinary tract symptoms. *Medicina* **2022**, *58*, 341. [CrossRef]
21. Manodoro, S.; Frigerio, M.; Barba, M.; Bosio, S.; de Vitis, L.A.; Marconi, A.M. Stem cells in clinical trials for pelvic floor disorders: A systematic literature review. *Reprod. Sci.* **2022**, *29*, 1710–1720. [CrossRef] [PubMed]
22. Serati, M.; Braga, A.; Salvatore, S.; Torella, M.; Di Dedda, M.C.; Scancarello, C.; Cimmino, C.; De Rosa, A.; Frigerio, M.; Candiani, M.; et al. Up-to-date procedures in female stress urinary incontinence surgery: A concise review on bulking agents procedures. *Medicina* **2022**, *58*, 775. [CrossRef] [PubMed]
23. Braga, A.; Castronovo, F.; Ottone, A.; Torella, M.; Salvatore, S.; Ruffolo, A.F.; Frigerio, M.; Scancarello, C.; De Rosa, A.; Ghezzi, F.; et al. Medium term outcomes of TVT-abbrevo for the treatment of stress urinary incontinence: Efficacy and safety at 5-year follow-up. *Medicina* **2022**, *58*, 1412. [CrossRef]
24. Frigerio, M.; Milani, R.; Barba, M.; Locatelli, L.; Marino, G.; Donatiello, G.; Spelzini, F.; Manodoro, S. Single-incision slings for the treatment of stress urinary incontinence: Efficacy and adverse effects at 10-year follow-up. *Int. Urogynecol. J.* **2021**, *32*, 187–191. [CrossRef] [PubMed]
25. Spelzini, F.; Manodoro, S.; Cola, A.; Palmieri, S.; Roselli, F.; Frigerio, M. Single-incision sling for stress urinary incontinence: A video tutorial. *Eur. J. Obstet. Gynecol. Reprod. Biol.* **2019**, *237*, 216–217. [CrossRef]
26. Cox, A.; Herschorn, S.; Lee, L. Surgical management of female SUI: Is there a gold standard? *Nat. Rev. Urol.* **2013**, *10*, 78–89, Erratum in *Nat. Rev. Urol.* **2013**, *10*, 188. [CrossRef]
27. Ulmsten, U.; Petros, P. Intravaginal slingplasty (IVS): An ambulatory surgical procedure for treatment of female urinary incontinence. *Scand. J. Urol. Nephrol.* **1995**, *29*, 75–82. [CrossRef]
28. Delorme, E. Transobturator urethral suspension: Mini-invasive procedure in the treatment of stress urinary incontinence in women. *Prog Urol.* **2001**, *11*, 1306–1313.
29. Milani, R.; Manodoro, S.; Cola, A.; Palmieri, S.; Frigerio, M. Management of unrecognized bladder perforation following suburethral tape procedure. *Int. J. Gynaecol. Obstet.* **2018**, *142*, 118–119. [CrossRef]
30. Milani, R.; Barba, M.; Manodoro, S.; Locatelli, L.; Palmieri, S.; Frigerio, M. Inability to walk and persistent thigh pain after transobturator tape procedure for stress urinary incontinence: Surgical management. *Int. Urogynecol. J.* **2021**, *32*, 1317–1319. [CrossRef]
31. Ruffolo, A.F.; Braga, A.; Torella, M.; Frigerio, M.; Cimmino, C.; De Rosa, A.; Sorice, P.; Castronovo, F.; Salvatore, S.; Serati, M. Vaginal laser therapy for female stress urinary incontinence: New solutions for a well-known issue—A concise review. *Medicina* **2022**, *58*, 512. [CrossRef] [PubMed]
32. Sun, K.; Zhang, D.; Wu, G.; Wang, T.; Wu, J.; Ren, H.; Cui, Y. Efficacy of magnetic stimulation for female stress urinary incontinence: A meta-analysis. *Ther. Adv. Urol.* **2021**, *13*, 17562872211032485. [CrossRef] [PubMed]
33. Lukanović, D.; Kunič, T.; Batkoska, M.; Matjašič, M.; Barbič, M. Effectiveness of Magnetic Stimulation in the Treatment of Urinary Incontinence: A Systematic Review and Results of Our Study. *J. Clin. Med.* **2021**, *10*, 5210. [CrossRef]
34. Frigerio, M.; Barba, M.; Cola, A.; Marino, G.; Volontè, S.; Melocchi, T.; De Vicari, D.; Maruccia, S. Flat Magnetic Stimulation for Stress Urinary Incontinence: A Prospective Comparison Study. *Bioengineering* **2023**, *10*, 295. [CrossRef]
35. Tubaro, A.; Zattoni, F.; Prezioso, D.; Scarpa, R.M.; Pesce, F.; Rizzi, C.A.; Santini, A.M.; Simoni, L.; Artibani, W.; Flow Study Group. Italian validation of the international consultation on incontinence questionnaires. *BJU Int.* **2006**, *97*, 101–108. [CrossRef]

36. Filocamo, M.T.; Serati, M.; Li Marzi, V.; Costantini, E.; Milanesi, M.; Pietropaolo, A.; Polledro, P.; Gentile, B.; Maruccia, S.; Fornia, S.; et al. The Female Sexual Function Index (FSFI): Linguistic validation of the Italian version. *J. Sex. Med.* **2014**, *11*, 447–453. [CrossRef] [PubMed]
37. Monticone, M.; Frigau, L.; Mola, F.; Rocca, B.; Giordano, A.; Foti, C.; Franchignoni, F. Italian versions of the Urogenital Distress Inventory-6 and Incontinence Impact Questionnaire-7: Translation and validation in women with urinary incontinence. *Disabil. Rehabil.* **2021**, *43*, 2930–2936. [CrossRef] [PubMed]
38. Srikrishna, S.; Robinson, D.; Cardozo, L. Validation of the patient global impression of improvement (PGI-I) for urogenital prolapse. *Int. Urogynecol. J.* **2010**, *21*, 523–528. [CrossRef]
39. Eisinga, R.; Heskes, T.; Pelzer, B.; Te Grotenhuis, M. Exact *p*-values for pairwise comparison of Friedman rank sums, with application to comparing classifiers. *BMC Bioinform.* **2017**, *18*, 68. [CrossRef]
40. Beasley, T.M.; Erickson, S.; Allison, D.B. Rank-based inverse normal transformations are increasingly used, but are they merited? *Behav. Genet.* **2009**, *39*, 580–595. [CrossRef]
41. Ross, T.D. Accurate confidence intervals for binomial proportion and Poisson rate estimation. *Comput. Biol. Med.* **2003**, *33*, 509–531. [CrossRef] [PubMed]
42. Fagerland, M.W.; Lydersen, S.; Laake, P. The McNemar test for binary matched-pairs data: Mid-p and asymptotic are better than exact conditional. *BMC Med. Res. Methodol.* **2013**, *13*, 91. [CrossRef]
43. Best, D.J.; Rayner, J.C. Conover's F Test as an Alternative to Durbin's Test. *J. Mod. Appl. Stat. Methods* **2014**, *13*, 76–83. [CrossRef]
44. Yount, S.M.; Fay, R.A.; Kissler, K.J. Prenatal and Postpartum Experience Knowledge, and Engagement with Kegels: A Longitudinal, Prospective, Multisite Study. *J. Womens Health* **2020**, *30*, 891–901. [CrossRef] [PubMed]
45. Greer, J.A.; Arya, L.A.; Smith, A.L. Urinary incontinence: Diagnosis and treatment in the elderly. *Curr. Transl. Geriatr. Exp. Gerontol. Rep.* **2013**, *2*, 66–75. [CrossRef]
46. Takahashi, S.; Kitamura, T. Overactive bladder: Magnetic versus electrical stimulation. *Curr. Opin. Obstet. Gynecol.* **2003**, *15*, 429–433. [CrossRef]
47. Leone, A.; Piccolo, D.; Conforti, C.; Pieri, L.; Fusco, I. Evaluation of safety and efficacy of a new device for muscle toning and body shaping. *J. Cosmet. Dermatol.* **2021**, *20*, 3863–3870. [CrossRef]
48. Lopopolo, G.; Salsi, B.; Banfi, A.; Isaza, P.G.; Fusco, I. Is It Possible to Improve Urinary Incontinence and Quality of Life in Female Patients? A Clinical Evaluation of the Efficacy of Top Flat Magnetic Stimulation Technology. *Bioengineering* **2022**, *9*, 140. [CrossRef]
49. Biondo, A.; Gonzalez Isaza, P.; Fusco, I. Efficacy of top flat magnetic stimulation technology for female stress and urge urinary incontinence: A clinical evaluation. *World J. Nephrol. Urol.* **2022**, *11*, 18–23. [CrossRef]
50. Swoboda, P.P.; Garg, P.; Levelt, E.; Broadbent, D.A.; Zolfaghari-Nia, A.; Foley, A.J.R.; Fent, G.J.; Chew, P.G.; Brown, L.A.; Saunderson, C.E.; et al. Regression of left ventricular mass in athletes undergoing complete detraining is mediated by decrease in intracellular but not extracellular compartments. *Circ. Cardiovasc. Imaging* **2019**, *12*, e009417. [CrossRef]
51. Narici, M.V.; Roi, G.S.; Landoni, L.; Minetti, A.E.; Cerretelli, P. Changes in force, cross-sectional area and neural activation during strength training and detraining of the human quadriceps. *Eur. J. Appl. Physiol.* **1989**, *59*, 310–319. [CrossRef] [PubMed]
52. Psilander, N.; Eftestøl, E.; Cumming, K.T.; Juvkam, I.; Ekblom, M.M.; Sunding, K.; Wernbom, M.; Holmberg, H.C.; Ekblom, B.; Bruusgaard, J.C.; et al. Effects of training, detraining, and retraining on strength, hypertrophy, and myonuclear number in human skeletal muscle. *J. Appl. Physiol.* **2019**, *126*, 1636–1645. [CrossRef] [PubMed]
53. Terzoni, S.; Ferrara, P.; Mora, C.; Destrebecq, A. Long-term effects of extracorporeal magnetic innervation for post-prostatectomy urinary incontinence: 1-year follow-up. *Int. J. Urol. Nurs.* **2021**, *16*, 26–31. [CrossRef]

Disclaimer/Publisher's Note: The statements, opinions and data contained in all publications are solely those of the individual author(s) and contributor(s) and not of MDPI and/or the editor(s). MDPI and/or the editor(s) disclaim responsibility for any injury to people or property resulting from any ideas, methods, instructions or products referred to in the content.

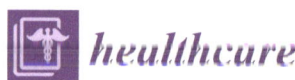

Review

Pelvic Organ Prolapse Syndrome and Lower Urinary Tract Symptom Update: What's New?

Gaetano Maria Munno, Marco La Verde, Davide Lettieri, Roberta Nicoletti, Maria Nunziata, Diego Domenico Fasulo, Maria Giovanna Vastarella, Marika Pennacchio, Gaetano Scalzone, Gorizio Pieretti, Nicola Fortunato, Fulvio De Simone, Gaetano Riemma and Marco Torella *

Obstetrics and Gynecology Unit, Department of Woman, Child and General and Specialized Surgery, University of Campania "Luigi Vanvitelli", 80138 Naples, Italy; gmm9401@gmail.com (G.M.M.); marco.laverde88@gmail.com (M.L.V.); davidelett@gmail.com (D.L.); roberta.nicoletti81@gmail.com (R.N.); maria.nunziata5@libero.it (M.N.); diegodomenico1993@gmail.com (D.D.F.); mariagiovannavastarella@hotmail.it (M.G.V.); marikapennacchio@gmail.com (M.P.); drgscalzone@gmail.com (G.S.); gorizio.pieretti@unicampania.it (G.P.); nicola.fortunato@libero.it (N.F.); fulviodesimone65@gmail.com (F.D.S.); gaetano.riemma@unicampania.it (G.R.)
* Correspondence: marcotorella@iol.it

Abstract: (1) Background: This narrative review aimed to analyze the epidemiological, clinical, surgical, prognostic, and instrumental aspects of the link between pelvic organ prolapse (POP) and lower urinary tract symptoms (LUTS), collecting the most recent evidence from the scientific literature. (2) Methods: We matched the terms "pelvic organ prolapse" (POP) and "lower urinary tract symptoms" (LUTS) on the following databases: Pubmed, Embase, Scopus, Google scholar, and Cochrane. We excluded case reports, systematic reviews, articles published in a language other than English, and studies focusing only on a surgical technique. (3) Results: There is a link between POP and LUTS. Bladder outlet obstruction (BOO) would increase variation in bladder structure and function, which could lead to an overactive bladder (OAB). There is no connection between the POP stage and LUTS. Prolapse surgery could modify the symptoms of OAB with improvement or healing. Post-surgical predictive factors of non-improvement of OAB or de novo onset include high BMI, neurological pathologies, age > 65 years, and the severity of symptoms; predictors of emptying disorders are neurological pathologies, BOO, perineal dysfunctions, severity of pre-surgery symptoms, and severe anterior prolapse. Urodynamics should be performed on a specific subset of patients (i.e., stress urinary incontinence, correct surgery planning), (4) Conclusions: Correction of prolapse is the primary treatment for detrusor underactivity and for patients with both POP and OAB.

Keywords: overactive bladder; pelvic organ prolapse; lower urinary tract symptoms; urodynamics

1. Introduction

In 1994, the term lower urinary tract symptoms (LUTS) was adopted to classify LUTS based on the presence of storage, voiding, and post-micturition symptoms [1]. The classification of LUTS included a wide range of clinical manifestations. Increased urinary frequency, nocturia, urinary urgency, and incontinence are included in the storage symptoms [1]. Slow/weak stream, hesitancy and terminal dribble, and immediate post-urination symptoms are included in voiding symptoms [2]. Following an evaluation of the patient's LUTS, physical findings, the results of urinalysis, and other necessary investigations, physicians may frequently make an empirical diagnosis as the basis for initial management. Several studies in Europe and North America found a LUTS prevalence of more than 60% in men and women over 40 years [3,4], with a higher prevalence in women over 70 [5]. Pelvic organ prolapse (POP) is defined as the herniation of the anterior vaginal wall, posterior vaginal wall, uterus, or vaginal apex into the vagina [6] and is commonly

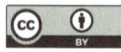

related to complex symptoms such as LUTS [7]. Even if a vast number of women over 50 is affected by POP, only 20% exhibit symptoms [7]. However, according to population projections from the United States Census Bureau, the number of patients who will develop POP is expected to increase by 46%, from the current 3.3 million to 4.9 million by 2050 [8]. To date, LUTS with POP are common but inconsistently reported, and there are few data on this relationship's incidence. Obstructive voiding is most frequently associated with POP [9]. Patients with isolated posterior POP should be examined for anorectal or bulging symptoms and LUTS [10]. The low severity of POP is typically asymptomatic [11].

Clinicians dealing with women with POP might choose between surgery, pessary usage, pelvic floor muscle training, or observation. Nonsurgical approaches are usually chosen first by both clinicians and women. Improvement of symptoms and, for conservative management, minimization of prolapse progression are the main objectives of all treatments [9]. Although the patient's preferences ultimately determine the course of therapy, people with symptomatic POP should be made aware that pessary usage is a feasible nonsurgical alternative. In case of unresponsiveness to non-invasive strategies, surgical correction of POP is often considered [1,3].

In order to provide a comprehensive evaluation of the clinical, surgical, instrumental, and prognostic aspects of the association between POP and LUTS, we divided this review into different sections. The main objective was to evaluate the newly studied and epidemiologic association between POP and LUTS; the grade of pop and severity of urinary symptoms; the role of urodynamics (UDS); and the influence of surgical and medical treatments on the symptoms and the patients' quality of life.

2. Materials and Methods

A literature search was performed using the Pubmed, Embase, Scopus, Google Scholar, and Cochrane databases to find correlations between POP and LUTS, using as mesh terms "pelvic organ prolapse" and "lower urinary tract symptoms". The literature review was conducted independently by two authors (GM and DL). Additional relevant articles that were cited in these original articles were added. Case reports, systematic reviews, non-human studies, and non-English articles were excluded. In addition, articles that focused on practical surgical techniques with no symptom evaluation were excluded. Figure 1 describes the search steps and screening procedure. In this narrative review, we focused on the topics in the subsequent sections:

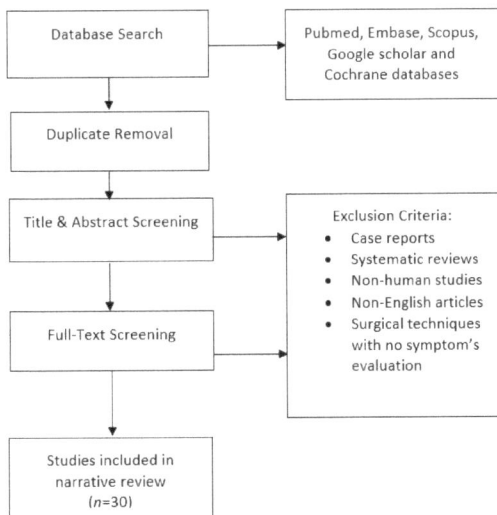

Figure 1. Summary of the search and screening methods applied in this narrative review.

3. What Is the Relationship between POP and LUTS?

Urinary problems, such as urgency, frequency, and difficulty of voiding, are prevalent in patients affected by uterine prolapse, although the link between prolapse and LUTS is unclear [12]. Cameron et al. evidenced a relationship between POP and LUTS, with a relative risk ranging from 1.2 to 5.8 [11]. It is unknown exactly why LUTS and POP occur together in a large percentage of women, but there is no plausible pathophysiological or anatomical explanation for why LUTS would produce POP [11]. There are, however, reasonable hypotheses for why POP could produce LUTS. POP is frequently associated with bladder outlet obstruction (BOO) and correlates with POP severity [13]. There is a consensus that POP-induced BOO may generate bladder alterations that result in overactive bladder (OAB) symptoms [13]. De Boer et al. [13] hypothesized three possible explanations for the correlation between POP and OAB:

- Neurological damage, with autonomic nerve and spinal micturition reflex;
- Alteration of the structure of the detrusor muscle;
- There is a the possibility that the stretching of the bladder causes stretch receptors in the urothelium to misfire and release neurotransmitters, such as acetylcholine and ATP [14,15]. Neurons detect neurotransmitters in the urothelium, which triggers the contraction of the bladder. However, many disorders may also share a common cause, including pelvic floor dysfunction, childbirth-related trauma, or ageing [16,17].

4. Is the POP Stage Related to OAB?

POP staging is currently reported using two major classifications, the Baden–Walker and the POP Quantification System (POP-Q) (Table 1).

Table 1. POP grading according to Baden–Walker and POP-Q classification systems.

Grade	Baden–Walker	POP-Q
0	Normal position for each respective site	No prolapse
1	Descent halfway to the hymen	Greater than 1 cm above the hymen
2	Descent to the hymen	1 cm or less proximal or distal to the plane of the hymen
3	Descent halfway past the hymen	Greater than 1 cm below the plane of the hymen, but protruding no further than 2 cm less than the total vaginal length
4	Maximum possible descent for each site	Eversion of the lower genital tract is complete

For the purposes of the Baden–Walker system, the vagina is separated into six sections: two anterior, two superior, and two posterior. Using the hymen as point 0, each is given a score between 0 and 4 based on how much descent is present while the patient is exerting themselves to the fullest [18].

Nine locations in the vagina are measured by the POP-Q evaluation technique. The hymen serves as a baseline against which all other points are measured. The prolapsed organs are measured in millimeters to the hymen. The measurements are made while the person is in the dorsal lithotomy position and the Valsalva technique is being performed. The cervix, hymen, perineal body, total vaginal length, posterior vaginal wall, and posterior fornix are the anatomical landmarks employed. The numbers at the proximal and distal ends are recorded on a three-by-three centimeter grid. The proper stage of prolapse is determined from the data on the grid [19].

It is unknown if the severity of POP and OAB are related [11]. However, contrary to expectations, Burrows et al. [20] discovered that urgency and urgency urinary incontinence (UUI) occurred more frequently in women with less advanced POP. It was confirmed by Kowalski et al. in a recent study [21]. Another ultrasound-based study indicated that women with a lower grade of prolapse bladder develop UUI more frequently [22]. In contrast, Miranne et al. found that a higher percentage of women with a more advanced stage of POP demonstrated urodynamic detrusor overactivity (DO) (35%) compared to women with an earlier stage of POP [23]. The severity of POP is related to obstructive symptoms but not necessarily to other urinary symptoms. Anterior and apical vaginal compartment prolapse had a stronger link to OAB symptoms than to posterior vaginal compartment prolapse [24]. OAB syndrome is prevalent in the early stages of anterior vaginal wall prolapse, while posterior compartment prolapse may reduce its incidence [25].

5. Is LUTS Relief Possible after a POP Repair?

Surgical repair is not required to alleviate symptoms. At four months, women using a pessary had a 38% reduction in urgency and a 26% reduction in UUI [26]. In another study on women with UUI and POP, effective pessary fitting led to a 46% improvement in symptoms [27]. Pessaries have the potential to be helpful instruments in decision making prior to the beginning of a surgical procedure [11]. The patient's LUTS were successfully treated with POP therapy, supporting the hypothesis that there is a connection between POP and LUTS [11].

Women who are concerned by their POP and have tried or refused nonsurgical therapies are candidates for surgical correction. There are several abdominal and vaginal surgical methods for treating POP [19]

The surgical management of POP depends on the localization of the defect. According to a vast survey, with or without the use of a synthetic graft, anterior colporrhaphy remained the most popular procedure for treating anterior compartment prolapse; vaginal hysterectomy with uterosacral suspension was used to treat uterine prolapse; posterior native tissue colporrhaphy was the most popular procedure for treating posterior compartment prolapse; and post-hysterectomy apical prolapse was repaired with abdominal sacrocolpopexy in 44% of cases [28].

In the past, a mesh material was employed in around one-third of urogynecological surgical operations for POP [29]. As many prosthetic operations, including urogynecological surgery, there have been documented cases of postoperative infection and migration problems with respect to prostheses [29].

6. Outcomes after Surgical POP Repair

De Boer et al. [13] collected 12 studies that examined OAB symptoms before and after POP repair. The duration of follow-up ranged from 2.5 to 60 months, and most studies reported a resolution rate of 90%. The RR of resolution was calculated by dividing the number of pre-operative symptoms by the number of post-operative symptoms. One trial revealed an RR of more than 1, with values ranging from 1.1 to 10.3 in 61% of patients [11,16]. Symptoms of OAB improve independently using the surgical method [11,30]. This is supported by Foster et al. [26], who showed how colpocleisis and reconstructive vaginal suspensions make no difference in OAB resolution one year after surgery. Following POP surgery, the majority of women who experience POP symptoms and have UI find that their UI is resolved or improved [31]. After correction, OAB symptoms improve independently from the POP severity [32].

7. POP Correction and OAB Improvement: Which Variables Influenced the Persistence of the Symptoms?

According to recent evidence, it is possible to identify clinical factors associated with the persistence of OAB symptoms following surgery. For example, in the current Cochrane review on POP surgical therapy, new or de novo OAB symptoms were reported in 12% of women in nine trials [33]. POP causes BOO, which leads to increased DO and OAB symptoms, but it may also cause permanent changes to the detrusor muscle, which may cause persistent bladder overactivity [11]. Patient factors that predicted persistent UUI included pre-operative urodynamic studies. Successful treatment of patients with DO and following POP surgery was the best therapeutic option for symptom improvement [34].

In another study, 24.5% of women with POP and DO showed persistent symptoms after prolapse surgical reduction (particularly with the mesh repair technique). At the same time, 3.5% of the patients had UDS evidence of DO only after surgery [35]. An age > 65 years, neurological diseases such as Parkinson's, BOO, or increased PVR > 200 mL were associated with persistent or de novo DO [35]. Pre-operative OAB is a risk factor for OAB persistence after POP reduction, while age and sling placement correlate with de novo OAB. Increased BMI is associated with post-operative OAB [36]. Patients with severe pre-operative symptoms, neurologic disease, pelvic floor dysfunction, bladder neck obstruction, or severe anterior wall prolapse are at risk of post-operative voiding dysfunction [37]. Many patients diagnosed with UI after POP reduction had no more symptoms. UI degree and previous anti-incontinence surgery are predictors of the persistence of UI after POP reduction [38]. Liedl B et al. demonstrate that moderate-to-severe OAB complaints could be associated with high degree POP and symptom relief occurred after adequate surgical reconstruction [39]. According to these results, Malanowska et al. demonstrated that surgery, including laparoscopic lateral suspension in patients with POP and OAB, could help relieve urinary symptoms [40]. Ling-Ying Wu et al., in their study, also confirmed the positive role in improving storage symptoms after reconstructive surgery [30]. OAB improved significantly after surgical correction of POP, according to Johnson et al., but age was connected with the persistence of storage symptoms, such as urgency [16]. Päivi K Karjalainen et al. evidenced that surgical repair of POP could relieve OAB, particularly after reconstructing anterior and apical compartments. They showed a correlation between apical and anterior POP and the severity of OAB symptoms. These patients had better relief after reconstructive surgery [24]. Ahmed M Tawfeek et al. performed a pre-operative and post-operative UDS in patients with LUTS. They showed that urinary symptoms improved after surgery, and DO was associated with the persistence of voiding symptoms [41].

Taking these findings together, even if the surgical correction of POP can improve OAB symptoms in most women, the presence of independent risk factors, including Parkinson's disease or other neurological pathologies, DO, advanced age, or increased BMI, might lead to the persistence of symptomatology even after successful reconstructive surgery.

8. Medical Treatment of LUTS?

According to OAB guidelines, antimuscarinics and 3-adrenoceptor agonists are second-line therapy for OAB [42]. The efficacy of medical therapy for OAB treatment has been limited and may also be associated with undesirable side effects. Following POP surgery, it can be used temporarily or as a therapy for persistent or new-onset OAB [11].

9. Urodynamics and POP Repair

Given the weak correlation between DO and UUI, preoperative DO is not always a good predictor of UUI after surgery. This finding aids in the prediction of postoperative outcomes, so routine preoperative pressure-flow UDS in women undergoing POP repair is not warranted [11]. Pressure-flow UDS could be proposed in patients with hydronephrosis, neurological disease, recurrent urinary tract infections (UTIs), and particularly for pre-surgery management [43]. If UDS is performed following the AUA/SUFU guidelines [44], the POP should be lowered to test detrusor dysfunction, and this procedure may differentiate between BOO and detrusor underactivity (DU). UDS should be performed on a subset of POP patients. This test can help us counsel POP patients with voiding symptoms, but it cannot provide additional information for patients with POP and UI [45]. UDS had no significant impact on preoperative management or counselling in POP surgery if occult stress urinary incontinence was not the indication for preoperative testing in women undergoing POP surgery [46]. Research, however, argues for UDS before surgery as a screening tool to prevent unnecessary concurrent continence treatments [47].

10. Sexuality after POP Repair

It is critical to incorporate sexual health into therapeutic practice. Evaluation of anatomical anomalies, lower urinary tract function, and anorectal function are sometimes given greater consideration in women with pelvic floor issues than sexual function.

The majority of women who have symptoms of POP and LUTS are still engaged in sexual activity. The possibility that female sexual dysfunctions will be identified may rise with the use of questionnaires and sexuality scales to help women and health care providers address sexual issues. The only questionnaires currently validated and created particularly to measure female sexual function in women with urine incontinence and/or pelvic organ prolapse are the Pelvic Organ Prolapse Incontinence Sexual Questionnaire (PISQ) and the PISQ-12-IR (IUGA-Revised). The PISQ-12-IR also enables examination of the results for urogynecologic care-requiring women who are not sexually active [48].

Ageing and menopause are linked to decreased sexual activity. However, the effects of surgery to cure LUTS and POP on female sexual function are still being debated.

Li et al. conducted a prospective observational study to determine the prevalence of female sexual dysfunction, relevant risk factors, and the effects of pelvic floor surgery in women who have POP, stress urinary incontinence, or both [48].

Prior to and following surgery, sexual activity and sexual function were examined together with potential risk factors. The Female Sexual Function Index and the PISQ-12 are two validated questionnaires that were used to assess sexual function. They showed that age and postmenopausal status were factors in the absence of sexual activity prior to surgery. Similarly, sexual dysfunction was linked with advancing age. Overall, there was no difference in the PISQ-12 score before and 12 months after surgery. Lubrication of the vagina was an unrelated feature that was linked to an improvement in sexual function following surgery. The improvement in the quality of sexual life following surgery was significantly impacted by menopause [48].

Similarly, Mattsson et al. evaluated the impact of female POP surgery on sexuality, patient satisfaction, and health-related quality of life; they also identified outcome predictors. Over a two-year follow-up period, 7 out of 10 patients with POP surgery reported an improvement in sexual habits and health-related quality of life; patient satisfaction was high. The most reliable indicators of improvement were vaginal bulging and apical prolapse beyond the hymen. They also highlighted that patients should be urged to give up smoking in order to prevent a negative outcome [49].

However, dyspareunia occurred in 26% of 53 women after posterior colporrhaphy and in 38% of women with both Burch colposuspension and posterior colporrhaphy, according to Weber et al.'s analysis of 81 women who underwent surgery for prolapse or urinary incontinence [50]. There were no site-specific procedures employed for posterior repair. Using general or non-pelvic floor disorder-specific questionnaires, others have discovered stable or declining sexual function. It is possible that some partners are concerned that sexual activity would affect the postoperative results because some patients had lower scores on the partner-related items. Therefore, it is likely necessary to know about favorable sexual outcomes [50].

According to Glavind et al. [51] the majority of women who receive surgical treatment for various forms of POP employing native tissue restoration and "site-specific" procedures report an improvement in their sexual lives thereafter. Preoperative urine incontinence was cured or improved in the majority of individuals [51].

In terms of how surgery effectively ameliorates sexual health rather than a different approach, several studies have been conducted.

Kinjo et al. compared the effectiveness of vaginal pessaries and modified transvaginal mesh (TVM) surgery in women with symptomatic POP [52].

They examined 130 symptomatic POP patients who had received either vaginal pessaries or modified TVM. Lower urinary tract, bowel, and sexual problems were evaluated together with the prolapse-related quality of life (QOL) using the prolapse QOL questionnaire. All questionnaires were completed before and a year after the therapy. One year following therapy, the prolapse and voiding symptoms as well as all the prolapse-related QOL categories were considerably better in the pessary group, with the exception of the personal connections and sleep/energy. The modified-TVM group saw a considerable improvement in all QOL categories as well as prolapse, urine storage, voiding, bowel, and sexual problems. They concluded that the vaginal pessary and modified TVM surgery both successfully cured prolapse and voiding symptoms and enhanced the majority of prolapse-related QOL variables. Modified TVM surgery was superior to pessary therapy in terms of relieving urine storage, bowel, and sexual complaints. However, compared to pessary insertion, modified TVM appeared to place the organs more effectively to enhance bowel, sexual, and bladder function [52].

Similarly, Van der Vaart et al. reported that surgery had a better effect on sexual function in sexually active POP patients than pessary treatment [53]. The improvement is mostly due to the POP symptoms' diminished influence on sexual performance. Sexually active women who declare that POP-related symptoms are bothering their sexual performance should be advised that surgery produces more notable relief. A superior course of therapy could not be proven for sexually inactive women. In contrast to pessary therapy, considerably more NSA women underwent surgery than pessary therapy, despite the fact that the differences in PISQ-IR scores between the two groups of NSA women were not statistically different. The patient must be given this information, which includes weighing the advantages and disadvantages of the surgery and the pessary, in order to make a balanced choice [53].

However, when performing surgery for POP, to avoid useless damages on sexual health, several considerations should be considered.

Giving realistic expectations of surgical results is crucial before undergoing pelvic floor disease surgery. In order to create a baseline, it is crucial to evaluate the patient's sexual orientation, attitude toward sexual activity, the effect of pelvic disease on sexual relations, the quality of orgasms, and desire. To prevent subsequent disappointment, patient expectations of the effects of pelvic floor surgery should be investigated and appropriate goals should be set. In the absence of pelvic disease, pre-existing sexual issues might indicate a worse than ideal outcome [54].

Sexual dysfunction in SUI patients may be exacerbated by damage to the vaginal innervation on the anterior and distal parts of the vaginal wall. To prevent such damage, excessive dissection should be avoided. Synthetic tape should not be placed too superficially while performing a mid-urethral sling surgery since this might cause discomfort during penetration and dyspareunia if the mesh gets exposed. When performing a mid-urethral sling surgery, excessive lateral positioning of the needles should be avoided in order to avoid serious vascular damage [54].

Vaginal length should be preserved whenever feasible in women having vaginal hysterectomy for prolapse or an anterior repair, and extensive vaginal mucosal excision should be avoided. Sexual function was unaffected by the vaginal cuff closure technique (vertical vs. horizontal closure). It is crucial to preserve introital caliber and vaginal length while doing a posterior repair. A suitable caliber would be 8–11 cm long and it should be possible to accommodate two or three fingers during vaginal reconstruction surgery. The likelihood of developing dyspareunia was significantly enhanced when an anterior colporrhaphy was combined with a posterior vaginal wall repair; therefore, there may be a purpose for doing the two operations independently when practical [55].

This would also suggest that in sexually active women, a prophylactic posterior repair should be avoided at the time of an anterior repair. A levator plication should be avoided in sexually active women because it results in a constriction ring inside the vagina. Whenever feasible, surgical methods should be used to prevent constriction of the vaginal introitus [55].

To maintain sexual function in sexually active women with a vaginal vault prolapse, a sacrocolpopexy should be recommended instead of a sacro-spinous fixation [54].

11. Conclusions

The link between OAB and POP in women is unclear. BOO due to POP and accompanying bladder muscle alterations appear to be the most probable explanation for how POP might induce OAB and explains why POP repair improves OAB symptoms in the majority of patients. This argument contradicts the idea that severe POP (which generates more BOO) does not induce worse OAB. A considerable proportion of women do not have OAB resolution following POP surgery, potentially due to permanent bladder alterations due to long-term BOO, or perhaps they are different conditions in particular women since OAB occurs without POP or BOO in many women. POP reduction should also be the first-line treatment for DU in women with coexisting POP, considering the limited treatment choices for this disorder. As this may be a unifying diagnosis and a single surgery might solve both conditions, it would appear wise to provide POP reduction surgically or with a pessary as the primary treatment choice for all women with OAB and POP. As the presence of DO, DU, or BOO does not alter surgical planning, UDS are not required before surgery unless the patient has a history of neurological disease, hydronephrosis, or recurrent UTIs. However, simple cystometrics with POP reduction are required prior to surgery to assess for occult SUI and to counsel patients on their risk of postoperative SUI to assist them in deciding whether to undergo a concomitant sling procedure. Women with bladder trabeculation, longer duration of OAB symptoms, age > 65 years, neurological disease, higher PVR > 200 mL, and greater degrees of BOO have a reduced likelihood of OAB remission following POP surgery. However, none of these risk factors significantly reduced the likelihood of resolution. Thus, they are not indicators against giving POP correction. The potential impact on sexual function should be discussed and used to guide decision making when counseling women with a prolapse or incontinence, especially prior to surgical treatment. It is essential to test sexual function before surgery in order to find any underlying sexual issues. This causes less disappointment when desired outcomes are not achieved and allows for more reasonable expectations from the therapies that are accessible. According to the most recent and reliable research, women should obtain counseling and management. It is important to understand the benefits and drawbacks of the procedure and how it can affect sexual function in sexually active women who are having pelvic floor surgery.

Author Contributions: Conceptualization, G.M.M. and M.L.V.; methodology, D.L.; data curation, R.N.; writing—original draft preparation, D.L., G.M.M., F.D.S. and G.P.; writing—review and editing, M.G.V., D.D.F., M.N., M.P., G.S. and N.F.; supervision, G.R. and M.T.; project administration, M.T. All authors have read and agreed to the published version of the manuscript.

Funding: This research received no external funding.

Institutional Review Board Statement: Not applicable.

Informed Consent Statement: Not applicable.

Data Availability Statement: No new data were created or analyzed in this study. Data sharing is not applicable to this article.

Conflicts of Interest: The authors declare no conflict of interest.

References

1. Abrams, P.; Cardozo, L.; Fall, M.; Griffiths, D.; Rosier, P.; Ulmsten, U.; Van Kerrebroeck, P.; Victor, A.; Wein, A. The standardisation of terminology of lower urinary tract function: Report from the Standardisation Sub-committee of the International Continence Society. *Am. J. Obstet. Gynecol.* **2002**, *187*, 116–126. [CrossRef] [PubMed]
2. Coyne, K.S.; Sexton, C.C.; Thompson, C.L.; Milsom, I.; Irwin, D.; Kopp, Z.S.; Chapple, C.R.; Kaplan, S.; Tubaro, A.; Aiyer, L.P.; et al. The prevalence of lower urinary tract symptoms (LUTS) in the USA, the UK and Sweden: Results from the Epidemiology of LUTS (EpiLUTS) study. *BJU Int.* **2009**, *104*, 352–360. [CrossRef] [PubMed]
3. Milsom, I.; Gyhagen, M. The prevalence of urinary incontinence. *Climacteric* **2019**, *22*, 217–222. [CrossRef] [PubMed]
4. Temml, C.; Heidler, S.; Ponholzer, A.; Madersbacher, S. Prevalence of the overactive bladder syndrome by applying the International Continence Society definition. *Eur. Urol.* **2005**, *48*, 622–627. [CrossRef]
5. Olsen, A.L.; Smith, V.J.; Bergstrom, J.O.; Colling, J.C.; Clark, A.L. Epidemiology of surgically managed pelvic organ prolapse and urinary incontinence. *Obstet. Gynecol.* **1997**, *89*, 501–506. [CrossRef]
6. Iglesia, C.B.; Smithling, K.R. Pelvic Organ Prolapse. *Am. Fam. Physician* **2017**, *96*, 179–185.
7. Digesu, G.A.; Chaliha, C.; Salvatore, S.; Hutchings, A.; Khullar, V. The relationship of vaginal prolapse severity to symptoms and quality of life. *BJOG: Int. J. Obstet. Gynaecol.* **2005**, *112*, 971–976. [CrossRef]

8. Wu, J.M.; Hundley, A.F.; Fulton, R.G.; Myers, E.R. Forecasting the prevalence of pelvic floor disorders in US Women: 2010 to 2050. *Obstet. Gynecol.* **2009**, *114*, 1278–1283. [CrossRef]
9. Harvey, M.-A.; Chih, H.J.; Geoffrion, R.; Amir, B.; Bhide, A.; Miotla, P.; Rosier, P.F.; Offiah, I.; Pal, M.; Alas, A.N. International Urogynecology Consultation Chapter 1 Committee 5: Relationship of pelvic organ prolapse to associated pelvic floor dysfunction symptoms: Lower urinary tract, bowel, sexual dysfunction and abdominopelvic pain. *Int. Urogynecol. J.* **2021**, *32*, 2575–2594. [CrossRef]
10. Kilic, D.; Guler, T.; Gokbel, I.; Gokbel, D.A.; Ceylan, D.A.; Sivaslioglu, A. Effects of isolated posterior vaginal wall prolapse on lower urinary tract symptoms. *J. Gynecol. Obstet. Hum. Reprod.* **2021**, *50*, 102095. [CrossRef]
11. Cameron, A.P. Systematic review of lower urinary tract symptoms occurring with pelvic organ prolapse. *Arab J. Urol.* **2019**, *17*, 23–29. [CrossRef] [PubMed]
12. Lowder, J.L.; Frankman, E.A.; Ghetti, C.; Burrows, L.J.; Krohn, M.A.; Moalli, P.; Zyczynski, H. Lower urinary tract symptoms in women with pelvic organ prolapse. *Int. Urogynecol. J.* **2010**, *21*, 665–672. [CrossRef] [PubMed]
13. De Boer, T.; Salvatore, S.; Cardozo, L.; Chapple, C.; Kelleher, C.; Van Kerrebroeck, P.; Kirby, M.G.; Koelbl, H.; Espuna-Pons, M.; Milsom, I. Pelvic organ prolapse and overactive bladder. *Neurourol. Urodyn. Off. J. Int. Cont. Soc.* **2010**, *29*, 30–39. [CrossRef] [PubMed]
14. Ferguson, D.; Kennedy, I.; Burton, T. ATP is released from rabbit urinary bladder epithelial cells by hydrostatic pressure changes—A possible sensory mechanism? *J. Physiol.* **1997**, *505*, 503. [CrossRef] [PubMed]
15. Sun, Y.; Chai, T.C. Up-regulation of P2X3 receptor during stretch of bladder urothelial cells from patients with interstitial cystitis. *J. Urol.* **2004**, *171*, 448–452. [CrossRef]
16. Johnson, J.R.; High, R.A.; Dziadek, O.; Ocon, A.; Muir, T.W.; Xu, J.; Antosh, D.D. Overactive bladder symptoms after pelvic organ prolapse repair. *Female Pelvic Med. Reconstr. Surg.* **2020**, *26*, 742–745. [CrossRef] [PubMed]
17. Villa, P.; Suriano, R.; Ricciardi, L.; Tagliaferri, V.; De Cicco, S.; De Franciscis, P.; Colacurci, N.; Lanzone, A. Low-dose estrogen and drospirenone combination: Effects on glycoinsulinemic metabolism and other cardiovascular risk factors in healthy postmenopausal women. *Fertil Steril* **2011**, *95*, 158–163. [CrossRef]
18. Vilos, G.A.; Reyes-MuNoz, E.; Riemma, G.; Kahramanoglu, I.; Lin, L.T.; Chiofalo, B.; Lordelo, P.; Della Corte, L.; Vitagliano, A.; Valenti, G. Gynecological cancers and urinary dysfunction: A comparison between endometrial cancer and other gynecological malignancies. *Minerva Med.* **2021**, *112*, 96–110. [CrossRef]
19. The American College of Obstetricians and Gynecologists; The American Urogynecologic Society. Pelvic Organ Prolapse. *Female Pelvic Med. Reconstr. Surg.* **2019**, *25*, 397–408. [CrossRef]
20. Burrows, L.J.; Meyn, L.A.; Walters, M.D.; Weber, A.M. Pelvic symptoms in women with pelvic organ prolapse. *Obstet. Gynecol.* **2004**, *104*, 982–988. [CrossRef]
21. Kowalski, J.T.; Wiseman, J.B.; Smith, A.R.; Helmuth, M.E.; Cameron, A.; DeLancey, J.O.; Hendrickson, W.K.; Jelovsek, J.E.; Kirby, A.; Kreder, K. Natural history of lower urinary tract symptoms in treatment-seeking women with pelvic organ prolapse; the Symptoms of Lower Urinary Tract Dysfunction Research Network (LURN). *Am. J. Obstet. Gynecol.* **2022**, *227*, 875.e1–875.e12. [CrossRef] [PubMed]
22. Dietz, H.; Clarke, B. Is the irritable bladder associated with anterior compartment relaxation? A critical look at the 'integral theory of pelvic floor dysfunction'. *Aust. N. Z. J. Obstet. Gynaecol.* **2001**, *41*, 317–319. [CrossRef] [PubMed]
23. Miranne, J.M.; Lopes, V.; Carberry, C.L.; Sung, V.W. The effect of pelvic organ prolapse severity on improvement in overactive bladder symptoms after pelvic reconstructive surgery. *Int. Urogynecol. J.* **2013**, *24*, 1303–1308. [CrossRef] [PubMed]
24. Karjalainen, P.K.; Tolppanen, A.-M.; Mattsson, N.K.; Wihersaari, O.A.; Jalkanen, J.T.; Nieminen, K. Pelvic organ prolapse surgery and overactive bladder symptoms—A population-based cohort (FINPOP). *Int. Urogynecol. J.* **2022**, *33*, 95–105. [CrossRef] [PubMed]
25. Liao, Y.-H.; Ng, S.-C.; Chen, G.-D. Correlation of severity of pelvic organ prolapse with lower urinary tract symptoms. *Taiwan J. Obstet. Gynecol.* **2021**, *60*, 90–94. [CrossRef]
26. Clemons, J.L.; Aguilar, V.C.; Tillinghast, T.A.; Jackson, N.D.; Myers, D.L. Patient satisfaction and changes in prolapse and urinary symptoms in women who were fitted successfully with a pessary for pelvic organ prolapse. *Am. J. Obstet. Gynecol.* **2004**, *190*, 1025–1029. [CrossRef]
27. Fernando, R.J.; Thakar, R.; Sultan, A.H.; Shah, S.M.; Jones, P.W. Effect of vaginal pessaries on symptoms associated with pelvic organ prolapse. *Obstet. Gynecol.* **2006**, *108*, 93–99. [CrossRef]
28. Jha, S.; Moran, P.A. National survey on the management of prolapse in the UK. *Neurourol. Urodyn.* **2007**, *26*, 325–331; discussion 332. [CrossRef]
29. Illiano, E.; Trama, F.; Crocetto, F.; Califano, G.; Aveta, A.; Motta, G.; Pastore, A.L.; Brancorsini, S.; Fabi, C.; Costantini, E. Prolapse Surgery: What Kind of Antibiotic Prophylaxis Is Necessary? *Urol. Int.* **2021**, *105*, 771–776. [CrossRef]
30. Wu, L.-Y.; Huang, K.-H.; Yang, T.-H.; Huang, H.-S.; Wang, T.-S.; Lan, K.-C.; Chuang, F.-C. The surgical effect on overactive bladder symptoms in women with pelvic organ prolapse. *Sci. Rep.* **2021**, *11*, 20193. [CrossRef]
31. Khayyami, Y.; Elmelund, M.; Klarskov, N. Urinary incontinence before and after pelvic organ prolapse surgery—A national database study. *Int. Urogynecol. J.* **2021**, *32*, 2119–2123. [CrossRef] [PubMed]
32. Kim, M.S.; Lee, G.H.; Na, E.D.; Jang, J.H.; Kim, H.C. The association of pelvic organ prolapse severity and improvement in overactive bladder symptoms after surgery for pelvic organ prolapse. *Obstet. Gynecol. Sci.* **2016**, *59*, 214–219. [CrossRef] [PubMed]

33. Maher, C.M.; Feiner, B.; Baessler, K.; Glazener, C. Surgical management of pelvic organ prolapse in women: The updated summary version Cochrane review. *Int. Urogynecol. J.* **2011**, *22*, 1445–1457. [CrossRef]
34. Foster, R.T., Sr.; Barber, M.D.; Parasio, M.F.R.; Walters, M.D.; Weidner, A.C.; Amundsen, C.L. A prospective assessment of overactive bladder symptoms in a cohort of elderly women who underwent transvaginal surgery for advanced pelvic organ prolapse. *Am. J. Obstet. Gynecol.* **2007**, *197*, 82.e1–82.e4. [CrossRef] [PubMed]
35. Lo, T.S.; Nagashu, S.; Hsieh, W.C.; Uy-Patrimonio, M.C.; Yi-Hao, L. Predictors for detrusor overactivity following extensive vaginal pelvic reconstructive surgery. *Neurourol. Urodyn.* **2018**, *37*, 192–199. [CrossRef]
36. Frigerio, M.; Manodoro, S.; Cola, A.; Palmieri, S.; Spelzini, F.; Milani, R. Risk factors for persistent, de novo and overall overactive bladder syndrome after surgical prolapse repair. *Eur. J. Obstet. Gynecol. Reprod. Biol.* **2019**, *233*, 141–145. [CrossRef]
37. Chen, A.; McIntyre, B.; De, E.J. Management of postoperative lower urinary tract symptoms (LUTS) after pelvic organ prolapse (POP) repair. *Curr. Urol. Rep.* **2018**, *19*, 74. [CrossRef]
38. Ugianskiene, A.; Kjærgaard, N.; Larsen, T.; Glavind, K. What happens to urinary incontinence after pelvic organ prolapse surgery? *Int. Urogynecol. J.* **2019**, *30*, 1147–1152. [CrossRef]
39. Liedl, B.; Goeschen, K.; Sutherland, S.E.; Roovers, J.P.; Yassouridis, A. Can surgical reconstruction of vaginal and ligamentous laxity cure overactive bladder symptoms in women with pelvic organ prolapse? *BJU Int.* **2019**, *123*, 493–510. [CrossRef]
40. Malanowska, E.; Starczewski, A.; Bielewicz, W.; Balzarro, M. Assessment of overactive bladder after laparoscopic lateral suspension for pelvic organ prolapse. *BioMed Res. Int.* **2019**, *2019*, 9051963. [CrossRef]
41. Tawfeek, A.M.; Osman, T.; Gad, H.H.; Elmoazen, M.; Osman, D.; Emam, A. Clinical and Urodynamic Findings Before and After Surgical Repair of Pelvic Organ Prolapse in Women with Lower Urinary Tract Symptoms. A Prospective Observational Study. *Urology* **2022**, *167*, 90–95. [CrossRef] [PubMed]
42. Gormley, E.A.; Lightner, D.J.; Faraday, M.; Vasavada, S.P. Diagnosis and treatment of overactive bladder (non-neurogenic) in adults: AUA/SUFU guideline amendment. *J. Urol.* **2015**, *193*, 1572–1580. [CrossRef] [PubMed]
43. Tran, H.; Chung, D.E. Incidence and management of de novo lower urinary tract symptoms after pelvic organ prolapse repair. *Curr. Urol. Rep.* **2017**, *18*, 87. [CrossRef] [PubMed]
44. Winters, J.C.; Dmochowski, R.R.; Goldman, H.B.; Herndon, C.A.; Kobashi, K.C.; Kraus, S.R.; Lemack, G.E.; Nitti, V.W.; Rovner, E.S.; Wein, A.J. Urodynamic studies in adults: AUA/SUFU guideline. *J. Urol.* **2012**, *188*, 2464–2472. [CrossRef] [PubMed]
45. Daneshpajooh, A.; Mirzaei, M.; Dehesh, T. Role of Urodynamic Study in the Management of Pelvic Organ Prolapse in Women. *Urol. J.* **2021**, *18*, 209–213.
46. Glass, D.; Lin, F.C.; Khan, A.A.; Van Kuiken, M.; Drain, A.; Siev, M.; Peyronett, B.; Rosenblum, N.; Brucker, B.M.; Nitti, V.W. Impact of preoperative urodynamics on women undergoing pelvic organ prolapse surgery. *Int. Urogynecol. J.* **2020**, *31*, 1663–1668. [CrossRef]
47. Sierra, T.; Sullivan, G.; Leung, K.; Flynn, M. The negative predictive value of preoperative urodynamics for stress urinary incontinence following prolapse surgery. *Int. Urogynecol. J.* **2019**, *30*, 1119–1124. [CrossRef]
48. Li, S.; Tan, C.; Yang, X. The effects of vaginal surgery and pelvic floor disorders on female sexual function. *J. Sex. Med.* **2023**, *20*, 645–650. [CrossRef]
49. Mattsson, N.K.; Karjalainen, P.K.; Tolppanen, A.M.; Heikkinen, A.M.; Sintonen, H.; Harkki, P.; Nieminen, K.; Jalkanen, J. Pelvic organ prolapse surgery and quality of life-a nationwide cohort study. *Am. J. Obs. Gynecol* **2020**, *222*, 588.e1–588.e10. [CrossRef]
50. Weber, A.M.; Walters, M.D.; Piedmonte, M.R. Sexual function and vaginal anatomy in women before and after surgery for pelvic organ prolapse and urinary incontinence. *Am. J. Obs. Gynecol* **2000**, *182*, 1610–1615. [CrossRef]
51. Glavind, K.; Larsen, T.; Lindquist, A.S. Sexual function in women before and after surgery for pelvic organ prolapse. *Acta Obs. Gynecol. Scand.* **2015**, *94*, 80–85. [CrossRef] [PubMed]
52. Kinjo, M.; Tanba, M.; Masuda, K.; Nakamura, Y.; Tanbo, M.; Fukuhara, H. Comparison of effectiveness between modified transvaginal mesh surgery and vaginal pessary treatment in patients with symptomatic pelvic organ prolapse. *Low. Urin. Tract Symptoms* **2022**, *14*, 64–71. [CrossRef] [PubMed]
53. van der Vaart, L.R.; Vollebregt, A.; Pruijssers, B.; Milani, A.L.; Lagro-Janssen, A.L.; Roovers, J.W.R.; van der Vaart, C.H. Female Sexual Functioning in Women with a Symptomatic Pelvic Organ Prolapse; A Multicenter Prospective Comparative Study Between Pessary and Surgery. *J. Sex. Med.* **2022**, *19*, 270–279. [CrossRef]
54. Jha, S. Maintaining sexual function after pelvic floor surgery. *Climacteric* **2019**, *22*, 236–241. [CrossRef]
55. Ucar, M.G.; Ilhan, T.T.; Sanlikan, F.; Celik, C. Sexual functioning before and after vaginal hysterectomy to treat pelvic organ prolapse and the effects of vaginal cuff closure techniques: A prospective randomised study. *Eur. J. Obs. Gynecol. Reprod. Biol.* **2016**, *206*, 1–5. [CrossRef] [PubMed]

Disclaimer/Publisher's Note: The statements, opinions and data contained in all publications are solely those of the individual author(s) and contributor(s) and not of MDPI and/or the editor(s). MDPI and/or the editor(s) disclaim responsibility for any injury to people or property resulting from any ideas, methods, instructions or products referred to in the content.

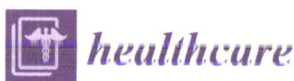

Review

From Clinical Scenarios to the Management of Lower Urinary Tract Symptoms in Children: A Focus for the General Pediatrician

Pier Luigi Palma, Pierluigi Marzuillo, Anna Di Sessa, Stefano Guarino, Daniela Capalbo, Maria Maddalena Marrapodi, Giulia Buccella, Sabrina Cameli, Emanuele Miraglia del Giudice, Marco Torella, Nicola Colacurci and Carlo Capristo *

Department of Woman, Child and General and Specialized Surgery, University of Campania "Luigi Vanvitelli", 80128 Naples, Italy
* Correspondence: carlo.capristo@unicampania.it

Abstract: Lower urinary tract symptoms (LUTS) are a relevant problem in the pediatric population, having a very high prevalence. Diurnal incontinence and nocturnal enuresis are surely the most frequent symptoms, presenting, respectively, in up to 30% of school-age children and up to 10% of children between 6 and 7 years. Stypsis is the most common comorbidity, and it must be considered in the management of LUTS; indeed, the treatment of constipation is curative in most cases for both incontinence and enuresis. The presence or absence of diurnal symptoms in nocturnal enuresis and urgency in diurnal incontinence helps in the differential diagnosis. Urotherapy is always the first-line treatment, while oxybutynin and desmopressin (where appropriate) may help if the first-line treatment is unsuccessful. It is essential to identify conditions that are potentially dangerous for kidney and urinary tract well-being, for which LUTS can be the first manifestation. Starting from a series of clinical scenarios, we will underline the diagnostic clues behind LUTS in children and we will summarize clinical and surgical approaches for the proper management of these conditions.

Keywords: overactive bladder; voiding dysfunctions; urinary incontinence; pediatric urogynaecology

Citation: Palma, P.L.; Marzuillo, P.; Di Sessa, A.; Guarino, S.; Capalbo, D.; Marrapodi, M.M.; Buccella, G.; Cameli, S.; Miraglia del Giudice, E.; Torella, M.; et al. From Clinical Scenarios to the Management of Lower Urinary Tract Symptoms in Children: A Focus for the General Pediatrician. *Healthcare* **2023**, *11*, 1285. https://doi.org/10.3390/healthcare11091285

Academic Editor: Paolo Cotogni

Received: 15 March 2023
Revised: 28 April 2023
Accepted: 29 April 2023
Published: 30 April 2023

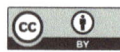

Copyright: © 2023 by the authors. Licensee MDPI, Basel, Switzerland. This article is an open access article distributed under the terms and conditions of the Creative Commons Attribution (CC BY) license (https://creativecommons.org/licenses/by/4.0/).

1. Introduction

Symptoms deriving from the lower urinary tract are grouped under the umbrella term "lower urinary tract symptoms" (LUTS). LUTS are classified by the International Children's Continence Society (ICCS) according to their relationship with the voiding or storage phase of the bladder cycle or a combination of both in changing severity. Mainly, the conditions are classified into either overactive bladder (OAB) or dysfunctional voiding. Storage symptoms are represented by increased (≥ 8 times/day) or decreased (≤ 3 times/day) number of diurnal voiding, daytime continuous or intermittent incontinence, enuresis, urgency, and nocturia. Voiding symptoms are classified as hesitancy, straining, weak stream, and intermittency [1].

LUTS are very frequent in the pediatric population, with daytime incontinence, defined as an uncontrollable leakage of urine, present in up to 30% of school-age children. Holding manoeuvres and urgency, which is a sudden and unexpected experience of an immediate need to void, are also highly prevalent [2]. Common holding manoeuvres are crossing legs, standing on tiptoe, or squatting with the heel pressed into the perineum. Enuresis, defined as intermittent incontinence while sleeping, has a prevalence of 10% in children aged between 6 and 7 years. It is subdivided into monosymptomatic (MNE), without daytime symptoms, and non-monosymptomatic enuresis (NMNE), with the presence of daytime symptoms usually associated with bladder dysfunction and less often with urinary anomalies [3]. Generally, LUTS are more frequent in girls aged between 6 and 8 years [2].

Nocturia is defined as when the child must wake during the night to void and is more frequent among school children [4].

Comorbidities are a relevant problem in these patients. ICCS suggested a list of comorbidities such as constipation, encopresis, urinary tract infection (UTI), vesicoureteral reflux (VUR), and neuropsychiatric conditions (attention deficit hyperactivity disorder, oppositional defiant disorder, learning disabilities, and disorders of sleep) that must be considered when studying LUTS properly. Stypsis is surely the commonest and most important comorbidity: up to 30% of children affected by stypsis have diurnal urinary incontinence and/or enuresis. On the other hand, proper stypsis management alone can resolve 90% of diurnal urinary incontinence cases and 60% of enuresis cases [5]. Holding manoeuvres, decreased voiding frequency, and urgency are associated with the presence of constipation [6]. The compression of the rectum on the bladder wall and the chronic external anal sphincter contraction are responsible for detrusor hyperactivity with frequent and forced contraction of the pelvic floor and anal sphincter itself, which, in turn, could "feed" constipation. This condition is known as bladder and bowel dysfunction (BBD) [7]. Moreover, children with bladder dysfunction are at risk of VUR as a consequence of urine retention in the bladder, with an increased risk of UTI and upper urinary tract damage [8].

LUTS diagnosis is not always easy to reach and so the treatment could be delayed. Firstly, LUTS are often underestimated by primary care paediatricians who tend to wait for a spontaneous resolution of the condition [3]. Secondly, the symptoms themselves are not always reported clearly by the child or his/her caregiver [1]. Voiding frequency is also hard to report precisely to caregivers until they have a chance to assess it with a complete bladder diary. School-age children may have a decreased voiding frequency related to poor hygienic conditions at school, and they could unconsciously suppress the needing of voiding through holding manoeuvres [2]. These problems may not help clinicians in taking an accurate anamnesis, which needs a lot of time to be well studied.

Starting from a series of "illustrative" case reports, we will underline the diagnostic issues and the diagnostic clues behind LUTS in children to help paediatricians in orienting toward the differential diagnosis and the proper management of these conditions.

2. Clinical Scenarios

2.1. Clinical Scenario 1

An 8-year-old girl was referred to our outpatient clinic for urgency, urge incontinence, and increased voiding frequency (12–14 times/day) in the last year. Before that, no urinary symptoms were described. Nocturnal and diurnal continence was attained at 2.5 years old and no UTI was reported by the mother. No malformations at the external genitalia examination were found. Urine analysis was normal. At the kidney and urinary tract ultrasound (KUS), both kidneys and bladder were normal and no post-void residual volume was found. The uroflowmetry revealed a tower-shaped curve. This clinical picture was suggestive of OAB. Standard urotherapy was the first line of treatment and an anticholinergic agent (oxybutynin) helped in the later management.

2.2. Clinical Scenario 2

A 7-year-old boy came to our outpatient clinic with increased daytime voiding frequency (more than 15–20 times) presenting in the last 5 months. No urinary urgency, nocturia, daytime incontinence, or nocturnal enuresis were reported. Stypsis was absent and urinalysis was normal. The clinical examination was unremarkable. The bladder voiding diary revealed 37 micturitions/day, with a volume void of each micturition between 10 and 40 mL. Based on this clinical presentation, the diagnosis of extraordinary daytime-only urinary frequency (EDOUF) was made. We reassured the parents about a benign prognosis and spontaneous resolution [9].

2.3. Clinical Scenario 3

A 4-year-old girl was observed for diurnal and nocturnal incontinence without urgency. The urinalysis was normal. The physical examination of external genitalia revealed a bifid clitoris, hypoplasia of minora labia, and patulous urethra due to a dorsal urethral defect. The diagnosis of female epispadias was found. Cystography was normal and the surgical correction of the defects determined the disappearance of the urinary incontinence [10]. At the postsurgical follow-up, no symptoms were reported.

2.4. Clinical Scenario 4

A 6-year-old girl presented with a history of daytime incontinence with increased daytime voiding frequency and enuresis. She also reported recurrent febrile UTIs since she was 18 months old. KUS showed bilateral hydronephrosis, with an anteroposterior diameter of the right pelvis of 21 millimetres and the left pelvis of 24 millimetres. The bladder wall was irregular and 6 millimetres thick (bladder fully filled). Moreover, she reported being styptic since she was 2 years old and recurrent nonfebrile UTIs in the last 6 months (about 3 episodes). Uroflowmetry revealed that a "staccato" pattern was present. An antibiotics prophylaxis with amoxicillin and a bowel regulation strategy (stool softeners plus lifestyle modification) were started. The girl was re-evaluated after 3 months, with normalizations of the symptoms, KUS, and uroflowmetry. In this case, the diagnosis was BBD, and all of the symptoms disappeared with proper urotherapy and stypsis management.

2.5. Clinical Scenario 5

An 8-year-old girl was observed for persistent urinary incontinence without urgency. She reached continence at 2.5 years old. At the physical examination, the genitalia were normal, but urine dripping was seen during the ostium vaginalis exploration. In the suspicion of an ectopic ureter, a KUS was performed, and a right kidney duplication with a megaureter of 8 mm of the upper pole was found. The Tc-99m MAG3 kidney scintigraphy revealed absent function (6%) of the right upper pole. In addition, we made a methylene blue test consisting of filling the vesical bladder with blue-coloured NaCl 0.9% by vesical catheterization. In this test, we found vaginal non-blue urine dropping, confirming that this dropping was derived from an ectopic ureter in the vagina and not from the vesical bladder. During cystoscopy, the ureteral orifice of the ureter of the upper pole was not found. The nephroureterectomy of the upper pole resolved the incontinence of the patient.

3. How to Clinically Orientate towards a Correct LUTS Diagnosis

An accurate anamnesis should be taken, focusing on symptoms reported by the child and confirmed by the caregiver. The paediatrician should investigate voiding patterns, frequency, bowel habits, fluid intake, and posturing taken during micturition. Moreover, a medical history of patients and relatives regarding nephro-urological diseases and other problems (diabetes, trauma, psychiatric diseases, psychosocial history, medications, and surgical history) should be considered. Asking for a history of constipation and recurrent UTIs should be the first step in the management of any urinary symptoms.

Physical examination is essential and sometimes enough to make a diagnosis. Any anomalies should be noted, including ear anomalies, which can be associated with urinary tract malformations [11]. Abdomen palpation could help in assessing stypsis by the presence of stool in the left iliac fossa. Most important is the evaluation of the genitalia in both males and females since continuous urinary incontinence without urgency and nocturnal enuresis could be caused by both hypospadias and epispadias [10,12]. Moreover, if genitalia is normal with urine dripping during an inspection, an ectopic ureter could be suspected, especially in the case of a duplex kidney without megaureter (or rarely with megaureter) of one of the two ureters draining that kidney [13]. In this case, a methylene blue test could be useful to confirm the clinical suspicion (please see clinical scenario 5). Another clinical entity to exclude is intravaginal micturition, which is frequently found in girls with overweight or obesity [14]. In this case, it could be useful to suggest micturition with a proper voiding position—spreading legs and voiding with feet supported—in order to prevent the intravaginal reflux of urines [14].

A urine analysis test is mandatory in excluding both mellitus (glycosuria), diabetes insipidus (low urinary density), and UTI (leukocyturia and/or nitrituria).

At first evaluation, it should always be asked that a bladder diary be completed by the caretaker or patient. ICCS recommends at least a 48 h daytime frequency and volume chart to well evaluate LUTS [7]. However, it depends on patients' compliance, and it is very subjective; therefore LUTS could be underestimated, and a 16% rate of false negatives for frequency has been seen [15]. Moreover, a bladder diary focusing on wet and dry night frequency could help. Additionally, nocturnal polyuria can be detected in enuretic children by collecting the urine volume produced during the night. To correctly measure night urinal volume, parents should sum the difference between wet diapers in the morning and dry diapers with the volume of the first micturition in the morning [16]. A urine production of >130% of the expected bladder capacity (EBC) is considered pathological [17].

KUS is a noninvasive and useful investigation tool that helps physicians in cases of kidney abnormalities, such as urinary tract dilatations or kidney duplications. Bladder thickness in healthy children should not overtake 3 and 6 millimetres in a full and empty bladder, respectively [18]. Bladder ultrasound is supportive in the diagnosis of bladder outlet obstruction (BOO) in males with increased bladder thickness. The latter could be present in OAB as well [19]. Residual postvoid volume should be assessed after a physiologic bladder filling, and a zero volume should be found in healthy children, while more than 20 mL on repeated measurements indicates voiding dysfunction [1]. Moreover, ultrasounds could be helpful in chronic stypsis diagnosis, since styptic children may have an increased rectum diameter (>3 cm) and a bladder dislocation [20]. Literature data show good reliability of urinary bladder ultrasound in children as far as bladder volume measurement is concerned. Given the variability in bladder wall thickness, a standardized methodology is desirable to increase its reliability [21].

Uroflowmetry is functional for a correct diagnosis. It is considered a noninvasive urodynamic test. Therefore, it is useful in approaching children with urinary symptoms. It consists in letting a toilet-trained child void their bladder into a toilet connected to a sensor that measures urine flow, and it is always associated with a residual postvoid volume measurement at ultrasonography. All of the adaptions possible for children should be taken to let them void their bladder in a position that is normal for them [22]. Uroflow is best performed when the bladder is at 50% of EBC [30 + (age in years $\times$ 30) up to age 12 years, after which it is considered 390 mL [23]. ICCS describes five patterns: a "bell-shaped" curve in normal voiding, a "tower-shaped" curve when an explosive detrusor contraction occurs, a "plateau-shaped" curve when there is an organic outlet tract obstruction, a "staccato" curve when there is sphincter overactivity during voiding, and "interrupted" curve when abdominal muscles are used for an acontractile detrusor [1]. Uroflowmetry has a diagnostic value and it could be used to screen children who need a more invasive test, such as cystometry [24]. Both cystometric and uroflowmetric techniques can be associated with pelvic floor electromyography (EMG), which assesses the degree of urethral contraction and relaxation.

Finally, cystometry is surely the most definitive test to diagnose voiding dysfunction and outlet obstruction. It allows paediatricians to measure bladder compliance during the filling phase, calculated by dividing the volume change by the change in detrusor pressure. Both transurethral and suprapubic routes can be used. In any case, cystometry is not mandatory, and most cases are diagnosed with uroflowmetry and KUS association. Indeed, cystometry is associated with adverse effects, e.g., UTI, macroscopic haematuria, and urinary retention in up to 20% of cases [25].

4. Therapeutic Approach

Generally, after the treatment of a possible underlying UTI, the first-line approach for any patient with LUTS is standard urotherapy. It is defined as a conservative-based therapy and treatment for LUTS that rehabilitates the low urinary tract [26]. It consists of giving patients and parents advice regarding the correct behaviour to partially or totally resolve the dysfunction. This includes information and demystification about pathology, lifestyle recommendations (increase daytime fluid intake, voiding regularly by day, and voiding before bed), and instructions and behavioural modifications to achieve optimal bladder and bowel habits (the child should relax pelvic floor muscles and sphincter during voiding) [26]. Moreover, if more than two nonfebrile UTIs occur in 6 months, or more than four in a year are reported, antibiotic prophylaxis and adequate hydration are recommended.

In the case that standard urotherapy is unsuccessful, a specific urotherapy is the method of choice. An example is "biofeedback", consisting in letting a child gain greater awareness of the pelvic floor and sphincter muscles by using external instruments [26]. Up to 80% of patients with a "dysfunctional voiding" diagnosis (defined by ICCS as a child who habitually contracts the urethral sphincter during voiding) could have improvement marked by a reduction in incontinence and UTI frequency using biofeedback [27]. Visual feedback of the uroflow curve and teaching perineal muscle identification by EMG electrodes are the best approaches [27]. Moreover, in the case of standard urotherapy and biofeedback failure, a clean intermittent self-catheterization may be helpful in children with high volumes of post-void residual fluid [28].

A postponing micturition exercise, as in clinical scenario 2, could be used in patients with EDUOF diagnosis for which effectiveness in 98.1% of patients who improved or normalized their voiding frequency has been shown [9]. However, we only recommend the postponing micturition exercise when the EDOUF affects the normal activities of either the children or parents. This recommendation had the scope to permit—for the months in which the EDOUF is more disturbing—normal daily activities for both children and parents. Moreover, with this suggestion, we did not aim to use retention control training, which is not recommended for any bladder dysfunction in childhood, but to give suggestions regarding correct micturition habits in order to establish a normal number of daily micturitions and to re-establish a cycle of routine bladder filling and emptying [29].

In patients with MNE, standard urotherapy is more effective than spontaneous cure by a rate of 15% per year [30]. Robson et al. saw a 50% reduction in bedwetting with urotherapy in 40% of the population, while 22% of children did not need any other treatments [31]. Moreover, ICCS recommend starting with urotherapy even in patients with NMNE [1].

MNE should be treated with a combination of urotherapy and desmopressin or alarm therapy. The latter consists in putting a sensor in the night clothes, which gives an auditory signal that wakes the child when it gets wet. The alarm should be preferred in children with a bladder capacity smaller than expected, who are likely to be resistant to desmopressin. It should be worn every night, and treatment should be continued until the patient is dry for 14 consecutive days or 2–3 months [32]. This approach is very family compliance-related since it could be very disturbing for parents and the child himself, and, therefore, it may not be accepted. In this case, treatment with desmopressin is preferable, available as a fast-melting oral lyophilization at a dosage of 120 µg increasing to 240 µg in the case of absent or only a partial response to the previous dosage [33]. Desmopressin is a vasopressin analogue, which, with its antidiuretic effect, concentrates urine, reducing the total volume of urine in the bladder. It is indicated in the case of nocturnal polyuria with a normal bladder capacity or when alarm therapy has failed [32]. Desmopressin is well tolerated; however, rarely, patients may, consequently, develop hyponatremia due to water intoxication, with symptoms including nausea, vomiting, headache, cerebral oedema, and convulsions (especially for the intranasal administration) [31]. To avoid side effects and to optimize the results, patients should reduce the fluid intake from 1 h before to 8 h after the desmopressin consumption. The response rate to desmopressin is higher in patients with frequently recurring nocturnal polyuria [17]. In the case of a partial response

(50–99% of wet nights) or the absence (<50% of wet nights) of a response to desmopressin alone, combination therapy with desmopressin plus oxybutynin can increase the response rate [34]. Alarm therapy and desmopressin treatment have similar efficacy in treating MNE [35].

In the case of OAB, urotherapy is still the first choice [36]. Anticholinergic agents, such as oxybutynin and tolterodine, should be used in the case of urgency persistence after standard urotherapy. They have antimuscarinic effects, blocking M_2 and M_3 receptors, which are predominantly expressed by bladder smooth muscle. Oxybutynin, at a dosage range from 0.3 to 0.5 mg/kg/day with a top dose of 10 mg [34], is preferred with its superior cost-effectiveness, and both immediate- and extended-release preparations can be used. Adverse effects are present in up to 30% of cases and include dry mouth, dizziness, constipation, somnolence, nausea, blurred vision, urinary hesitation, urinary retention, and dyspepsia, with less incidence of the extended-release preparations. Tolterodine is preferred in the case of serious or disturbing adverse effects to oxybutynin since it is more selective for the bladder and thus there are fewer adverse effects and greater efficacy [37]. Moreover, in the case of bladder-neck dysfunction, an α-blocker treatment may be useful in reducing the voiding dysfunction [38].

In case of unresponsiveness, transcutaneous electrical nerve stimulation (TENS) could be considered. It consists of inhibiting the presynaptic afferent neurons carrying impulses from the bladder by stimulating the nerves of the peripheral segmental dermatome [39]. Finally, an intravesical injection of botulinum toxin A may help to reach complete continence, despite a few adverse effects reported [38].

In conclusion, BBD and recurrent cystitis should be always excluded and eventually treated, as in scenario 4. In the case of the persistence of LUTS, a diagnosis revaluation with deeper diagnostic tools is required.

5. When a Surgical Approach Is Needed

Clinical scenarios 3 and 5 represent examples in which a clinical approach is not enough. In the case of female epispadias, an accurate genitalia examination is sufficient, and early surgical intervention is fundamental to let the patient achieve continence and preserve the urinary tract.

An ectopic ureter is a more complex condition, and the diagnosis could not be as immediate as epispadias. The term "ectopic ureter" describes a ureter that inserts at or distal to the bladder neck, and it is more frequent in females [40]. Frequently, the ectopic ureter drains the upper pole of a duplex kidney, and, while rare, it drains a hypoplastic or dysplastic kidney [40]. In 35% of cases, the insertion is in the urethra, in 34% of cases, it is in the vestibule, and in 25% of cases, it is in the vagina [13]. Clinically, patients describe not being able to reach dryness during the daytime or night, with persistent continuous incontinence. KUS may be able to detect a duplex kidney, while DMSA scintigraphy is useful in detecting poorly functioning renal tissue. A vaginoscopy and a cystoscopy may help in the identification of the ectopic ureter orifice [40]. Patients may undergo many diagnostic procedures and the diagnosis may take a long time with a 5.7-year delay from symptoms presentation to diagnosis [40]. Despite its rarity, an ectopic ureter may be found in male children as well, where it drains a hypoplastic kidney more frequently [41].

A surgical approach is needed in the case of posterior urethral valves (PUV), which are the most common congenital cause of lower urinary tract obstruction. PUV is usually diagnosed during routine prenatal ultrasounds with the detection of hydronephrosis, a thick-walled bladder, and a keyhole sign in the bladder neck of males (dilated prostatic urethra) [42]. In the case of a misdiagnosis, mild PUV could present in older children with recurrent UTIs and LUTS such as delayed voiding and weak stream. Moreover, PUV may be identified in children with renal failure, proteinuria, or through hydronephrosis studies [42]. A voiding cystourethrography (VCUG) is the gold standard imaging for diagnosis [43], and renal scintigraphy is needed to evaluate both kidneys' differential function. Catheter drainage (when appropriate) and plan endoscopic valve ablation, if the child is stable, seem to be the best approach [42].

6. Potential Long-Term Impact on Health and Quality of Life of Children

Proper management, with rapid diagnosis and treatment, is critical in children with LUTS because of the negative influence that LUTS can have on the quality of life. Both enuresis and daytime incontinence affect children and their families socially, behaviourally, and emotionally, with a risk of social isolation, peer conflict, and classroom challenges. Moreover, LUTS affect the individual in terms of development, self-esteem, and performance, as well as the relationship within the family, causing a high level of stress. Rangel et al. concluded that enuretic children have a low quality of life compared to non-enuretic children, without any differences in gender or age [44].

Additionally, it is known that children with both OABs have a prevalence of VUR between 14% and 47%. On the same line, the treatment of overactivity has a positive effect on the resolution and downgrading of VUR [8].

Moreover, the chronic obstruction caused by PUV can lead to hypertrophy of the bladder wall and detrusor muscle, with changes in bladder compliance. The consequent increment in intravesical pressure can cause VUR, and, thus, recurrent infection and progressively impaired renal function [42].

Finally, dysfunctional voiding can present indistinguishably from the classical neurogenic bladder, and such patients may encounter bilateral hydronephrosis and renal failure [45]. Both conditions are associated, as well as PUV, with a bladder pressure increase, with a risk of VUR, hydronephrosis, recurrent UTIs, and end-stage renal insufficiency.

7. Conclusions

LUTS are very common conditions in the pediatric population. They are usually underestimated and their diagnosis is not always immediate, with a frequent need to reevaluate patients. Many diagnostic tools are available to help clinicians orientate through clinical issues of LUTS. A clinical approach starting with urotherapy is usually sufficient for the management, while a few conditions need a surgical approach. In brief, urinary incontinence should be divided into nocturnal and diurnal incontinence. In the former, the co-presence of diurnal symptoms makes for a diagnosis of NMNE, while their absence makes for a diagnosis of MNE. In the case of diurnal incontinence, the presence or absence of urgency should be considered when making a differential diagnosis between OAB and other conditions that could require surgical intervention, such as an ectopic ureter. Medications, such as oxybutynin (in the case of NMNE or OAB) and desmopressin (MNE), are mostly used in the case of unsuccessful urotherapy. Figure 1 synthetizes the diagnostic clues and the proper therapeutic approach for LUTS. LUTS should never be underestimated since they can hide pathologies that could put a child's health in trouble.

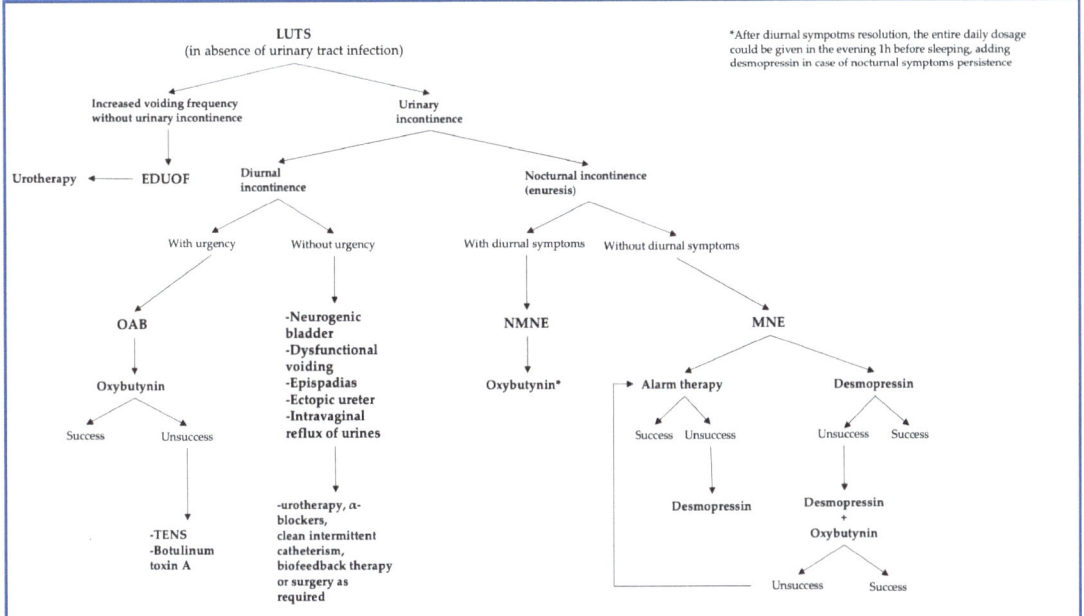

Figure 1. The diagnostic clues and the proper therapeutic approach for LUTS. Abbreviations: EDUOF, extraordinary daytime-only urinary frequency; MNE, monosymptomatic nocturnal enuresis; NMNE, non-monosymptomatic nocturnal enuresis; OAB, overactive bladder; and TENS, transcutaneous electrical nerve stimulation.

Author Contributions: Conceptualization, P.L.P. and P.M.; methodology, A.D.S. and S.G.; data curation, D.C., M.M.M., G.B. and S.C.; writing—original draft preparation, E.M.d.G. and M.T.; writing—review and editing, N.C. and C.C.; supervision, C.C.; project administration, P.L.P. All authors have read and agreed to the published version of the manuscript.

Funding: This research received no external funding.

Institutional Review Board Statement: Not applicable.

Informed Consent Statement: Not applicable.

Data Availability Statement: The data presented in this study are available upon request from the corresponding author.

Conflicts of Interest: The authors declare no conflict of interest.

References

1. Nevéus, T.; von Gontard, A.; Hoebeke, P.; Hjälmås, K.; Bauer, S.; Bower, W.; Jørgensen, T.M.; Rittig, S.; Walle, J.V.; Yeung, C.K.; et al. The Standardization of Terminology of Lower Urinary Tract Function in Children and Adolescents: Report from the Standardisation Committee of the International Children's Continence Society. *J. Urol.* **2006**, *176*, 314–324. [CrossRef]
2. Vaz, G.T.; Vasconcelos, M.M.; Oliveira, E.A.; Ferreira, A.L.; Magalhães, P.G.; Silva, F.M.; Lima, E.M. Prevalence of Lower Urinary Tract Symptoms in School-Age Children. *Pediatr. Nephrol.* **2012**, *27*, 597–603. [CrossRef] [PubMed]
3. Walle, J.V.; Rittig, S.; Tekgül, S.; Austin, P.; Yang, S.S.D.; Lopez, P.J.; Van Herzeele, C. Enuresis: Practical Guidelines for Primary Care. *Br. J. Gen. Pract.* **2017**, *67*, 328–329. [CrossRef] [PubMed]
4. Mattsson, S.H. Voiding Frequency, Volumes and Intervals in Healthy Schoolchildren. *Scand. J. Urol. Nephrol.* **1994**, *28*, 1–11. [CrossRef] [PubMed]
5. Loening-Baucke, V. Urinary Incontinence and Urinary Tract Infection and Their Resolution with Treatment of Chronic Constipation of Childhood. *Pediatrics* **1997**, *100*, 228–232. [CrossRef]

6. Sampaio, C.; Sousa, A.S.; Fraga, L.G.A.; Veiga, M.L.; Netto, J.M.B.; Barroso, U. Constipation and Lower Urinary Tract Dysfunction in Children and Adolescents: A Population-Based Study. *Front. Pediatr.* **2016**, *4*, 1–6. [CrossRef] [PubMed]
7. Austrin, P.F.; Bauer, S.B.; Bower, W.; Chase, J.; Franco, I.; Hoebeke, P.; Rittig, S.; Walle, J.V.; von Gontard, A.; Wright, A.; et al. The standardization of terminology of lower urinary tract function in children and adolescents: Update report from the standardization committee of the International Childrens Continence Society. *Neurourol. Urodyn.* **2016**, *35*, 471–481. [CrossRef] [PubMed]
8. Sillén, U. Bladder Dysfunction and Vesicoureteral Reflux. *Adv. Urol.* **2008**, *2008*, 815472. [CrossRef] [PubMed]
9. Marzuillo, P.; Diplomatico, M.; Marotta, R.; Perrone, L.; Miraglia del Giudice, E.; Polito, C.; La Manna, A.; Guarino, S. Extraordinary Daytime Only Urinary Frequency in Childhood: Prevalence, Diagnosis, and Management. *J. Pediatr. Urol.* **2018**, *14*, 177.e1–177.e6. [CrossRef] [PubMed]
10. Apicella, A.; Marzuillo, P.; Marotta, R.; La Manna, A. Female Epispadias. *J. Pediatr.* **2015**, *167*, 1164. [CrossRef]
11. Wang, R.Y.; Earl, D.L.; Ruder, R.O.; Graham, J.M. Syndromic Ear Anomalies and Renal Ultrasounds. *Pediatrics* **2001**, *108*, e23. [CrossRef]
12. Mario, L.; Niel Di, S.; Tommaso, G.; Giovanni, R. Female Hypospadias and Urinary Incontinence: Surgical Solution of a Little-Known Entity. *Int. Arch. Urol. Complicat.* **2018**, *4*, 2–5. [CrossRef]
13. Ellerker, A.G. The extravescical ectopic ureter. *Br. J. Surg.* **1958**, *45*, 344–353. [CrossRef]
14. Bernasconi, M.; Borsari, A.; Garzoni, L.; Siegenthaler, G.; Bianchetti, M.G.; Rizzi, M. Vaginal Voiding: A Common Cause of Daytime Urinary Leakage in Girls. *J. Pediatr. Adolesc. Gynecol.* **2009**, *22*, 347–350. [CrossRef] [PubMed]
15. Lopes, I.; Veiga, M.L.; Braga, A.A.N.M.; Brasil, C.A.; Hoffmann, A.; Barroso, U. A Two-Day Bladder Diary for Children: Is It Enough? *J. Pediatr. Urol.* **2015**, *11*, 348.e1–348.e4. [CrossRef] [PubMed]
16. Mangani, S.; Sauro, F.; Ponticelli, A. Nocturia in Mothers and Enuresis in Children: Possible Links. *Türk Üroloji Dergisi/Turkish J. Urol.* **2020**, *46*, 146–151. [CrossRef] [PubMed]
17. Marzuillo, P.; Marotta, R.; Guarino, S.; Fedele, M.C.; Palladino, F.; Capalbo, D.; Della Vecchia, N.; Miraglia del Giudice, E.; Polito, C.; La Manna, A. 'Frequently Recurring' Nocturnal Polyuria Is Predictive of Response to Desmopressin in Monosymptomatic Nocturnal Enuresis in Childhood. *J. Pediatr. Urol.* **2019**, *15*, 166.e1–166.e7. [CrossRef]
18. Jequier, S.; Rousseau, O. Sonographic Measurements of the Normal Bladder Wall in Children. *Am. J. Roentgenol.* **1987**, *149*, 563–566. [CrossRef]
19. Farag, F.F.; Heesakkers, J. Imaging Assessments of Lower Urinary Tract Dysfunctions: Future Steps. *Turk. Urol. Derg.* **2014**, *40*, 78–81. [CrossRef]
20. Joensson, I.M.; Siggaard, C.; Rittig, S.; Hagstroem, S.; Djurhuus, J.C. Transabdominal Ultrasound of Rectum as a Diagnostic Tool in Childhood Constipation. *J. Urol.* **2008**, *179*, 1997–2002. [CrossRef]
21. Marzuillo, P.; Guarino, S.; Capalbo, D.; Acierno, S.; Menale, F.; Prisco, A.; Arianna, V.; La Manna, A.; Miraglia del Giudice, E. Interrater Reliability of Bladder Ultrasound Measurements in Children. *J. Pediatr. Urol.* **2020**, *16*, 219.e1–219.e7. [CrossRef] [PubMed]
22. Hoebeke, P.; Bower, W.; Combs, A.; De Jong, T.; Yang, S. Diagnostic Evaluation of Children With Daytime Incontinence. *J. Urol.* **2010**, *183*, 699–703. [CrossRef] [PubMed]
23. Koff, S.A. Estimating Bladder Capacity in Children. *Urology* **1983**, *21*, 248–252. [CrossRef] [PubMed]
24. Wen, J.G.; Djurhuus, J.C.; Rosier, P.F.W.M.; Bauer, S.B. ICS Educational Module: Cystometry in Children. *Neurourol. Urodyn.* **2018**, *37*, 2306–2310. [CrossRef]
25. Klingler, H.C.; Madersbacher, S.; Djavan, B.; Schatzl, G.; Marberger, M.; Schmidbauer, C.P. Morbidity of the Evaluation of the Lower Urinary Tract with Transurethral Multichannel Pressure-Flow Studies. *J. Urol.* **1998**, *159*, 191–194. [CrossRef]
26. Nieuwhof-Leppink, A.J.; Hussong, J.; Chase, J.; Larsson, J.; Renson, C.; Hoebeke, P.; Yang, S.; von Gontard, A. Definitions, Indications and Practice of Urotherapy in Children and Adolescents: A Standardization Document of the International Children's Continence Society (ICCS). *J. Pediatr. Urol.* **2021**, *17*, 172–181. [CrossRef]
27. Sinha, S. Dysfunctional Voiding: A Review of the Terminology, Presentation, Evaluation and Management in Children and Adults. *Indian J. Urol.* **2011**, *27*, 437–447. [CrossRef]
28. Oakeshott, P.; Hunt, G.M. Intermittent Self Catheterization for Patients with Urinary Incontinence or Difficulty Emptying the Bladder. *Br. J. Gen. Pract.* **1992**, *42*, 253–255.
29. Marzuillo, P.; Polito, C.; La Manna, A.; Guarino, S. Response to "Re. Extraordinary Daytime Only Urinary Frequency in Childhood: Prevalence, Diagnosis and Management". *J. Pediatr. Urol.* **2018**, *14*, 180–181. [CrossRef]
30. Forsythe, W.I.; Redmond, A. Enuresis and Spontaneous Cure Rate Study of 1129 Enuretics From the Royal Belfast Hospital for Sick Children, Belfast. *Arch. J Dis. Child.* **1974**, *49*, 259–263. [CrossRef]
31. Robson, W.L.; Leung, A.K. Side Effects and Complications of Treatment with Desmopressin for Enuresis. *J. Natl. Med. Assoc.* **1994**, *86*, 775–778. [PubMed]
32. Walle, J.V.; Rittig, S.; Bauer, S.; Eggert, P.; Marschall-Kehrel, D.; Tekgul, S. Practical Consensus Guidelines for the Management of Enuresis. *Eur. J. Pediatr.* **2012**, *171*, 971–983. [CrossRef]
33. Woo, S.H.; Park, K.H. Enuresis Alarm Treatment as a Second Line to Pharmacotherapy in Children with Monosymptomatic Nocturnal Enuresis. *J. Urol.* **2004**, *171*, 2615–2617. [CrossRef]

34. Capalbo, D.; Guarino, S.; Di Sessa, A.; Esposito, C.; Grella, C.; Papparella, A.; Miraglia del Giudice, E.; Marzuillo, P. Combination Therapy (Desmopressin plus Oxybutynin) Improves the Response Rate Compared with Desmopressin Alone in Patients with Monosymptomatic Nocturnal Enuresis and Nocturnal Polyuria and Absence of Constipation Predict the Response to This Treatment. *Eur. J. Pediatr.* **2023**. [CrossRef] [PubMed]
35. Cakiroglu, B.; Arda, E.; Tas, T.; Senturk, A.B. Alarm Therapy and Desmopressin in the Treatment of Patients with Nocturnal Enuresis. *Afr. J. Paediatr. Surg.* **2018**, *15*, 131–134. [CrossRef] [PubMed]
36. Geoffrion, R.; Lovatsis, D.; Walter, J.E.; Chou, Q.; Easton, W.; Epp, A.; Harvey, M.A.; Larochelle, A.; Maslow, K.; Neustaedter, G.; et al. Treatments for Overactive Bladder: Focus on Pharmacotherapy. *J. Obstet. Gynaecol. Canada* **2012**, *34*, 1092–1101. [CrossRef] [PubMed]
37. Koç, B.; Canpolat, N.; Adaletli, İ.; Sever, L.; Emir, H.; Çalışkan, S. Efficacy of Tolterodine in Children with Overactive Bladder. *Turkish Arch. Pediatr.* **2020**, *55*, 284–289. [CrossRef]
38. Franco, I. Overactive Bladder in Children. *Nat. Rev. Urol.* **2016**, *13*, 520–532. [CrossRef]
39. Sharma, N.; Rekha, K.; Srinivasan, K.J. Efficacy of Transcutaneous Electrical Nerve Stimulation in the Treatment of Overactive Bladder. *J. Clin. Diagn. Res.* **2016**, *10*, QC17–QC20. [CrossRef]
40. Borer, J.G.; Bauer, S.B.; Peters, C.A.; Diamond, D.A.; Decter, R.M.; Shapiro, E. A Single-System Ectopic Ureter Draining an Ectopic Dysplastic Kidney: Delayed Diagnosis in the Young Female with Continuous Urinary Incontinence. *Br. J. Urol.* **1998**, *81*, 474–478. [CrossRef]
41. Williams, D.I.; Royle, M. Ectopic Ureter in the Male Child. *Br. J. Urol.* **1969**, *41*, 421–427. [CrossRef] [PubMed]
42. Hodges, S.J.; Patel, B.; McLorie, G.; Atala, A. Posterior Urethral Valves. *Sci. World J.* **2009**, *9*, 1119–1126. [CrossRef] [PubMed]
43. Casella, D.P.; Tomaszewski, J.J.; Ost, M.C. Posterior Urethral Valves: Renal Failure and Prenatal Treatment. *Int. J. Nephrol.* **2012**, *2012*, 351067. [CrossRef] [PubMed]
44. Rangel, R.A.; Seabra, C.R.; Ferrarez, C.E.P.F.; Soares, J.L.; Choi, M.; Cotta, R.G.; De Figueiredo, A.A.; De Bessa, J.; Netto, J.M.B. Quality of Life in Enuretic Children. *Int. Braz. J. Urol.* **2021**, *47*, 535–541. [CrossRef] [PubMed]
45. Adams, J.; Mehls, O.; Wiesel, M. Pediatric Renal Transplantation and the Dysfunctional Bladder. *Transpl. Int.* **2004**, *17*, 596–602. [CrossRef] [PubMed]

Disclaimer/Publisher's Note: The statements, opinions and data contained in all publications are solely those of the individual author(s) and contributor(s) and not of MDPI and/or the editor(s). MDPI and/or the editor(s) disclaim responsibility for any injury to people or property resulting from any ideas, methods, instructions or products referred to in the content.

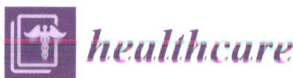

Article

Prevalence and Severity of Pelvic Floor Disorders during Pregnancy: Does the Trimester Make a Difference?

Yoav Baruch [1,*], Stefano Manodoro [2,*], Marta Barba [3], Alice Cola [3], Ilaria Re [3] and Matteo Frigerio [3]

1. Urogynecology and Pelvic Floor Unit, Department of Obstetrics and Gynecology, Tel Aviv Medical Center, Tel Aviv University, Tel Aviv 6997801, Israel
2. Department of Obstetrics and Gynecology, ASST Santi Paolo e Carlo, San Paolo Hospital, 20132 Milano, Italy
3. Department of Obstetrics and Gynecology, Fondazione IRCCS San Gerardo dei Tintori, University Milano Bicocca, 20900 Monza, Italy; m.barba8792@gmail.com (M.B.)
* Correspondence: yoavi100@gmail.com (Y.B.); stefano.manodoro@gmail.com (S.M.)

Abstract: (1) Background: Women experience pelvic floor dysfunction symptoms during pregnancy. This study is the first to investigate and compare variances in the prevalence and severity of pelvic floor symptoms between trimesters using a valid pregnancy-targeted questionnaire. (2) Methods: A retrospective cohort study was conducted between August 2020 to January 2021 at two university-affiliated tertiary medical centers. Pregnant women (*n* = 306) anonymously completed the Pelvic Floor Questionnaire for Pregnancy and Postpartum with its four domains (bladder, bowel, prolapse, and sexual). (3) Results: Thirty-six women (11.7%) were in the 1st trimester, eighty-three (27.1%) were in the 2nd trimester, and one hundred and eighty-seven (61.1%) were in the 3rd trimester. The groups were similar in age, pregestational weight, and smoking habits. A total of 104 (34%) had bladder dysfunction, 112 (36.3%) had bowel dysfunction, and 132 (40.4%) reported sexual inactivity and/or sexual dysfunction. Least prevalent (33/306; 10.8%) were prolapse symptoms. Increased awareness of prolapse and significantly higher rates of nocturia and the need to use pads due to incontinence were recorded in the 3rd trimester. Sexual dysfunction or abstinence were equally distributed in all three trimesters. (4) Conclusions: Bladder and prolapse symptoms, equally frequent throughout pregnancy, significantly intensified in the 3rd trimester. Bowel and sexual symptoms, equally frequent throughout pregnancy, did not intensify in the third trimester.

Keywords: PFQPP; pregnancy; pelvic floor disorders; sexual dysfunction; quality of life; stress urinary incontinence; pelvic organ prolapse; urge urinary incontinence

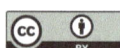

1. Introduction

Pelvic floor dysfunction (PFD) is a common multifactorial heterogeneous condition mainly consequent to weakening of the pelvic floor following vaginal or operative delivery. Otherwise, PFD can be related to genetic, structural and or hormonal factors [1]. PFD symptoms include vaginal, bowel, lower urinary tract, and sexual impairments such as urinary and anal incontinence, overactive bladder, pelvic organ prolapse, and sexual discomfort. PFD symptoms are widespread and are known to affect millions of women worldwide. Almost a quarter of women in the United States suffer from at least one pelvic floor disorder whether urinary incontinence, fecal incontinence, or pelvic organ prolapse [2]. It remains difficult, however, to determine the true prevalence of PFD because many women who suffer from FFD symptoms choose not to seek medical assistance and some are even reluctant to discuss PFD symptoms with their caregivers. The prevalence of PFD increases with older age and elevated body mass index [3,4]. Other than age and obesity, risk factors for PFD include smoking, mode of delivery, familial predisposition, race, and connective tissue disorders [5]. It has been shown that familial cases tend to portray more than one pelvic floor defect suggesting that underlying genetic factors may enhance PFD morbidity [6]. PFD negatively affects the social and physical functions of women, restricts their daily activities, impairs sexual function, and ultimately reduces their overall quality of life (QoL) [7]. The widespread prevalence of PFD symptoms, although far from being life threatening, results in lost productivity and a considerable economic burden on healthcare resources.

Women experience an increase in urinary incontinence, pelvic floor organ prolapse, sexual handicaps, and colorectal symptoms during pregnancy [8,9]. Involuntary loss of urine upon sneezing or coughing in pregnant women is detrimental to the quality of life. The quality of life of women with PFD symptoms is expected to decrease with increasing gestational age.

The use of validated QoL questionnaires rather than clinical interviews is effective and useful for the assessment of PFD symptoms as regards to their presence, severity, and their impact on patients' quality of life, bringing to light conditions that may otherwise remain unrevealed [10]. The German "Pelvic Floor Questionnaire for pregnant and postpartum women" (PFQPP) is a self-completed questionnaire that was recently constructed to cover all four essential domains of pelvic floor function (bladder, bowel, prolapse, and sexual function) and to assess PFD symptoms' severity, their prevalence, and their impact on quality of life [11]. The questionnaire, which differentiates between women who report bothersome symptoms and those who do not, is a reliable and valid tool that incorporates 42 recognized items, and its original German version can be downloaded using the link in the Supplementary Material section [11]. The questionnaire integrates five ascertained risk factors: age over 35 years, familial predisposition, body mass index > 25 kg/m^2, cigarette smoking, and a subjective inability to voluntarily contract the pelvic floor muscles [11,12].

The PFQPP translated into and validated in the Italian language [13] was recently submitted to 1048 pregnant women predominantly in the 3rd trimester ($n = 927$) recruited at eight hospitals in Italy. Almost half of the pregnant women suffered from PFD symptoms, one-third abstained from sexual activity, and half of them suffered from dyspareunia [14].

Pelvic floor distress symptoms have been adequately investigated in the third trimester of pregnancy whereas their presence in early pregnancy has been rather overlooked. We hypothesized that pelvic distress remains underreported in early and mid-pregnancy until symptoms worsen in the third trimester. Our objective was to delineate variances in PFD symptomatology between the three trimesters of pregnancy. We thus compared the prevalence and severity of PFD symptoms in a subset of women who anonymously completed the Italian PFQPP at different stages of pregnancy.

2. Materials and Methods

This study relays a secondary analysis from a cross-sectional study that was originally conducted in eight hospitals in Italy and Italian-speaking Switzerland [8].

The research protocol was approved by the local Institutional Review Board (n. 3116/2019) before the study began. Two tertiary medical centers namely, Santi Paolo e Carlo, San Paolo Hospital, Milan, Italy, and San Gerardo Hospital, Monza, Italy, who recruited women in all three trimesters, undertook this analysis. The PFQPP (validated in the Italian language), completed by 306 pregnant women, was used to evaluate and compare pelvic floor distress symptoms at different stages of pregnancy. The investigators distributed and collected the surveys from August 2020 to January 2021. Routine statistical methods were used to interpret the results.

Women with singleton pregnancies, 18 years and older, fluent in the Italian language, and recruited at antenatal outpatient clinics during routine pregnancy visits were asked to anonymously complete the Italian PFQPP. The exclusion criteria included: insufficient Italian language proficiency, diabetes mellitus, neurological disorders, and any other substantial co-morbidity. The women were subdivided between the pregnancy trimesters. Prevalence, severity, and risk factors were evaluated using the PFQPP.

2.1. The Pelvic Floor Questionnaire for Pregnancy and Postpartum—PFQPP

The Italian Pelvic Floor Questionnaire for Pregnancy and Postpartum embraces four domains of pelvic floor function (bladder, bowel, prolapse, and sexual function). The PFQPP weighs PFD symptoms' severity and their impact on quality of life during pregnancy and postpartum. The patients were asked to consider how much their bowel, bladder, prolapse, and sexual issues bothered them. Responses that range from "not at all"; "a little"; "quite a lot"; and "very much" were deemed applicable. "I don't have any symptom" was deemed not applicable. The total score in each domain defined the severity of PFD. The prevalence was calculated by the presence of bothersome symptoms when at least one point was granted.

The following items in the PFQPP were selected to assess the prevalence of specific PFD symptoms: Bladder question 5 was used to assess the prevalence of urge urinary incontinence re: "Do you leak urine before reaching the toilet when you have the desire to urinate?". Bladder question 6 was used to assess the prevalence of stress incontinence re: "Do you leak urine when you laugh, sneeze, cough, or engage in sports?". Bladder question 9 was used to assess the prevalence of incomplete bladder voiding re: "Do you feel like your bladder hasn't completely emptied?". Bowel question 4 was used to assess the prevalence of constipation re: "Do you experience constipation?". Bowel question 8 was used to assess the prevalence of fecal incontinence re: "Do you have trouble maintaining stools or do you experience fecal leaks?". Prolapse question 1 was used to assess the prevalence of prolapse symptoms re: "Do you experience a bulging sensation in the vagina?". Sexual question 5 was used to assess the prevalence of dyspareunia: "Do you feel pain during intercourse?". The magnitude of related symptoms was scored on a 5-point Likert Scale with the following choice of answers: "0 = not applicable—I do not have symptoms", "1—not at all"; "2—a little"; "3—quite a lot" and "4—very much".

The relationship between PFD symptoms and known risk factors including age over 35 years, familial predisposition (a family member with PFD symptoms), body mass index > 25 kg/m^2, cigarette smoking, and a subjective inability to voluntarily contract the pelvic floor muscles was examined. Pelvic floor contraction (PFC) inability outlines the "subjective ability to voluntarily contract the pelvic floor muscles". The question posed by the PFQPP "Are you capable to contract the muscles in the pelvic floor?" was used to assess PFC inability and the answers proposed are "yes", "I do not know" and "no" [10]. The answer "no" designates pelvic floor contraction (PFC) inability.

2.2. Statistical Analysis

Categorical variables were summarized as frequency and percentage. Normally distributed continuous variables were reported as mean and standard deviation (SD) while skewed variables were reported as median and interquartile range. The Chi-square test and Fisher's exact tests were applied to compare categorical variables between the three trimesters of pregnancy, while ANOVA and Kruskal Wallis tests were used to compare continuous variables between the three trimesters. All statistical tests were two-sided and a p-value of less than 0.05 was considered statistically significant. The Statistical Package for the Social Sciences (IBM SPSS software for windows), version 28, IBM Corporation, Armonk, New York, NY, USA, 2021) was used for all statistical analyses.

3. Results

The study cohort included 306 women. Thirty-six (11.8%) women were in the 1st trimester of pregnancy, 83 (27.1%) were in 2nd trimester, and one hundred and eighty-seven (61.1%) were in the 3rd trimester of pregnancy. The mean age at recruitment was 32.6 ± 4.6 years. The groups were comparable in age at recruitment and did not differ as regards to age, pregestational weight, and cigarette smoking (Table 1).

Table 1. General characteristics and risk factors in pregnancy trimesters. PFC = pelvic floor contraction; PFDs = pelvic floor dysfunction symptoms.

Characteristics and Risk Factors	All Patients n = 306	1st Trimester n = 36	2nd Trimester n = 83	3rd Trimester n = 187	p
Maternal Age	32.6 (±4.6)	33.4 (±4)	32.8 (±4.7)	32.4 (±4.8)	0.481
Gestational Age	30.5 (±20)	10.25 (±1.7)	19.9 (±4.4)	34.8 (±3.6)	<0.001 [b]
Pregestational weight (kg)	62 (±12.4)	61.1 (±11)	61.8 (±12)	62.8 (±12)	0.607
Current weight (kg)	70 (±12.8)	62.2 (±11)	67.1 (±12)	72.7 (±12)	<0.010 [a]
Age > 35	75 (25.9%)	11 (31.4%)	19 (25%)	45 (25.1%)	0.725
Familiarity with PFDs (n = 304)	34 (11.2%)	3 (8.6%)	14 (16.9%)	17 (9.1%)	0.156
Smoking (n = 306)	14 (4.6%)	2 (5.6%)	1 (1.2%)	11 (5.9%)	0.206
Pelvic floor contraction inability (n = 304)	15 (4.9%)	2 (5.6%)	5 (6.1%)	8 (4.3%)	0.671

Age at interview was not provided by 16 participants. [a] Denotes a significant difference between all three trimesters. [b] Denotes a significant difference between the 3rd trimester and either the 2nd or 1st trimester, with no significant difference calculated between the 1st and 2nd trimesters.

All women who gave consent to participate in the study completed at least part of the questionnaire (none were left blank) and the rate of missing items was 1%. Bladder, bowel, and sexual symptoms were frequent (reported by 34%, 36.3%, and 36.4% of participants, respectively) whereas prolapse symptoms were reported by only 10.8% of participants (Table 2).

Table 2. Prevalence of PFD symptoms in the three pregnancy trimesters.

PFD Symptoms (n = 306)	All Trimesters	1st Trimester (n = 36)	2nd Trimester (n = 83)	3rd Trimester (n = 187)	p
No symptoms	120 (39.2%)	19 (52.7%)	35 (42.1%)	66 (35.3%)	0.117
Vesical Dysfunction	104 (34%)	9 (25%)	24 (28.9%)	71 (38%)	0.716
Bowel Dysfunction	112 (36.3%)	11 (30.6%)	30 (36.1%)	71 (38%)	0.691
Pelvic Support Dysfunction	33 (10.8%)	2 (5.6%)	6 (7.2%)	25 (13.4%)	0.182
Sexual Dysfunction	65 (21.2%)	6 (16.7%)	16 (19.3%)	43 (23%)	0.611
Sexual Inactivity	55 (18.4%)	3 (8.3%)	15 (18.5%)	37 (20%)	0.352

3.1. Sexual Domain

Fifty-five women (55/306; 18.0%) reported absent sexual activity. Motives for sexual inactivity were a lack of a partner (21/55; 38.2%); partner-related inactivity (health-related, lack of desire, or fear of harming pregnancy) (22/55; 40%); a lack of sexual desire (9/55; 16.4%); and unpleasant or painful intercourse (3/55; 5.4%). These were equally distributed between the trimesters ($p = 0.302$). Of the remaining women, 65 (65/251; 25.9%) reported sexual dysfunction defined by answers "2—a little," "3—quite a lot," and "4—very much" to the question "How much do your sexual symptoms bother you?". Sexual dysfunction was equally distributed in the 1st, 2nd, and 3rd trimesters of pregnancy ($p = 0.611$). The total sexual domain scores were 1.04, 1.25, and 1.25 in the 1st, 2nd, and 3rd trimesters, respectively ($p = 0.382$).

3.2. Bladder Domain

A total of 104/306 (34%) participants reported bladder dysfunction with overall rates equally distributed in the 1st, 2nd, and 3rd trimesters of pregnancy ($p = 0.168$). Symptoms related to urinary distress were more intense in the 3rd trimester of pregnancy compared to the 1st and 2nd trimesters of pregnancy. As seen in Table 3, total bother scores distinguished a significant difference between the 3rd trimester [1.46 (1.04–2.3)] and the 2nd [1.25 (0.62–1.87)] and 1st trimester [1.15 (0.67–1.82)] with no significant difference between the 1st and 2nd trimesters, ($p = 0.004$).

Table 3. Bother scores calculated for each trimester separately.

Bother Scores	1st Trimester	2nd Trimester	3rd Trimester	p
Urinary domain score	1.15 (0.67–1.82)	1.25 (0.62–1.87)	1.46 (1.04–2.3)	0.004 [b]
Intestinal domain score	1.61 (0.64–2.5)	1.29 (0.97–2.25)	1.61 (0.97–2.25)	0.709
Pelvic domain score	0.24 (0–0.8)	0.38 (0–0.94)	0.65 (0–1.29)	0.012 [b]
Sexual domain score	1.04 (0.41–2.08)	1.25 (0.41–2.08)	1.25 (0.42–2.5)	0.382
TOTAL score	3.99 (2.87–5.44)	4.41 (3.14–5.98)	5.31 (3.62–7.12)	0.005 [b]

[b] Denotes a significant difference between the scores calculated for the 3rd trimester and either the 2nd or 1st trimester, with no significant difference calculated between the 1st and 2nd trimesters.

Significantly higher rates of nocturia, the need for pads due to incontinence, and a false sensation of UTI (presented by answers to bladder question 2, question 11, and question 14, respectively) were recorded in the 3rd trimester compared to the 1st and 2nd trimesters (Table 4).

Table 4. Specific items in the questionnaire that were significant between the trimesters.

Significant PFQPP Items	1st Trimester	2nd Trimester	3rd Trimester	p
V2 Presence of nocturia	16 (44.4%)	36 (43.9%)	119 (63.6%)	0.004 [b]
V11 Use of pads due to urinary leakage	5 (13.9%)	13 (15.7%)	53 (28.3%)	0.028 [b]
V14 False sensation of UTI	3 (8.3%)	14 (17.1%)	48 (25.7%)	0.037 [c]
P2 Sensing prolapse of uterus or vagina at rest	2 (5.6%)	11 (13.3%)	40 (21.5%)	0.035 [c]
P3 Sensing prolapse during physical effort.	2 (5.6%)	15 (18.1%)	49 (26.3%)	0.014 [c]

[b] Denotes a significant difference between the 3rd trimester and either the 2nd and 1st trimester, with no significant difference calculated between the 1st and 2nd trimesters. [c] Denotes a significant difference only between the 3rd trimester and 1st trimester.

3.3. Bowel Domain

A total of 112/306 (36.3%) participants reported intestinal dysfunction with overall rates equally distributed in the 1st, 2nd, and 3rd trimesters of pregnancy ($p = 0.691$). Bother scores calculated for 1st [1.61 (0.64–2.5)], 2nd [1.29 (0.97–2.25)], and 3rd trimesters [1.61 (0.97–2.25)] were compared, with no significant differences observed between the three trimesters ($p = 0.709$).

3.4. Prolapse Domain

Thirty-three women (33/306; 10.8%) reported prolapse symptoms with overall rates equally distributed in the 1st, 2nd, and 3rd trimesters of pregnancy. However, when the bother scores were computed, a significant difference between the scores calculated for the 3rd trimester [0.65 (0–1.29)] and those calculated for the 2nd [0.38 (0–0.94)] and 1st trimesters [0.24 (0–0.8) was noted ($p = 0.012$) with no significant difference between the 1st and 2nd trimesters. A significantly higher rate of bulging symptoms either at rest or during effort (presented by answers to prolapse question 2 and prolapse question 3, respectively) was recorded in the 3rd trimester compared to the 1st and 2nd trimesters of pregnancy (Table 4).

3.5. Pelvic Floor Total Burden

There were no significant differences in prevalence between the groups when the domain items were counted in total. When the bother scores of all four domains were summed, a significant difference between the scores calculated for the 3rd trimester [5.31 (3.62–7.12)] and those calculated for the 2nd [4.41 (3.14–5.98)] and 1st trimester [3.99 (2.87–5.44)] was noted ($p = 0.005$), with no significant difference between the 1st and 2nd trimesters of pregnancy.

3.6. Risk Factors

Five related risk factors were explored: age over 35 years, familial predisposition, body mass index > 25 kg/m^2, cigarette smoking, and a subjective inability to voluntarily contract the pelvic floor muscles. Overall, 69.6% of the participants demonstrated either one (48.4%), two (17.3%), or three (3.9%) risk factors that were equally distributed among the groups.

4. Discussion

Pelvic floor distress symptoms have been sufficiently studied in the third trimester of pregnancy whereas their presence in early pregnancy has been sparsely investigated. To the best of our knowledge, this is the first study that investigates the frequency and assortment of pelvic floor dysfunction complaints throughout pregnancy and examines the degree of bother they cause using a valid questionnaire for pregnant women. To define the prevalence and severity of PFD symptoms all along, rather than in the 3rd trimester of pregnancy, we employed a self-completed, validated, and reliable tool created to assess all four domains of pelvic floor function (bladder, bowel, prolapse, and sexual function) [13]. Pelvic floor outcomes, including stress incontinence, anal incontinence, prolapse, and sexual dysfunction were measured at different stages of pregnancy using the PFQPP. We found that 60.8% of the study cohort endured at least one PFD symptom during pregnancy and that specific PFD symptoms intensified in the third trimester of pregnancy.

Previous studies have underlined that sexual dysfunction is extremely common in the third trimester of pregnancy, with it overwhelmingly impacting women's quality of life [14,15]. Several studies report a significant decline in sexual desire and sexual activity during the third trimester of pregnancy [14–17]. Sexual dysfunction, in the 3rd trimester, is mediated by a lack of adequate information about sex in pregnancy and the worry that intercourse may harm the pregnancy by inducing preterm labor or premature rupture of membranes. A recent survey using the Italian PFQPP revealed that in the third trimester of pregnancy, one-third of women abstained from sexual activity and half of them had dyspareunia [14]. The decline in sexual activity is also due to a lack of sexual desire [14]. Sexual dysfunction can lead to depression, anxiety, hypervigilance to pain, negative body image, and low self-esteem and is strongly correlated with urinary incontinence [18]. Our study discloses that sexual inactivity and/or dysfunction, reported by as many as 39.2% of participants, were equally dispersed in the first, second, and third trimesters of pregnancy and did not intensify in the third trimester denoting that sexual dysfunction is promoted by the pregnancy condition itself.

A trend towards Increased rates (5.6%, 7.2%, and 13.4% in the 1st, 2nd, and 3rd trimesters, respectively) of prolapse symptoms did not reach significance probably due to the small number of women experiencing prolapse symptoms (n = 33; 10.8%). However, when the bother scores were computed, a significant difference between the scores calculated for the 3rd trimester and those calculated in the 1st and 2nd trimesters was obtained denoting that bulging symptoms were more disturbing in the 3rd trimester of pregnancy (Table 4). Urinary complaints reported by as many as 34% of participants showed significantly higher rates for nocturia and the need to use pads in the 3rd trimester compared to the 1st and 2nd trimesters which is in line with previous observations that hold that the bother instigated by urinary tract symptoms is most frequent in the 3rd trimester [19]. The rate and magnitude of bowel complaints, reported by 36.3% of participants, were similar in the three groups.

Well-established risk factors for PFD, although expected to be more salient among women experiencing PFD symptoms in early pregnancy, were found to be equally distributed within the three groups (Table 1). Smokers were scarce in the cohort as a whole (n = 11; 4.6%).

Pelvic floor rehabilitation for pregnant women, displaying PFD symptoms, is hindered by underdiagnosis, embarrassment, fear of stigma, high costs, long waiting periods, or restricted access to medical services. PFD symptoms even though over-expressed during pregnancy remain at large underdiagnosed and undertreated. Pregnant women tend to regard PFD symptoms as a common and transient discomfort associated with pregnancy and do not consider themselves liable to still suffer from PFD symptoms later in life and generally do not seek medical attention. Urinary incontinence and the sensation of pelvic organs bulging through the vagina impede daily functions and depress self-image. These distressing symptoms certainly merit medical attention, sound counselling, and prompt management. A care plan for PFD prevention or treatment during pregnancy is lacking and the need to increase women's knowledge of PFD and motivate them to engage in PFD prevention is delayed by time constraints during prenatal visits. Women should be intentionally informed and counseled about PFD symptoms so that those who are overweight, smokers, or unable to actively contract their pelvic floor muscles can receive targeted counseling about their increased risk and take preventive action [20].

Intervention strategies that can reduce and lessen PFD symptoms include weight reduction, participation in sports, and pelvic floor muscle training (PFMT) [21]. PFMT is a conservative intervention that can improve bladder, bowel, prolapse, and sexual function. PFMT proven effective to treat stress and urge incontinence [21,22] and employed before or as of early pregnancy is expected to prevent or alleviate PFD symptoms. It has been reported that PFMT improves sexual function in postmenopausal women and when introduced postnatally [23,24]. However, studies describing the effect of PFMT on sexual function and other PFD symptoms during pregnancy are lacking. Obviously, such studies are difficult to achieve since most PFD symptoms are rather mild and remain underreported in early pregnancy. Pelvic floor muscle training which is devoid of serious adverse effects and has been recommended as a first-line treatment in the general population may prove essential to pregnant women.

Lately, eHealth (digital health) intervention programs have been mounted to provide information about pelvic floor ailments and management. A thorough meta-analysis conducted by Xu et al. [25] shows that eHealth intervention is useful in recovering PFD symptoms, especially as regards to outcomes such as stress and urinary incontinence, quality of life, pelvic floor muscle strength, and sexual function. Due to their anonymity, flexibility, and accessibility, eHealth interventions can reduce women's sense of embarrassment, reduce cost and time, and simplify access to healthcare services. eHealth intervention programs should be made accessible to women during pregnancy and after birth. Treatment of PDF following delivery remains the principle considering that two-thirds of women are still bothered by PFD symptoms one year after delivery [26]. PFD symptoms which are not considered life-threatening overwhelmingly disturb women's life and are associated with decreased body image and postpartum depression [27–30].

Our results show that marginal PFD symptoms emerge early in pregnancy and intensify throughout pregnancy. It remains mandatory to screen pregnant women early in pregnancy and to offer them sound counseling and treatment.

Strengths and Limitations

Anonymous questionnaires, especially in sensitive areas such as sexual incompetence, are more likely to uncover symptoms that might otherwise remain hidden. Anonymity, however, hampers the assessment of potential influencers and confounders not investigated by the questionnaire itself. We acknowledge the need for a longitudinal study that queries and assesses responses from the same participant at different stages of pregnancy. This again may be hindered by anonymity. The PFQPP has been fundamental in the early diagnosis of PFDs in pregnancy, and, to the best of our knowledge, this is the first study to examine differences between trimesters using a valid pregnancy-targeted questionnaire.

5. Conclusions

Sixty percent of the participants suffered from at least one pelvic floor disorder. Our study shows that bladder and prolapse symptoms are frequent throughout pregnancy but significantly intensify in the 3rd trimester. Sexual dysfunction remains equally distressing throughout pregnancy, thereby mearing quality of life and self-esteem. Bowel dysfunction is less prevalent compared to other PDF symptoms and the recorded trend towards increased severity during pregnancy that did not reach significance merit further investigation. The preponderance of PDF symptoms, although subtle in early pregnancy, requires that pregnant women be aware of such symptoms early. Healthcare professionals need to adopt a proactive approach and motivate pregnant women to indulge in PFMT. PFQPP emerges as a precious, easy use, risk estimate tool that awards early detection of PDF.

Supplementary Materials: The following supporting information can be downloaded at: https://www.mdpi.com/article/10.3390/healthcare11081096/s1, The original German version of the Pelvic Floor Questionnaire for pregnant and postpartum women.

Author Contributions: Conceptualization, M.F. and S.M.; formal analysis, Y.B.; validation, M.B.; data collection, A.C. and I.R.; supervision, M.F. and S.M.; writing—original draft preparation, Y.B.; writing—review and editing, M.B., A.C. and I.R. All authors have read and agreed to the published version of the manuscript.

Funding: This research received no external funding.

Institutional Review Board Statement: The study was conducted in accordance with the Declaration of Helsinki and approved by the Institutional Review Board of Monza San Gerardo (n. 3116/March 2019).

Informed Consent Statement: Informed consent was obtained from all subjects involved in the study.

Data Availability Statement: Data supporting the reported results can be found in a specific archived database generated during the study and they are available upon reasonable request.

Conflicts of Interest: The authors declare no conflict of interest.

References

1. Rortveit, G.; Subak, L.L.; Thom, D.H.; Creasman, J.M.; Vittinghoff, E.; Eeden, S.K.V.D.; Brown, J.S. Urinary Incontinence, Fecal Incontinence and Pelvic Organ Prolapse in a Population-Based, Racially Diverse Cohort. *Urogynecology* **2010**, *16*, 278–283. [CrossRef]
2. Wu, J.M.M.; Vaughan, C.P.M.; Goode, P.S.; Redden, D.T.; Burgio, K.L.; Richter, H.E.; Markland, A.D.D. Prevalence and Trends of Symptomatic Pelvic Floor Disorders in U.S. Women. *Obstet. Gynecol.* **2014**, *123*, 141–148. [CrossRef] [PubMed]
3. Kenne, K.A.; Wendt, L.; Jackson, J.B. Prevalence of pelvic floor disorders in adult women being seen in a primary care setting and associated risk factors. *Sci. Rep.* **2022**, *12*, 9878. [CrossRef] [PubMed]
4. Nygaard, I. Prevalence of Symptomatic Pelvic Floor Disorders in US Women. *JAMA* **2008**, *300*, 1311–1316. [CrossRef]
5. Hallock, J.L.; Handa, V.L. The Epidemiology of Pelvic Floor Disorders and Childbirth. *Obstet. Gynecol. Clin. N. Am.* **2016**, *43*, 1–13. [CrossRef]
6. Norton, P.A.; Allen-Brady, K.; Wu, J.; Egger, M.; Cannon-Albright, L. Clinical characteristics of women with familial pelvic floor disorders. *Int. Urogynecology J.* **2014**, *26*, 401–406. [CrossRef] [PubMed]
7. Coyne, K.S.; Sexton, C.C.; Irwin, D.E.; Kopp, Z.S.; Kelleher, C.J.; Milsom, I. The impact of overactive bladder, incontinence and other lower urinary tract symptoms on quality of life, work productivity, sexuality and emotional well-being in men and women: Results from the EPIC study. *BJU Int.* **2008**, *101*, 1388–1395. [CrossRef]
8. Palmieri, S.; De Bastiani, S.S.; Degliuomini, R.; Ruffolo, A.F.; Casiraghi, A.; Vergani, P.; Gallo, P.; Magoga, G.; Cicuti, M.; Parma, M.; et al. Prevalence and severity of pelvic floor disorders in pregnant and postpartum women. *Int. J. Gynecol. Obstet.* **2021**, *158*, 346–351. [CrossRef]
9. Yohay, D.; Weintraub, A.Y.; Mauer-Perry, N.; Peri, C.; Kafri, R.; Yohay, Z.; Bashiri, A. Prevalence and trends of pelvic floor disorders in late pregnancy and after delivery in a cohort of Israeli women using the PFDI-20. *Eur. J. Obstet. Gynecol. Reprod. Biol.* **2016**, *200*, 35–39. [CrossRef]
10. Braga, A.; Barba, M.; Serati, M.; Soligo, M.; Marzi, V.L.; Agrò, E.F.; Musco, S.; Caccia, G.; Castronovo, F.; Manodoro, S.; et al. Update on Italian-validated questionnaires for pelvic floor disorders. *Minerva Obstet. Gynecol.* **2023**, *75*, 62–68. [CrossRef]
11. Metz, M.; Junginger, B.; Henrich, W.; Baeßler, K. Development and Validation of a Questionnaire for the Assessment of Pelvic Floor Disorders and Their Risk Factors During Pregnancy and Post Partum. *Geburtshilfe Frauenheilkd.* **2017**, *77*, 358–365. [CrossRef]
12. Durnea, C.M.; Khashan, A.S.; Kenny, L.C.; Durnea, U.A.; Dornan, J.C.; O'Sullivan, S.M.; O'Reilly, B.A. What is to blame for postnatal pelvic floor dysfunction in primiparous women—Pre-pregnancy or intrapartum risk factors? *Eur. J. Obstet. Gynecol. Reprod. Biol.* **2017**, *214*, 36–43. [CrossRef]
13. Palmieri, S.; Cola, A.; Ceccherelli, A.; Manodoro, S.; Frigerio, M.; Vergani, P. Italian validation of the German Pelvic Floor Questionnaire for pregnant and postpartum women. *Eur. J. Obstet. Gynecol. Reprod. Biol.* **2020**, *248*, 133–136. [CrossRef] [PubMed]

14. Frigerio, M.; Barba, M.; Palmieri, S.; Ruffolo, A.F.; Gallo, P.; Magoga, G.; Manodoro, S.; Vergani, P. On the behalf of the Urogynecology-Pelvic Floor Working Group (GLUP) Prevalence and severity of sexual disorders in the third trimester of pregnancy. *Minerva Obstet. Gynecol.* **2022**. [CrossRef]
15. Cassis, C.; Mukhopadhyay, S.; Morris, E.; Giarenis, I. What happens to female sexual function during pregnancy? *Eur. J. Obstet. Gynecol. Reprod. Biol.* **2021**, *258*, 265–268. [CrossRef]
16. Daud, S.; Zahid, A.Z.M.; Mohamad, M.; Abdullah, B.; Mohamad, N.A.N. Prevalence of sexual dysfunction in pregnancy. Trimester of pregnancy was found to have a significant association with the incidence of sexual dysfunction. *Arch. Gynecol. Obstet.* **2019**, *300*, 1279–1285. [CrossRef] [PubMed]
17. Ozerdogan, N.; Sahin, B.M.; Gursoy, E.; Zeren, F. Sexual dysfunction in the third trimester of pregnancy and postpartum period: A prospective longitudinal study. *J. Obstet. Gynaecol.* **2022**, *42*, 2722–2728. [CrossRef]
18. Frigerio, M.; Barba, M.; Cola, A.; Braga, A.; Celardo, A.; Munno, G.M.; Schettino, M.T.; Vagnetti, P.; De Simone, F.; Di Lucia, A.; et al. Quality of Life, Psychological Wellbeing, and Sexuality in Women with Urinary Incontinence—Where Are We Now: A Narrative Review. *Medicina* **2022**, *58*, 525. [CrossRef] [PubMed]
19. Franco, E.M.; Parés, D.; Colomé, N.L.; Paredes, J.R.M.; Tardiu, L.A. Urinary incontinence during pregnancy. Is there a difference between first and third trimester? *Eur. J. Obstet. Gynecol. Reprod. Biol.* **2014**, *182*, 86–90. [CrossRef]
20. Bugge, C.; Strachan, H.; Pringle, S.; Hagen, S.; Cheyne, H.; Wilson, D. Should pregnant women know their individual risk of future pelvic floor dysfunction? A qualitative study. *BMC Pregnancy Childbirth* **2022**, *22*, 161. [CrossRef]
21. Dumoulin, C.; Cacciari, L.P.; Hay-Smith, E.J.C. Pelvic floor muscle training versus no treatment, or inactive control treatments, for urinary incontinence in women. *Cochrane Database Syst. Rev.* **2018**, *2018*, CD005654. [CrossRef] [PubMed]
22. Hagen, S.; Glazener, C.; McClurg, D.; Macarthur, C.; Elders, A.; Herbison, P.; Logan, J. Pelvic floor muscle training for secondary prevention of pelvic organ prolapse (PREVPROL): A multicentre randomised controlled trial. *Lancet* **2017**, *389*, 393–402. [CrossRef] [PubMed]
23. Sobhgol, S.S.; Priddis, H.; Smith, C.A.; Dahlen, H.G. The Effect of Pelvic Floor Muscle Exercise on Female Sexual Function during Pregnancy and Postpartum: A Systematic Review. *Sex. Med. Rev.* **2018**, *7*, 13–28. [CrossRef]
24. Franco, M.M.; Pena, C.C.; de Freitas, L.M.; Antônio, F.I.; Lara, L.A.; Ferreira, C.H.J. Pelvic Floor Muscle Training Effect in Sexual Function in Postmenopausal Women: A Randomized Controlled Trial. *J. Sex. Med.* **2021**, *18*, 1236–1244. [CrossRef] [PubMed]
25. Xu, P.; Wang, X.; Guo, P.; Zhang, W.; Mao, M.; Feng, S. The effectiveness of eHealth interventions on female pelvic floor dysfunction: A systematic review and meta-analysis. *Int. Urogynecology J.* **2022**, *33*, 3325–3354. [CrossRef]
26. Lipschuetz, M.; Cohen, S.M.; Liebergall-Wischnitzer, M.; Zbedat, K.; Hochner-Celnikier, D.; Lavy, Y.; Yagel, S. Degree of bother from pelvic floor dysfunction in women one year after first delivery. *Eur. J. Obstet. Gynecol. Reprod. Biol.* **2015**, *191*, 90–94. [CrossRef]
27. Jelovsek, J.E.; Barber, M.D. Women seeking treatment for advanced pelvic organ prolapse have decreased body image and quality of life. *Am. J. Obstet. Gynecol.* **2006**, *194*, 1455–1461. [CrossRef]
28. Swenson, C.W.; DePorre, J.A.; Haefner, J.K.; Berger, M.B.; Fenner, D.E. Postpartum depression screening and pelvic floor symptoms among women referred to a specialty postpartum perineal clinic. *Am. J. Obstet. Gynecol.* **2018**, *218*, 335.e1–335.e6. [CrossRef]
29. Hullfish, K.L.; Fenner, D.E.; Sorser, S.A.; Visger, J.; Clayton, A.; Steers, W.D. Postpartum depression, urge urinary incontinence, and overactive bladder syndrome: Is there an association? *Int. Urogynecology J.* **2007**, *18*, 1121–1126. [CrossRef]
30. Vrijens, D.; Berghmans, B.; Nieman, F.; van Os, J.; Van Koeveringe, G.; Leue, C. Prevalence of anxiety and depressive symptoms and their association with pelvic floor dysfunctions—A cross sectional cohort study at a Pelvic Care Centre. *Neurourol. Urodyn.* **2017**, *36*, 1816–1823. [CrossRef]

Disclaimer/Publisher's Note: The statements, opinions and data contained in all publications are solely those of the individual author(s) and contributor(s) and not of MDPI and/or the editor(s). MDPI and/or the editor(s) disclaim responsibility for any injury to people or property resulting from any ideas, methods, instructions or products referred to in the content.

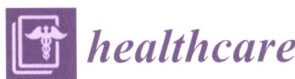

Article

Functional Exercise Versus Specific Pelvic Floor Exercise: Observational Pilot Study in Female University Students

Esther Díaz-Mohedo [1], Itxaso Odriozola Aguirre [2], Elena Molina García [3], Miguel Angel Infantes-Rosales [1,*] and Fidel Hita-Contreras [4]

1. Department of Physiotherapy, University of Málaga, 29016 Málaga, Spain
2. Freelance Physiotherapist, 31000 Pamplona, Spain
3. Freelance Physiotherapist, 29000 Málaga, Spain
4. Department of Physiotherapy, University of Jaén, 23071 Jaén, Spain
* Correspondence: mainfantes@uma.es

Abstract: Objectives: To evaluate the electromyographic (EMG) activity of the pelvic floor musculature (PFM) that takes place when performing the functional movement screen (FMS) exercise, comparing it with the activation in the maximum voluntary contraction of PFM in the supine position (MVC-SP) and standing (MVC-ST). Material and Methods: A descriptive, observational study conducted in two phases. In the first study phase, the baseline EMG activity of PFM was measured in the supine position and standing during MVC-SP and MVC-ST and during the execution of the seven exercises that make up the FMS. In the second phase of the study, the baseline EMG activity of PFM was measured in the supine position and standing during MVC-SP and MVC-ST and during the FMS exercise that produced the most EMG in the pilot phase: trunk stability push-up (PU). ANOVA, Friedman's and Pearson's tests were used. Results: All FMS exercises performed in the pilot phase showed a value below 100% maximum voluntary contraction (MVC) except PU, which presented an average value of 101.3 μv (SD = 54.5): 112% MVC (SD = 37.6). In the second phase of the study, it was observed that there were no significant differences ($p = 0.087$) between the three exercises performed: MVC-SP, MVC-ST and PU (39.2 μv (SD = 10.4), 37.5 μv (SD = 10.4) and 40.7 μv (SD = 10.2), respectively). Conclusions: There is no evidence of the existence of significant differences in EMG activation in PFM among the three exercises analysed: MVC-SP, MVC-ST and PU. The results show better EMG values in the functional exercise of PU.

Keywords: pelvic floor; functional exercise; Kegel exercise; electromyography; women; push-up

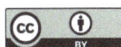

1. Introduction

Urinary incontinence is very common in women of all ages; its prevalence in Europe and America varies between 5% and 42% [1,2]. Currently, the non-pharmacological and non-surgical treatment of urinary incontinence includes PFM training as first-line therapy (recommendation level A) [3,4], demonstrating its short-term efficacy [5–10]. However, the long-term efficacy of these exercises largely depends on adherence to the treatment [2]. Different systems have been used, such as electromyographic biofeedback [11,12] and mobile applications, with the aim of improving this aspect, showing a good but insufficient potential result [13]. Thus, it is still necessary to propose new therapeutic strategies that improve treatment adherence.

Nowadays, due to changes in lifestyle, so-called functional exercise or training is gaining special relevance due to its numerous benefits, and it has attracted a considerable part of the population to practice this type of training [14–16] in sports centres, which includes deep squats and trunk stability push-ups, among many others. These exercises are gathered in the FMS, which is a popular set of tests that evaluate the functionality and quality of movement; it consists of seven basic mobility tests that require a balance between mobility and stability (including motor control) [17]. Its inter- and intra-observer reliability has been demonstrated, and it is used to explore the functional asymmetries of the locomotor system and stability deficits [18–20]. In some cases, FMS exercises have been combined with diagnostic techniques, such as EMG, to identify the degree of activation of a specific muscle group during the execution of a certain movement [21].

The pelvic floor in women may be the only area of the body where the positive effect of physical activity and exercise has been questioned: exercising women have three times the risk of experiencing urinary incontinence [22,23]. In a recent review [24], Bø brought to light the existing controversy, describing two opposing and possible hypotheses on the effect of physical activity on the pelvic floor: (a) general exercise training strengthens the pelvic floor: exercise could lead to a co-contraction of the PFM, creating an indirect training effect, and (b) general exercise training overloads, stretches and weakens the pelvic floor: physical activity increases intra-abdominal pressure (IAP) and the PFM is not able to activate and co-contract quickly or strongly enough to counteract this increased pressure.

Regarding Theory (b), two exercise modalities may increase IAP to a greater extent than others and, thus, possibly affect the pelvic floor and contribute to the incidence, progression or recurrence of pelvic floor disorders [25]: strength training and high-impact activities.

It is important to consider FMS exercise as a strength exercise; understanding whether FMS exercise might predispose to, or prevent, dysfunction of the pelvic floor and, thus, these conditions is important. The aim of this exploratory study is to evaluate, through EMG, the degree of activation of PFM that takes place when performing the PU exercise included in FMS in nulliparous and continent women, comparing it with the activation that occurs in MVC-SP and MVC-ST.

2. Material and Methods

2.1. Study Design

The design of this study corresponds to an observational approach with a descriptive aim and a prospective, cross-sectional, temporal sequence performed in two phases: the pilot phase and the execution phase. The study was approved by the Andalusian Biomedical Research Ethics Portal (Ref: 1103-N-20), and the data were gathered in the Faculty of Health Sciences of the University of Málaga (Spain) between October 2021 and December 2021, following the principles of the Declaration of Helsinki and the rules of good clinical practice.

2.2. Participants and Inclusion Criteria

The participants were recruited by opportunistic sampling among the postgraduate physiotherapy students of the University of Málaga (Spain); 37 women, who represented 34.9% of the selected population, volunteered to participate in the study without receiving any economic or academic compensation. The candidates were supplied with a comprehensive description of the aim and methods of each type of study.

The inclusion criteria were: women aged between 18 and 40 years, nulliparous, continent (0 points in the ICIQ-SF), with a body mass index (BMI) between 18 and 30 kg/m^2, medically healthy, capable of performing the exercises included in the FMS and a good understanding of the Spanish language. The exclusion criteria were: pain, PFM strength below 3 according to the Modified Oxford Scale, a history of urogynecological or lumbopelvic surgery and/or pelvic floor or lumbopelvic dysfunctions, acute urinary or vaginal infection, pregnancy, menopause and neurological alterations.

After obtaining their informed consent, a personal history was taken from each participant. Six women were excluded (2 participants for presenting pain during the vaginal exploration, 2 for having a score above 0 in ICIQ-SF, 1 for the muscular balance of PFM < 3 according to the Modified Oxford Scale, and 1 for acute vaginal infection). Lastly, 31 women who met the inclusion criteria participated in the study: 6 of them in the first phase of the pilot study and 25 in the second phase of the definitive intervention (Figure 1).

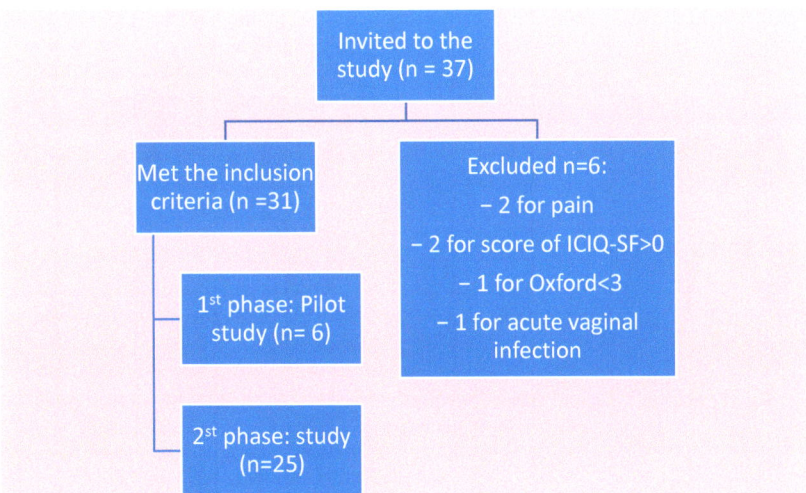

Figure 1. Flowchart of the participants of the study.

2.3. Study Variables

The demographic data included age, height, weight, level of physical activity, use of contraceptives and smoking. To evaluate PFM strength and the level of physical activity, the Oxford Modified Scale and the International Physical Activity Questionnaire (IPAQ) (short version) [26] were used, respectively.

In the first (pilot) phase of the study, 6 women had their PFM baseline EMG activity measured in the supine position (BASP) and standing (BAST), during MVC-SP and MVC-ST, as well as during the execution of the 7 exercises that make up the FMS: overhead squat, hurdle step, in-line lunge, shoulder mobility, rotatory stability, active straight leg raise and trunk stability push-up.

In the second phase of the study, the remaining 25 women had their PFM baseline EMG activity measured in the supine position (BASP) and standing (BAST) during MVC-SP and MVC-ST and during the execution of the FMS exercise that produced the most EMG activity in the pilot phase: trunk stability push-up (PU).

The EMG measurements were carried out using an intravaginal Periform® probe (Neen Performance Health International Ltd., Sutton-in-Ashfield, UK), and the EMG signals were gathered through wireless PODs connected to the intravaginal probe, which allowed the transmission and visualisation of the data instantaneously at the central unit (PHENIX® Liberty, VIVALTIS, Montpellier, France).

Surface EMG (sEMG) amplitude data are strongly influenced by detection conditions. One solution for this problem is the normalisation of the sEMG signal to a reference value. The most common method is referred to as MVC-normalisation, referring to a maximum voluntary contraction performed both in the supine position (MVC-SP) and standing (MVC-ST). The sEMG level is then expressed as % MVC [27]. The mean of the peak values obtained in each repetition of FMS, divided by the reference value of MVC-SP and MVC-ST, determines the PFM activation level during the exercise (% MVC-SP and % MVC-ST, respectively).

2.4. Study Protocol

All measurements were performed to create only one set of data by two physiotherapists specialised in urogynecology. The participants did not perform any intense physical exercise within 24 h before the recordings in order to prevent possible alterations in the execution of the exercises, conducting the test in the first morning hours to minimise the potential impact of fatigue on the results.

Prior to the recording of the measurements through EMG, the participants were asked to empty their bladders and were briefed on how to contract their PFM correctly, controlling the parasite contraction of the neighbouring muscles (adductors, glutei and superficial abdominal wall) and/or the reversal of the perineal order through vaginal bidigital palpations in the supine position in triple flexion, using nitrile gloves with a small amount of water-based hypoallergenic lubricant. The briefing they received for the contraction of PFM was "squeeze and lift my fingers as strongly as you can", and they did not receive any feedback about the test. Once the correct contraction was ensured, they were asked to perform an MVC, and PFM strength was classified according to the Oxford Modified Scale [21].

Subsequently, the superficial EMG of PFM was measured, placing the intravaginal probe with water-based hypoallergenic lubricant and verifying its correct position to prevent EMG signal noise [25].

In the pilot phase of the study, 6 women were randomly selected among the participants. Firstly, measurements were recorded in the supine position (with the feet of the participant leaning on the stretcher): (a) BASP for 30 s, and (b) the EMG activity of MVC-SP in 3 contractions of 5 s each, leaving 1 min of rest between each repetition. Then, the same procedure was repeated with the participant standing: (a) BAST of PFM in the orthostatic position for 30 s, and (b) the EMG activity of MVC-ST in 3 contractions of 5 s each, leaving 1 min of rest between each repetition. Once these values were recorded, the maximum EMG activity of PFM was measured during the execution of the 7 exercises that make up the FMS. It is important to mention that the participants were not asked to contract PFM directly, but to perform the different tests correctly, taking the FMS guidelines as a reference [26]. A total of three repetitions of each exercise were recorded, followed by 1 min of rest between each of the exercises included in the FMS.

In the second phase of the study, the rest of the sample (25 women) had their EMG activity of PFM measured in 3 exercises, executed in a randomised order: MVC-SP, MVC-ST and the FMS exercise that produced the most EMG activity in the previous pilot phase: PU. As in the pilot phase, the participants were not directly asked to contract their PFM but to perform the PU exercise correctly, with the same references and repetitions as in the previous phase (Figure 2).

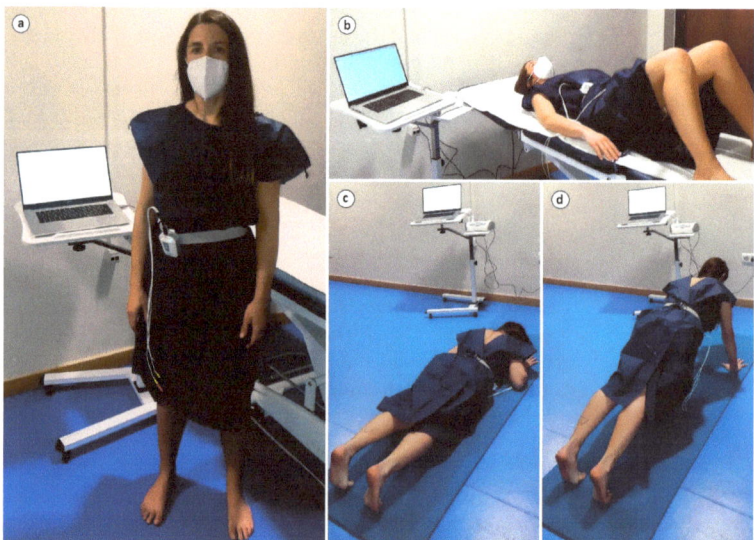

Figure 2. EMG activity measured in (**a**) the supine position (BASP), (**b**) standing (BAST) and (**c**,**d**) trunk stability push-up (PU).

2.5. Statistical Analysis

The repeated measures ANOVA test and Friedman's test were used to identify differences in the measurements of the three exercises. To explore the correlation between numerical variables, Pearson's correlation coefficient was used. All the statistical analyses were carried out using the statistical software Jamovi v1.6 (The Jamovi Project. Sydney, Australia) [28–30].

3. Results

The demographic data of all participants are shown in Table 1. The average age of the participants was 26 years ($SD = 3.2$), the mean BMI was 22.3 kg/m^2 ($SD = 3.3$) and the average muscle balance in the exploration was 4.3 ($SD = 0.7$).

Table 1. Demographic data of the participants.

Demographic Data (n = 31)		
	Mean (SD)	Range
Age	25.9 (3.0)	23.0–38.0
BMI	22.3 (3.1)	18.3–29.7
Muscular balance (Oxford)	4.3 (0.7)	(3–5)
Hormonal contraceptives (yes, no (%))	2 (6.4%)	
Smoking (yes, no (%))	4 (12.9%)	
Moderate physical activity level	20 (64.5%)	

All the tests and exercises of the FMS performed by the six participants in the pilot phase showed a value under 100% MVC (both SP and ST) except PU, which obtained a mean value of 101.3 µv ($SD = 54.5$), that is, 112% MVC ($SD = 37.6$); therefore, this exercise was selected for the next phase of the study.

In the second phase, the remaining 25 women continued with the study protocol, performing only PU from the FMS. The results are presented in Table 2.

Table 2. Electromyographic values (µV and % MVC) of baseline activity in the supine position (BASP) and standing (BAST), and maximum voluntary contraction in the supine position (MVC-SP), standing (MVC-ST) and during the push-up (PU) exercise.

EMG Activity of PFM (µV) (n = 25)		
Measures	Mean (SD)	Range
BASP	4.0 (3.2)	1.0–16.0
BAST	6.8 (3.7)	2.0–17.0
MVC-SP	39.2 (10.4)	21.7–57.3
MVC-ST	37.5 (10.4)	18.0–57.3
PU	40.7 (10.2)	17.3–55.7
PU/MVC-SP Ratio (%)	112 (42.6)	33.8–225
PU/MVC-ST Ratio (%)	118 (45.0)	41.9–236

Abbreviations: baseline activity in the supine position (BASP), baseline activity standing (BAST), maximum voluntary contraction in the supine position (MVC-SP), maximum voluntary contraction standing (MVC-ST), push-up (PU), the ratio of push-up/maximum voluntary contraction in the supine position (Ratio PU/MVC-SP) and the ratio of push-up/maximum voluntary contraction standing (Ratio PU/MVC-ST).

We used Shapiro–Wilk tests and Q-Q graphs and found no evidence against normality in any of the main variables: MVC-SP, MVC-ST, PU, PU/MVC-SP and PU/MVC-ST ($p > 0.274$ in all cases).

Neither the parametric ANOVA test of repeated measures ($p = 0.365$) nor Friedman's non-parametric test ($p = 0.087$) revealed differences between the three exercises (MVC-SP, MVC-ST and PU). The data did not deviate from normality.

A 95% confidence interval for PU/MVC-SP and PU/MVC-ST ratios with respect to MVC were [99–136] and [94–129], respectively.

The PU exercise does not appear to be inferior in terms of MSP activation with respect to MVC-SP and MVC-ST.

Among the biometric variables, a significant correlation was only found for BMIs with an MVC-SP/PU ratio of $r = 0.473$, $p = 0.017$ and with an MVC-ST/PU ratio of $r = 0.426$, $p = 0.034$.

4. Discussion

The present study has analysed and compared the EMG activity of PFM during the PU exercise of the FMS in 25 nulliparous and continent women with maximum voluntary contractions of PFM in the supine position and standing (MVC-SP and MVC-ST, respectively). The results show no evidence of significant differences between the three analysed exercises. Despite the fact that the participants were not asked to voluntarily activate their PFM during the execution of the PU exercise, the latter presented better EMG values than MVC-SP and MVC-ST.

With the aim of justifying the influence of exercise on the integrity of the pelvic floor, two exercise modalities have been reported to increase IAP to a greater extent than others, and thus they may have a negative effect on the pelvic floor: extenuating strength training (e.g., weight lifting), and high-impact activities, such as jumping and running [24]. The habitual practice of the PU exercise, often included in current training and physical activity programmes (similar to the typical "planking"), is not contemplated within such group; therefore, its recommendation in healthy women should not be banished.

The PU exercise is defined as an exercise for the training and valuation of lumbopelvic stability. Thus, it is logical that, during its correct execution, given the direct activation of the transverse abdominal muscle (whose fibres are directly connected to those of the transverse perineal muscle) [31], PFM participates by playing one of its main functions: lumbopelvic stabilisation [32–34]. During its execution, a pattern of global trunk stability is required, connecting the lower and upper parts of the body, thereby producing an unconscious and/or reflex co-contraction of the PFM [35], which could explain the EMG activation achieved. Such a result, in our opinion, creates an indirect training effect that contributes to reducing the levator ani hiatal area by causing the hypertrophy and shortening of the surrounding muscles, thus lifting the pelvic floor and the internal organs to a higher pelvic location. Theoretically, such morphological changes could reduce the risk of urinary incontinence, faecal incontinence and pelvic organ prolapse [24].

Moreover, the correlation between % MVC in the supine and standing positions and BMI could be due to the generation of a greater increase of IAP at higher BMI values, which would be in line with previous studies [36–38]. This increase in IAP would generate a greater PFM activity, with the aim of maintaining pelvic visceral statics and guaranteeing continence.

In any case, the IAP generated and managed during the exercise is still a controversial topic. Different studies clearly show that the maximum values of IAP have a wider range among women who perform the same standardised activity [39], and the maximum IAPs vary among studies for the same activity, partly due to the instruments used to measure IAP, the way in which maximum IAP is created, and the differences between populations [24]. In the same line, an interesting study questioned the idea that "safe" exercises for the pelvic floor generate lower IAPs than conventional exercises since no differences were found in the IAP values between the recommended and ill-advised versions of half of the exercises [21]. Another study highlights that the activities that are generally restricted after surgery may generate lower IAP values than non-restricted activities (e.g., the maximum average IAP was higher when the participant stood up from a chair than climbing stairs, doing crunches and lifting weights) [25].

However, EMGs do not provide information about the real effect of IAP increase on the statics and displacement of intra-pelvic structures. In this sense, the possible development of imaging techniques that allow observing, in real-time, the displacement of the pelvic organs in situations of IAP increase or muscular activation is in the hands of bioengineering.

It is fundamental to consider the fact that the EMG values in the three types of contraction tests were similar in a young sample capable of performing a high activation of their PFM. The reproduction of this study in a larger and more representative sample, as well as the comparison of the results with women in whom the pelvic floor function can be affected by age, high BMI values, vaginal births and the habitual practice of risk exercises (extenuating strength training, running or jumping), will be an interesting aspect to explore in future studies [40].

It is widely accepted that the effectiveness of exercises for PFM depends on the adherence of the patient to them, essentially derived from self-efficacy, finding a positive correlation between the two factors (effectiveness–self-efficacy) [2,41,42]. In healthy and nulliparous women, this could be a good strategy to prevent pelvic floor dysfunction (especially urinary incontinence), encouraging them to practise this type of functional exercise in sports centres, where there may be greater self-efficacy due to the belief about the benefits derived from it (general and indirect benefits on the pelvic floor), as well as a better capacity to execute them and the social support received. This could generate behavioural changes in the attitude of women, which will make them participate more actively and with greater commitment in their preventive treatment, minimising the dropout rates in PFM training derived from the responsibility of performing the Kegel exercises on their own without receiving any feedback.

In any case, due to the existing knowledge gaps and the lack of further research, it is not possible to draw solid conclusions about the effect of physical activity on the rate of pelvic floor dysfunctions, highlighting the need for more high-quality studies that clarify this aspect [24].

Limitations of the Study

Although EMG is a method that allows us to evaluate muscle activity in an objective and reliable manner, it is necessary to mention the cross-talk phenomenon. This is defined as the recorded EMG activity that comes from the neighbouring muscles rather than exclusively from the study target muscles [43,44], which could alter the final results and lead to erroneous interpretations. During functional exercises, large muscle groups are activated, such as the gluteus maximus, and although its influence on the EMG result has not been demonstrated yet, this factor should be taken into account.

It is also important to consider motion artifacts, which can distort the EMG signal. This study used a wireless system and a Periform® probe, due to its pear shape and the longitudinal placement of the metallic plates, with the aim of reducing such phenomenon, although it is necessary to develop new intravaginal EMG probe designs in order to improve EMG measurements in research and in clinical practice [25].

Moreover, three repetitions of each exercise were used, which does not guarantee a good activation of the musculature with the increase in repetitions. That is, further information is required about the fatigability of PFM, both in a session and in the long term between sessions.

The data provided by this pilot study "tend" to explain that PU can activate PFM muscles; however, it is necessary to carry out more robust methodological and statistical research with larger samples to advance such statements.

In addition to expanding the sample, it is also necessary to include other symptomatic and/or older populations in order to continue defining new prevention and treatment protocols for perineal health and new types of training that increase the adherence of users.

5. Conclusions

In the nulliparous and continent women of our sample, there was no evidence of significant differences in the EMG activation of PFM between the three exercises analysed: MVC-SP, MVC-ST and PU. The results show better EMG values in PFM for the functional exercise of PU. This functional exercise, which is often included in current functional training programmes, may be, on one hand, training the PFM indirectly and, on the other hand, promoting behavioural changes in the attitude of women that could encourage them to participate more actively and with greater commitment in their preventive treatment, thus minimising the dropout rates that occur with classic PFM training.

Author Contributions: Conceptualization, E.D.-M. and F.H.-C.; methodology, E.D.-M. and M.A.I.-R.; software, E.M.G. and I.O.A.; validation, E.D.-M. and E.M.G.; formal analysis, F.H.-C.; investigation, E.D.-M. and I.O.A.; resources, I.O.A. and E.M.G.; data curation, M.A.I.-R.; writing—original draft preparation, E.D.-M. and I.O.A.; writing—review and editing, F.H.-C.; visualization, M.A.I.-R.; supervision, F.H.-C. and E.M.G.; project administration, E.D.-M. All authors have read and agreed to the published version of the manuscript.

Funding: This research received no external funding.

Institutional Review Board Statement: The study was approved by the Andalusian Biomedical Research Ethics Portal (Ref: 1103-N-20).

Informed Consent Statement: Informed consent was obtained from all subjects involved in the study.

Data Availability Statement: Data sharing not applicable.

Acknowledgments: PHENIX® Liberty, VIVALTIS, for their support and the equipment provided for this study.

Conflicts of Interest: The authors declare no conflict of interest.

References

1. Chiaffarino, F.; Parazzini, F.; Lavezzari, M.; Giambanco, V. Gruppo Interdisciplinare di Studio Incontinenza Urinaria (GISIU) Impact of urinary incontinence and overactive bladder on quality of life. *Eur. Urol.* **2003**, *43*, 535–538. [CrossRef] [PubMed]
2. Medrano Sánchez, E.M.; Suárez Serrano, C.M.; De la Casa Almeida, M.; Díaz Mohedo, E.; Chillón Martínez, R. Spanish version of the broome pelvic muscle self-efficacy scale: Validity and reliability. *Phys. Ther.* **2013**, *93*, 1696–1706. [CrossRef]
3. Abrams, P.; Cardozo, L.; Fall, M.; Griffiths, D.; Rosier, P.; Ulmsten, U.; van Kerrebroeck, P.; Victor, A.; Wein, A. Standardisation Sub-committee of the International Continence Society. The standardisation of terminology of lower urinary tract function: Report from the Standardisation Sub-committee of the International Continence Society. *Neurourol. Urodyn.* **2002**, *21*, 167–178. [CrossRef] [PubMed]
4. Díaz-Mohedo, E. *Guía de Práctica Clínica para Fisioterapeutas en la Incontinencia Urinaria Femenina*; Colegio Profesional de Fisioterapeutas de Andalucía: Sevilla, Spain, 2011.
5. Bø, K.; Talseth, T.; Holme, I. Single blind, randomised controlled trial of pelvic floor exercises, electrical stimulation, vaginal cones, and no treatment in management of genuine stress incontinence in women. *BMJ* **1999**, *318*, 487–493. [CrossRef]
6. Laycock, J.; Brown, J.; Cusack, C.; Green, S.; Jerwood, D.; Mann, K.; McLachlan, Z.; Schofield, A. Pelvic floor reeducation for stress incontinence: Comparing three methods. *Br. J. Community Nurs.* **2001**, *6*, 230–237. [CrossRef] [PubMed]
7. Bø, K.; Talseth, T. Long-term effect of pelvic floor muscle exercise 5 years after cessation of organized training. *Obstet. Gynecol.* **1996**, *87*, 261–265. [CrossRef]
8. Glazener, C.M.A.; Herbison, G.P.; MacArthur, C.; Grant, A.; Wilson, P.D. Randomised controlled trial of conservative management of postnatal urinary and faecal incontinence: Six year follow up. *BMJ* **2005**, *330*, 337. [CrossRef] [PubMed]
9. Bø, K.; Kvarstein, B.; Nygaard, I. Lower urinary tract symptoms and pelvic floor muscle exercise adherence after 15 years. *Obstet. Gynecol.* **2005**, *105*, 999–1005. [CrossRef]
10. Soltero González, A.; Campoy Martínez, P.; Barrero Candau, R.; Medrano Sánchez, E.; Pérez Pérez, M.; Rodríguez Pérez, A. Rehabilitation in female stress urinary incontinence. *Arch. Esp. Urol.* **2002**, *55*, 1035–1046.
11. Nunes, E.F.C.; Sampaio, L.M.M.; Biasotto-Gonzalez, D.A.; Nagano, R.C.D.R.; Lucareli, P.R.G.; Politti, F. Biofeedback for pelvic floor muscle training in women with stress urinary incontinence: A systematic review with meta-analysis. *Physiotherapy* **2019**, *105*, 10–23. [CrossRef] [PubMed]

12. Zhang, Q.; Wang, L.; Zheng, W. Surface electromyography of pelvic floor muscles in stress urinary incontinence. *Int. J. Gynaecol. Obstet. Off. Organ Int. Fed. Gynaecol. Obstet.* **2006**, *95*, 177–178. [CrossRef] [PubMed]
13. Latorre, G.F.S.; de Fraga, R.; Seleme, M.R.; Mueller, C.V.; Berghmans, B. An ideal e-health system for pelvic floor muscle training adherence: Systematic review. *Neurourol. Urodyn.* **2019**, *38*, 63–80. [CrossRef]
14. Thompson, W. Worldwide Survey of Fitness Trends for 2018 The CREP Edition Apply It. *ACSM Health Fit. J.* **2017**, *21*, 10–19. [CrossRef]
15. Thompson, W. Worldwide Survey of Fitness Trends for 2019. *ACSM's Health Fit. J.* **2018**, *22*, 10–17. [CrossRef]
16. Thompson, W. Worldwide Survey of Fitness Trends for 2020. *ACSM's Health Fit. J.* **2019**, *23*, 10–18. [CrossRef]
17. Teyhen, D.S.; Shaffer, S.W.; Lorenson, C.L.; Halfpap, J.P.; Donofry, D.F.; Walker, M.J.; Dugan, J.L.; Childs, J.D. The Functional Movement Screen: A reliability study. *J. Orthop. Sports Phys. Ther.* **2012**, *42*, 530–540. [CrossRef]
18. Cook, G.; Burton, L.; Hoogenboom, B.J.; Voight, M. Functional movement screening: The use of fundamental movements as an assessment of function—Part 1. *Int. J. Sports Phys. Ther.* **2014**, *9*, 396–409.
19. Minick, K.I.; Kiesel, K.B.; Burton, L.; Taylor, A.; Plisky, P.; Butler, R.J. Interrater reliability of the functional movement screen. *J. Strength Cond. Res.* **2010**, *24*, 479–486. [CrossRef]
20. Bonazza, N.A.; Smuin, D.; Onks, C.A.; Silvis, M.L.; Dhawan, A. Reliability, Validity, and Injury Predictive Value of the Functional Movement Screen: A Systematic Review and Meta-analysis. *Am. J. Sports Med.* **2017**, *45*, 725–732. [CrossRef]
21. Tian, T.; Budgett, S.; Smalldridge, J.; Hayward, L.; Stinear, J.; Kruger, J. Assessing exercises recommended for women at risk of pelvic floor disorders using multivariate statistical techniques. *Int. Urogynecol. J.* **2018**, *29*, 1447–1454. [CrossRef]
22. Teixeira, R.V.; Colla, C.; Sbruzzi, G.; Mallmann, A.; Paiva, L.L. Prevalence of urinary incontinence in female athletes: A systematic review with meta-analysis. *Int. Urogynecol. J.* **2018**, *29*, 1717–1725. [CrossRef] [PubMed]
23. de Mattos Lourenco, T.R.; Matsuoka, P.K.; Baracat, E.C.; Haddad, J.M. Urinary incontinence in female athletes: A systematic review. *Int. Urogynecol. J.* **2018**, *29*, 1757–1763. [CrossRef] [PubMed]
24. Bø, K.; Nygaard, I.E. Is Physical Activity Good or Bad for the Female Pelvic Floor? A Narrative Review. *Sports Med. Auckl. N. Z.* **2020**, *50*, 471–484. [CrossRef] [PubMed]
25. Weir, L.F.; Nygaard, I.E.; Wilken, J.; Brandt, D.; Janz, K.F. Postoperative activity restrictions: Any evidence? *Obstet. Gynecol.* **2006**, *107*, 305–309. [CrossRef]
26. Puig-Ribera, A.; Martín-Cantera, C.; Puigdomenech, E.; Real, J.; Romaguera, M.; Magdalena-Belio, J.F.; Recio-Rodríguez, J.I.; Rodriguez-Martin, B.; Arietaleanizbeaskoa, M.S.; Repiso-Gento, I.; et al. Screening Physical Activity in Family Practice: Validity of the Spanish Version of a Brief Physical Activity Questionnaire. *PLoS ONE* **2015**, *10*, e0136870. [CrossRef] [PubMed]
27. Burden, A.; Bartlett, R. Normalisation of EMG amplitude: An evaluation and comparison of old and new methods. *Med. Eng. Phys.* **1999**, *21*, 247–257. [CrossRef]
28. PMCMR.pdf. Available online: https://cran.r-project.org/web/packages/PMCMR/PMCMR.pdf (accessed on 5 February 2022).
29. R: The R Project for Statistical Computing. Available online: https://www.r-project.org/ (accessed on 5 February 2022).
30. Dunn, P.K. Statistical Software I Science Research Methods: Software. Available online: https://bookdown.org/pkaldunn/SRM-software/statistical-software.html (accessed on 5 February 2022).
31. Pereira, L.C.; Botelho, S.; Marques, J.; Amorim, C.F.; Lanza, A.H.; Palma, P.; Riccetto, C. Are transversus abdominis/oblique internal and pelvic floor muscles coactivated during pregnancy and postpartum? *Neurourol. Urodyn.* **2013**, *32*, 416–419. [CrossRef]
32. Sapsford, R.R.; Hodges, P.W.; Richardson, C.A.; Cooper, D.H.; Markwell, S.J.; Jull, G.A. Co-activation of the abdominal and pelvic floor muscles during voluntary exercises. *Neurourol. Urodyn.* **2001**, *20*, 31–42. [CrossRef]
33. Capson, A.C.; Nashed, J.; Mclean, L. The role of lumbopelvic posture in pelvic floor muscle activation in continent women. *J. Electromyogr. Kinesiol. Off. J. Int. Soc. Electrophysiol. Kinesiol.* **2011**, *21*, 166–177. [CrossRef]
34. Madill, S.J.; McLean, L. Quantification of abdominal and pelvic floor muscle synergies in response to voluntary pelvic floor muscle contractions. *J. Electromyogr. Kinesiol. Off. J. Int. Soc. Electrophysiol. Kinesiol.* **2008**, *18*, 955–964. [CrossRef]
35. Stüpp, L.; Resende, A.P.M.; Petricelli, C.D.; Nakamura, M.U.; Alexandre, S.M.; Zanetti, M.R.D. Pelvic floor muscle and transversus abdominis activation in abdominal hypopressive technique through surface electromyography. *Neurourol. Urodyn.* **2011**, *30*, 1518–1521. [CrossRef]
36. Altman, D.; Cartwright, R.; Lapitan, M.C.; Milsom, I.; Nelson, R.; Sjöström, S.; Tikkinen, K.A.O. Epidemiology of urinary incontinence (UI) and other lower urinary tract symptoms (LUTS), pelvic organ prolapse (POP) and anal incontinence (AI). In *Incontinence*; Abrams, P., Cardozo, L., Wagg, A., Wein, A.J., Eds.; International Continence Society: Bristol, UK, 2017; pp. 1–141, ISBN 978-0-9569607-3-3.
37. Aboseif, C.; Liu, P. Pelvic Organ Prolapse. In *StatPearls*; StatPearls Publishing: Treasure Island, FL, USA, 2022. Available online: http://www.ncbi.nlm.nih.gov/books/NBK563229/ (accessed on 5 February 2022).
38. Noblett, K.L.; Jensen, J.K.; Ostergard, D.R. The relationship of body mass index to intra-abdominal pressure as measured by multichannel cystometry. *Int. Urogynecol. J. Pelvic Floor Dysfunct.* **1997**, *8*, 323–326. [CrossRef]
39. Nygaard, I.E.; Hamad, N.M.; Shaw, J.M. Activity restrictions after gynecologic surgery: Is there evidence? *Int. Urogynecol. J.* **2013**, *24*, 719–724. [CrossRef]
40. Chmielewska, D.; Stania, M.; Sobota, G.; Kwaśna, K.; Błaszczak, E.; Taradaj, J.; Juras, G. Impact of different body positions on bioelectrical activity of the pelvic floor muscles in nulliparous continent women. *BioMed Res. Int.* **2015**, *2015*, 905897. [CrossRef]

41. Chen, S.-Y.; Tzeng, Y.-L. Path analysis for adherence to pelvic floor muscle exercise among women with urinary incontinence. *J. Nurs. Res. JNR* **2009**, *17*, 83–92. [CrossRef]
42. Messer, K.L.; Hines, S.H.; Raghunathan, T.E.; Seng, J.S.; Diokno, A.C.; Sampselle, C.M. Self-efficacy as a predictor to PFMT adherence in a prevention of urinary incontinence clinical trial. *Health Educ. Behav. Off. Publ. Soc. Public Health Educ.* **2007**, *34*, 942–952. [CrossRef]
43. Keshwani, N.; McLean, L. State of the art review: Intravaginal probes for recording electromyography from the pelvic floor muscles. *Neurourol. Urodyn.* **2015**, *34*, 104–112. [CrossRef]
44. Flury, N.; Koenig, I.; Radlinger, L. Crosstalk considerations in studies evaluating pelvic floor muscles using surface electromyography in women: A scoping review. *Arch. Gynecol. Obstet.* **2017**, *295*, 799–809. [CrossRef]

Disclaimer/Publisher's Note: The statements, opinions and data contained in all publications are solely those of the individual author(s) and contributor(s) and not of MDPI and/or the editor(s). MDPI and/or the editor(s) disclaim responsibility for any injury to people or property resulting from any ideas, methods, instructions or products referred to in the content.

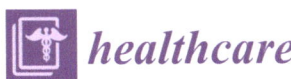

Review

Microbiota Ecosystem in Recurrent Cystitis and the Immunological Microenvironment of Urothelium

Mattia Dominoni [1,2], Annachiara Licia Scatigno [1,2,*], Marco La Verde [3], Stefano Bogliolo [4], Chiara Melito [1,2], Andrea Gritti [1,2], Marianna Francesca Pasquali [1,2], Marco Torella [3] and Barbara Gardella [1,2]

1. Department of Clinical, Surgical, Diagnostic and Paediatric Sciences, University of Pavia, 27100 Pavia, Italy
2. Department of Obstetrics and Gynecology, IRCCS Foundation Policlinico San Matteo, 27100 Pavia, Italy
3. Department of Woman, Child and General and Specialized Surgery, Obstetrics and Gynecology Unit, University of Campania "Luigi Vanvitelli", 81100 Naples, Italy
4. Department of Obstetrics and Gynecological Oncology, P.O del Tigullio" Hospital-ASL4, Metropolitan Area of Genoa, 16034 Genoa, Italy
* Correspondence: annachiara.scatigno@gmail.com; Tel.: +39-038-250-3267; Fax: +39-038-250-3146

Abstract: Urinary tract infections (UTIs) represent one of the most frequent low genital tract diseases in the female population. When UTIs occur with a frequency of at least three times per year or two times in the last six month, we speak of recurrent UTI (rUTI) and up to 70% of women will have rUTI within 1 year. It was previously thought that antibiotic resistance was principally responsible for the recurrence of UTIs, but nowadays new diagnostic technologies have shown the role of microbiota in the pathophysiology of these diseases. Much research has been conducted on the role of gut microbiome in the development of rUTI, while little is known yet about vaginal and urinary microbiome and the possible immunological and microscopical mechanisms through which they trigger symptoms. New discoveries and clinical perspectives are arising, and they all agree that a personalized, multi-modal approach, treating vaginal and urinary dysbiosis, may reduce rUTIs more successfully.

Keywords: recurrent urinary tract infection; vaginal microbiota; urinary microbiota; dysbiosis

1. Introduction

A total of 1.5 million people suffers from urinary tract infections (UTIs) every year, making it one of the most prevalent health problems [1]. Women experience UTIs eight times more often than men [2], and 50–60% of adult women will have at least one UTI in their lifetime, affecting their quality of life and psychological wellbeing [3,4].

Anatomical characteristics, sexual behaviour, urogenital aging, pelvic organ prolapse, urethral diverticula, vescico-vaginal fistula, urinary incontinence, menopause, and pregnancy all represent possible risk factors for women [5].

In clinical practice it may be useful to distinguish between uncomplicated and complicated UTIs. Complicated UTIs are caused by urological anomalies, including indwelling catheters, renal insufficiency, neurogenic bladder, pregnancy, previous urological surgery, and conditions causing an immunocompromised state [6], and these may also progress to sepsis and other systemic illnesses, which mostly impact the kidneys [6].

Recurrent UTIs (rUTIs) are characterised as complicated and/or uncomplicated UTIs that happen at least three times yearly or twice over six months [7,8], differently from persistent infections in which the pathogen is not eradicated but instead persists in some of the infected people's cells [9]. Recurrent UTIs are common; after getting one, 24% of women will get another within 6 months, and up to 70% will get another within a year [10,11]. Six or more episodes of rUTIs occur in at least 35 million women worldwide each year (1% of all women) [10–12].

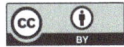

The pathophysiology of rUTIs is not well understood. However, in the 80s, it was already clear that recurrence of UTIs was closely linked to antibiotic resistance [13–15]. The increased use of antibiotics globally, along with prophylactic therapy, contributed to the development of multiresistant bacteria, such as extended-spectrum beta-lactamase-producing bacteria, carbapenemase-resistant organisms, and pan-resistant bacteria [16,17].

Furthermore, the myth that urine is sterile has been dispelled only in recent years by developments in technology and molecular biology, concomitantly with the discovery of the role of microbiota of the bladder, vagina, and gut in the pathophysiology of rUTIs [18–20]. While little is known about the vaginal and urinary microbiomes, a great deal of study has been done on the function of the gut microbiome in the development of rUTIs [21].

The purpose of this review is to highlight potential mechanisms by which the vaginal and urinary microbiomes, as well as the potential role of the urothelial immunological microenvironment, contribute to rUTIs onset in women of different ages (Figure 1).

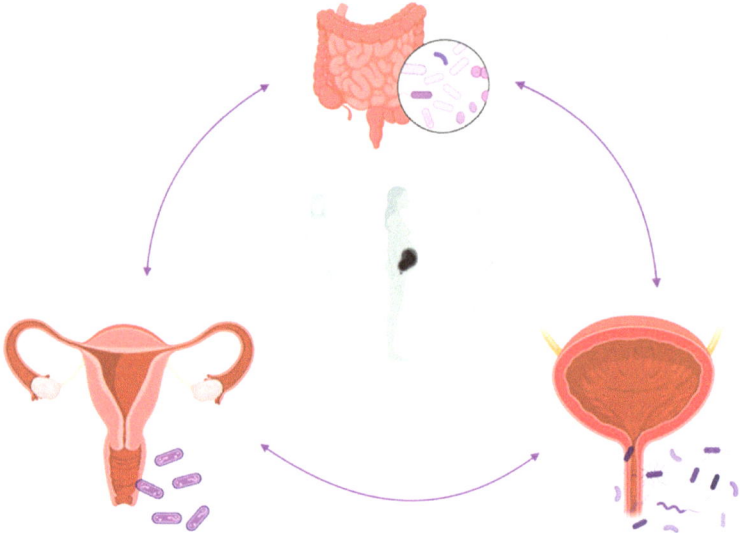

Figure 1. Abstract figure. The interplay between the gut, vaginal, and urinary microbiome in the onset of rUTIs during woman different ages. Figure created with BioRender.com (accessed on 29 January 2023).

2. Materials and Methods

The most significant medical databases, including PubMed, Cochrane Database of Systematic Reviews, EMBASE, and Web of Science, were consulted, according to a combination of the following keywords: "recurrent urinary tract infection, recurrent cystitis, vaginal microbiome, vaginal microbiota, urinary microbiota, urinary microbiome, urobiome, dysbiosis, urinary bladder disease", including pluralization and English spelling variations and suffixes/prefixes. From 2000 until 11 November 2022, we collected all publications, including case studies, literature reviews, and prospective or retrospective trials. Two authors (MD and ALS) independently evaluated the references to incorporate the literature data into the review. Preferred reporting items for systematic reviews and meta-analyses (PRISMA) method was applied to conduct a systematic search (Figure 2).

In the first step, the authors considered the title of the paper, then the abstract, and finally the manuscript. Consequently, the data obtained was collected. Studies were considered qualified if they met the following criteria: (I) the involvement of the vaginal microbiota and microbiome in the onset of rUTIs in female population, (II) the role of the urinary microbiota and microbiome in rUTIs in women, (III) dysbiosis as a cause of recurrent cystitis, and (IV) novel therapeutics approaches in the field of study. Instead, the following were considered exclusion criteria: (I) case reports; (II) conference abstracts, editorials, and pre-prints manuscripts; (III) multimedia; and (IV) papers written in languages other than English.

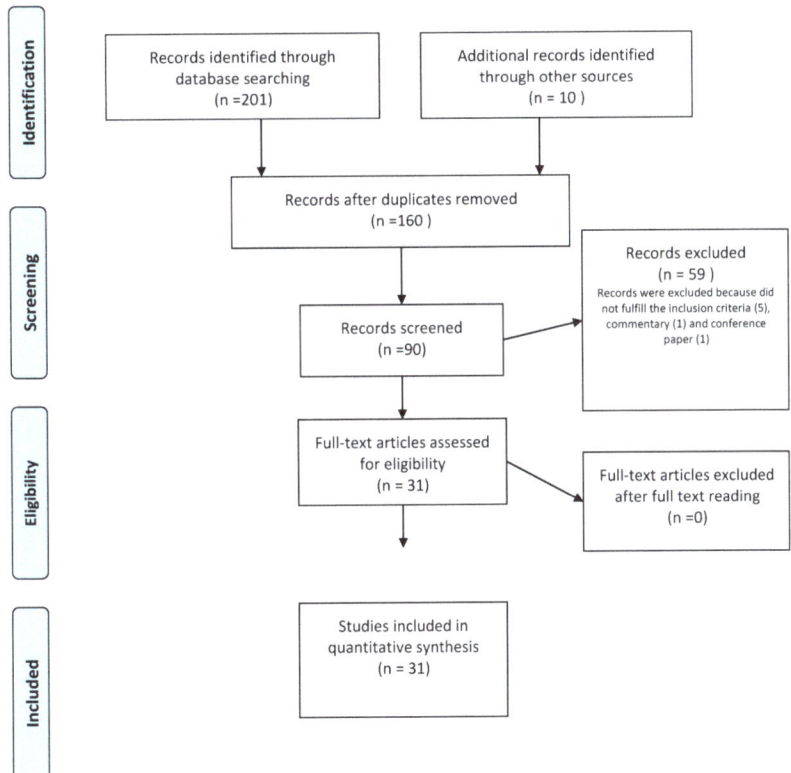

Figure 2. PRISMA flow diagram of study selection process.

To ensure validity and prevent any selection, performance, detection, attrition, and reporting bias, two researchers (MD and ALS) independently assessed the risk of bias for each selected study, in accordance with the Cochrane Handbook for Systematic Reviews of Interventions [22,23]. Conflicts were resolved through discussion between researchers. Finally, the two researchers examined and extracted data separately.

3. Results

The search method provided 201 papers in total and another 10 studies were included through the references. In total, 90 publications were screened by title and/or abstract following the elimination of articles not published in English or published before 2000. Duplicate papers, and irrelevant works were excused from the analysis. In the end, 31 research articles were included and analysed (Figure 1). Table 1 reports the main findings derived from the literature data about the internship between microbiota, immunology, and rUTIs.

3.1. Vaginal Microbiome and rUTIs

The pathogenesis of rUTIs is significantly influenced by the vaginal microenvironment, in contrast to widespread assumption, which attested that bacteria causing UTIs typically originate from the gut altered microbiota, as the only way of infection [24].

Community state types (CSTs) represents a classification used to describe at least five major subcategories of cervico-vaginal bacterial species involved in the maintenance of vaginal balancing between physiological and pathological flora. Each group has a unique mix of bacteria, each with a different relative characteristic. Four of these are dominated by one of the following four species: *L. crispatus* (CST I), *L. gasseri* (CST II), *L. iners* (CST III), or *L. jensenii* (CST V) [25,26].

Instead, CST IV predominantly contains anaerobic bacteria, such *G. vaginalis*, *Atopobium vaginae*, and *Megasphaera spp.*, similar to the vaginal microbiota in bacterial vaginosis [25,26]. Interestingly, a recent meta-analysis reported that *Prevotella bivia*, *G. vaginalis*, *Chlamydia trachomatis*, and *Human Papillomavirus* infections are more common in women with lower levels of *Lactobacillus* in their CST IV cervico-vaginal microbiota than in women with higher levels of *Lactobacillus* [27].

Several *Lactobacillus* species, such as *L. crispatus*, *L. jensenii*, *L. gasseri*, and *L. iners*, constitute most of the vaginal microbiota in women of reproductive age [28–30]. These bacteria produce lactic acid, helping the maintenance of the vaginal acidic pH [31,32].

By creating bacteriocins and hydrogen peroxide, vaginal lactobacilli perform a protective function, inhibiting the colonisation of other potential pathogens, particularly *E. coli* [28,33–36]. For this reason, lower lactobacilli levels promote the insurgence of bacterial vaginosis or vaginal *E. coli* colonisation, which increase the risk of UTI insurgence [30,37–39].

The vagina also represents a reservoir for pathogens: The literature data underlines that women with a history of UTI exhibit more *E. coli* colonisation in the vaginal introitus (>105 CFU/mL), highlighting the importance of vaginal microenvironment in the pathogenesis of rUTIs [40].

S. saprophyticus is the most frequent gram-positive bacterial source of community-acquired UTI. *S. saprophyticus* virulence in in vitro and rat UTI model is based on the following components: Secreted surface-associated proteins Aas (hemagglutinin) and Ssp (lipase), the proteins UafA of cell wall, SdrI, SssF, and UafB, which mediate adherence, and the ureases [30].

By contrast, *S. aureus* and *S. epidermidis* can also cause UTI, especially during catheterization or pregnancy: Experimental models highlighted that the nickel ABC-transporters Opp2 and Opp5a are involved in the pathogenesis of *S. aureus* urinary infection [30,41–44].

Finally, vaginal bacteria, such as *Actinobacteria*, other *Firmicutes*, and gram-negative anaerobic organisms, which are not common uropathogens, may colonise the urinary system, alter the physiological microbiota, and change the immunological assessment of vaginal and bladder mucosa. In other words, even if specific vaginal bacteria do not colonise the bladder or are eliminated by the host prior to the diagnosis of a UTI, brief contact with these bacteria in the urinary tract can still have a significant impact on UTI pathogenesis [30]. This phenomenon is called "covert pathogenesis" [30,45]. For instance, group *B streptococcus* and *G. vaginalis* promote the survival of *E. coli* in the bladder, permitting the development of UTIs [46–48]. Numerous studies have connected *Streptococcus agalactiae* (GBS) colonisation to vulvo-vaginitis [49] and urinary tract infections [50], but none have looked at the connection between vaginal GBS and GBS UTI [30]. GBS colonisation is typically asymptomatic. By contrast, *Gardnerella vaginalis* can also cause UTI and is connected to sepsis, renal disease, and urgency incontinence [30,51], as we better described later (Section 4.2).

3.2. Urinary Microbiome and rUTIs

Modern urine culture techniques have shown that several bacteria allow the maintenance of urothelium homeostasis [52–54]. The host characteristics, which change across people, life, and geographical areas, as well as environmental exposure and behavioural factors, are the most important factors for maintaining the balance of this microbial ecosystem [55].

The most often identified colonising microorganisms in the urine microbiome are *Lactobacillus* and *Streptococcus*, which constitute a barrier against infections, producing factors, which inhibit the adhesion of pathogens to epithelium, such as lactic acid. *Alloscardovia*,

Burkholderia, Jonquetella, Klebsiella, Saccharofermentans, Rhodanobacter, and *Veillonella* are less often identified bacteria [56]. *Proteobacteria* (35.6%), *Firmicutes* (31.3%), *Actinobacteria* (22.4%), *Bacteroidetes* (6.4%), and others (4.3%) are the key phyla of the human urinary tract, according to Morand et al. [57]. The authors attested that the urine microbiota ordinarily contains several uropathogens, but pathogenicity results from an imbalance in their relative percentages and from the host immunological response [58].

From 435 urine samples, Dubourg et al. identified 450 different bacterial species, of which 256 had never been discovered before in urine, while 18 were entirely new [58].

Other recent research suggests that many urinary system diseases, including UTIs and rUTIs, may be influenced by the urine microbiome (or urobiome), which plays a key role in the maintenance of the homeostasis of urothelial microenvironment [59]. Urinary microbiota abnormalities precede UTI onset, and the urobiome normalizes following therapy, as Bossa et al. demonstrated [60].

The knowledge of the urobiome is fundamental in clinical practice because different clinical manifestations are probably connected to a specific urine microbiota modification, as attested by Burnett et al. [61]. Additionally, non-infectious urologic conditions, such as neurogenic bladder dysfunction, interstitial cystitis, and urgency urine incontinence have been associated to changes in the urinary microbiota spectrum [54].

It is interesting to consider in the knowledge of a UTI's pathology and in the importance of health urobiome is the evidence that uropathogenic Escherichia coli (UPEC) has a reservoir also in the bladder epithelium; many investigations in both adults and children, as well as in bladder biopsies, demonstrated intracellular UPEC in bladder epithelial cells that release in urine [62–66]. In addition, 82% of rUTIs are brought on by the same UPEC strain as in the prior infection, even when the proper antibiotic therapy is administered [24,67–71]. The pathogenesis of UPEC is described in Section 4.2.

4. Discussion and Conclusions

4.1. Risk Factors for rUTIs in Women

Hormonal fluctuations have a significant role in the changes in vaginal and urine microbiomes composition; oestrogen promotes *Lactobacillus* development in the bladder and vagina, increasing their defensive role against pathogens and infections. Consequently, loss of oestrogen in postmenopausal women causes a reduction in vaginal lactobacilli and an increase in rUTIs [72,73]. The genitourinary syndrome of menopause is constituted by vaginal epithelium thinning, a decrease in extracellular matrix, proteoglycans and collagens synthesis, and vulvovaginal atrophy [74], which facilitate the penetration of bacteria in urothelium and vaginal epithelium.

For this reason, post-menopausal women are more prone to develop rUTIs, with a rate of 8–11% [75–78]. Regarding vaginal and urinary microbiome composition after menopause, some authors demonstrated that post-menopausal women present fewer distinct bacterial species [79–81], while others supported the development of an increased diversity of species [82].

UTIs are also a common problem among pregnant women, representing the most common infection during this period of life, particularly asymptomatic bacteriuria, affecting 2 to 7% of pregnant women [83]. As we all know, pregnancy is characterized by physiological changes in immune response, the vaginal microbiome also undergoes major changes. Indeed, pregnancy reduces the differences in microbiome diversity across women; particularly, pregnancy-related vaginal alterations result in an increased *Lactobacillus* dominance and a reduced species diversity [84]. These changes are protective regarding a preterm birth rate because they boost infection resistance and support the production of anti-inflammatory cytokines [85]. Furthermore, they regard also racioethnic differences in the vaginal microbiome, so particularly in women of African ancestry, the configuration of the vaginal microbiome during pregnancy may have predictive value for premature birth [86].

Other factors that influence vaginal microbiome composition are:

1. Contraceptive methods: Spermicidal products containing nonoxynol-9 deplete lactobacilli and favor *E. coli* colonization [87–92]. Instead, oral contraceptives seem to decrease the rate of bacterial vaginosis [93], but they do not influence the risk of rUTIs;
2. Sexual activity: Vaginal activity either promotes the entry of possible germs into the urethral meatus from the vagina or facilitates the transfer of potential uropathogens to the vagina [10,48,94–98];
3. New antimicrobial treatments (oral or topical) for the risk of the development of antibiotic resistance [16,17].

4.2. NGS as a Better Diagnostic Tool

Nowadays, several studies and research articles have re-written the idea that most UTI bacteria originate in the gut [99], and recent research has clarified the role that urine and vaginal bacteria play in the onset and recurrence of these diseases [100,101]. The microbiomes of the vagina and urinary tract are inextricably related and together participate in the maintenance of a healthy balance in the genital and urinary tracts [19]. In addition, from a microbiological perspective, around one-third of the bladder microbiota only resides in the vagina [102]. Mechanical transfer is one of the main risk factors for UTIs and rUTIs [10,48,94–98,103] because it enables vaginal bacteria to enter the urinary system, such as during sexual activity [33,70].

In this new perspective, the myth that urine is sterile was disproved also thanks to the development of new analytical techniques, such as NGS and metagenomic approaches [18], which allowed for the detection of a microbiome in the healthy urogenital tract [104–106]. Microbial ecologists created the culture-independent DNA-based identification of microorganisms with the aim of identifying bacterial species without the need for culture. Particularly, NGS employs PCR amplification and high-throughput sequencing of essential 16S rRNA genes, using polymorphisms of the 16S rRNA gene amplicon to distinguish bacterial species, even those that are closely related [19,107]. A urine sample is sequenced using a multi-step process that starts with the isolation and purification of microbial DNA, follows with 16S rRNA amplification and sequencing, and ends with bioinformatic analysis through a variety of software database platforms. As a result, there are still a lot of restrictions with this technology, particularly in terms of its clinical uses [18].

Yoo et al. demonstrated that the clinical application of urine NGS in cases of acute uncomplicated cystitis and rUTIs reported a better sensitivity than the application of conventional urine culture [82], which is consistent with prior research [108–111]. Indeed, it appears that a typical urine culture misses roughly 90% of non-UPEC pathogens [110], and anaerobic bacteria or a multi-microbial illness may be to blame for negative findings in routine urine cultures [107,112,113].

Most importantly, NGS is not greatly impacted by antibiotic usage, because bacteria do not need to be alive as for a traditional culture method [114]. Furthermore, NGS is highly sensitive to atypical bacteria, anaerobes, or multimicrobial urinary tract infections [113]. Another crucial element that facilitates prompt clinical decision-making and medication is represented by the faster NGS technique for the detection of pathogens with respect to culture; this reduces testing times from several days to just 24 h [114].

4.3. Pathophysiology and Immunology in rUTIs

While analysing the immunological assessment of urinary infections, data in the literature reported that intracellular bacterial communities (IBCs) and quiescent intracellular reservoirs (QIRs) are two methods that allow pathogens to survive antibiotic treatment and to host an immune response in the bladder, developing a chronic colonization [63,66].

Regarding UPEC, adhesive organelles, such as type 1, P, S, and F1C pili, are used to first infiltrate the host cells in the urothelium. Then, UPEC creates IBCs, which consist of the development of a biofilm formed of a polysaccharide matrix wrapped in a uroplakin coating, enabling UPEC to proliferate and thrive in a secure manner [64,115–119]. As opposed to this, QIRs are made up of a subgroup of bacteria that have remained undetected by the host immune system for a considerable amount of time in cells after receiving antibiotics [120,121]. Dormant bacteria may begin to reproduce and lead to reinfection because of the urothelium's turnover. IBCs are transitory, developing within a few hours in the cytosol as opposed to QIRs, which might spend months quiescent within the endosomes [122].

Lipopolysaccharide (LPS), a key component of UPEC pathogenicity, affects UPEC life cycles and promotes reservoir development [123] by activating intracellular signalling pathways and innate and adaptive immune responses [124]. By raising cytosolic calcium through a Toll-like receptor (TRL 4-mediated increase), LPS suppresses the synthesis of cytokines [125]. Additionally, NLRP3 inflammasome activation by pathogen-associated molecules, such as flagellin and hemolysin as well as LPS can cause urothelial cells to exfoliate and let UPEC to enter deeply [126,127].

Regarding the relationship between the innate and adaptive immune systems and rUTIs, this is not completely understood yet [122].

The functions of pentraxin 3 (PTX3) and uroplakin IIIa (UPIIIa) signalling have received little attention in the literature. A crucial function of PTX3 is that polymorphisms or a deficit in it may impair the body's capacity to control infection, which may promote infection spread [128]. The endocytic process is instead induced by UPIIIa signalling, which enters the intracellular space [129].

Instead, particular attention has been paid to the relation between vaginal microenvironment and urinary tract inflammatory diseases. The assumption that the vagina is the main source of bladder colonising pathogens was made since women have UTIs at a greater rate than males [115,116]. The vaginal canal can operate as a reservoir for *E. coli* and other bacteria, becoming a significant player in the pathogenesis of UTI.

E. coli can penetrate vaginal cells and remain in the vagina during UTI, according to preliminary research in murine UTI models [117]. Regarding this, more research has been conducted on the relationship between *Gardenerella vaginalis* and *E. coli.*

Animal experiments that exposed the urinary system to different common vaginal bacteria (especially *Gardnerella*) in the setting of *E. coli* UTI corroborate the previous reported theory of "covert pathogenesis" [30,71].

Gardnerella can frequently be found in urine samples from healthy, asymptomatic women. Three patterns of patients who tested positive for *Gardnerella* were proposed by Yoo et al. [71]: (I) the *Escherichia*-dominant group; (II) the *Gardnerella*-dominant group; and (III) the *Lactobacillus*-dominant group. They emphasised that all *Escherichia* dominant groups were linked to rUTI, but *Gardnerella*- and *Lactobacillus*-dominant groups might be linked to rUTI but not necessarily be symptomatic. This supported the idea that bladder dysbiosis can cause various symptoms by altering the immune system's reaction to bacterial colonisation [71]. Furthermore, it was shown that *Gardnerella* may be a "covert" pathogen that causes *E. coli* activation [69], and UTI can also happen in the *Lactobacillus*-dominant group even if a minor amount of *Gardnerella* is present, if *Lactobacillus* has a poor protective effect [71].

Other research confirmed that the development of UPEC from bladder reservoirs is significantly influenced by *Gardnerella*. Indeed, it influences urothelial apoptosis and exfoliation and other mucosal immune system-related activities as demonstrated in a mouse model [130,131]. Among these, immediate-early (IE) genes, including the orphan nuclear receptor Nur77 (also known as Nr4a1), are increased in mice exposed to *Gardnerella* [131,132]; at the same time, animals lacking Nur77 are not at risk from recurrent UPEC UTI after *Gardnerella* exposure.

Numerous cellular functions are controlled by Nur77, including apoptosis in various tissues [133,134]. Additionally, Nur77 regulates inflammation [135] and has a specific impact on T-cell responses [136] and Ly6C-monocytes [137]. As a result, the IE response could play a role in the *Gardnerella*-related recurrent UPEC UTI [138].

Instead, KEGG pathways and GO keywords are significantly changed after several *Gardnerella* exposures [138]. IL-12, IFN-g, and RANTES levels rise in bladder homogenates after exposure to *Gardnerella* [48], and pathways associated to T and B cells are also activated.

Finally, Kirjavainen et al. investigated immune defence anomalies in women with rUTIs and discovered that peripheral monocytes and myeloid dendritic cells (DCs) produced elevated level of interleukin-12 and did not induce the T cell activation. In the case of rUTIs, the T cell polarisation is avoided. In addition, there was a decrease in levels of vascular endothelial growth factor (VEGF) related with tissue healing and a reduction in concentrations of monocyte chemotactic protein 1, the main chemoattractant for DC and monocytes [139].

All these factors may promote the insurgence of urinary infection and chronic colonisation due to the deficiency of immune response and the imbalance of host response to bacterial injuries. It is likely that the host immune response depends on the phenotypic and behaviour characteristics (such as smoking, sexual activity, alcohol abuse, and menopausal status) of a host as previous described.

4.4. New Perspectives of Therapy and Prevention

Recurrent UTIs are strictly associated with urinary tract dysbiosis [18,104]. The importance of lactobacilli and oestrogens in the prevention of rUTIs was confirmed by Neugent et al., who described the correlations between *Bifidobacterium*, *Lactobacillus*, and urinary oestrogens in women with no history of UTIs [140]. According to this theory, some researchers suggested that administering probiotics may be more beneficial in treating rUTIs [141,142] as opposed to administering antibiotics or taking antibiotics prophylactically at low doses to prevent recurrent infections, both of which promote the evolution of pathogenic resistance by causing bacterial persister cells [143].

A considerable decrease in rUTIs is linked to the use of Lactobacillus vaginal suppositories [38,55,144]. Sadahira et al. showed that the administration GAI 98,322 strain of *L. crispatus* had a significant effect in reducing the recurrent cystitis in 86% of patients. However, more importantly, the suppressive effect persisted in 77% of patients for at least a year after the end of the therapy, with a significant decrease in the mean number of cystitis episodes both during and after administration [145]. The oral treatment with *Lactobacillus reuteri RC-14* and *Lactobacillus rhamnosus GR-1* also improved the population profiles of vaginal lactobacilli and reduced the colonisation of potentially dangerous bacteria [146].

In order to support the host's immunological assessment against bacterial invasion and prevent recurrent infection, functional restoration should be the main focus of therapy, according to the recent literature data on the urinary tract urobiome and the importance the local and systemic immune system response in the prevention of UTIs recurrence [147].

As was already mentioned, oestrogen regulates the balance of the urogenital microbiome; it promotes lactobacilli growth, whereas oestrogen insufficiency results in a decrease in vaginal lactobacilli, which raises the risk of rUTIs [72,73]. Therefore, rUTIs may be decreased by oestrogen replacement treatment [73,94,148–151], and intravaginal oestrogen may provide great benefit with less risk when compared to oral oestrogen [152].

Recently, research has been conducted on the use of natural sources for therapy and prevention of rUTIs. For example, Mehta et al. studied the potential antibacterial role of the oroxindin from *Bacopa monnieri* against UTIs caused by *Klebsiella pneumoniae* and *Proteuns mirabilis*. *B. monnieri* is a medicinal plant growing in the world's wetlands and warmer regions; the authors demonstrated that *K. pneumoniae* and *P. mirabilis* can be effectively eliminated by *B. monnieri*, also establishing its safety [153].

5. Conclusions

In conclusion the complex correlation among microbiota, low genital tract, and urinary system is based on the balance between host characteristics, immunological microenvironment and pathogens. Further investigation may provide an accurate analysis of the urogenital microbiome, especially to promote a tailoring therapy in order to reduce antibiotic resistance and increase the physiological mechanism of urothelium response.

Table 1. Main findings from the studies included in the review.

Variables	Main Findings
Role of vaginal microbiome [30,37,44,59,71,72,101,131,138,142]	The vaginal microbiome is involved in rUTIs pathogenesis: if its balance is maintained, it constitutes a barrier against pathogens. However, every change, which we know as bacterial vaginosis, is an important risk factor for the development of urinary tract infections.
	This may be a consequence of the decrease in vaginal lactobacilli, which seems to allow the growth of gram-positive bacteria, (especially *Staphylococcus saprophyticus*, *Escherichia coli*, *Enterococcus faecalis*, and *Streptococcus agalactiae*) or *Gardnerella vaginalis*.
	These vaginal bacteria may be present in the vaginal canal and colonize the urinary system, avoiding the immune response and allowing the formation of *E.coli* reservoirs.
Role of urinary microbiome [61,77,141]	Urinary system microbiota has a key role in preserving urinary health. So, the pathophysiology of rUTI is influenced by urobiome.
	Indeed, urinary microbiome composition differs between healthy and rUTIs subjects. Specific urine microorganisms are linked to distinct clinical features in women with rUTI.
Risk factors of rUTIs and dysbiosis [10,76–79]	Risk factors for the development of symptoms include host variables, host behaviours, and bacterial features. Among these, menopause influences the urine microbiota composition following aging and the decrease in oestreogens protection. First of all, it brings altered Lactobacillus composition, increasing the risk of rUTIs.
Possible immunological pathways [48,66,122,130,139]	Several microscopic pathways have been identified, including the intracellular bacterial community, QIR, LPS, multimicrobial infection, and urothelial mucosal remodelling. These mechanisms allow uropathogens to persist in the bladder and survive antibiotic therapy and host immune response. Furthermore, immunological defences show some abnormalities in UTI-prone women, such as increased levels of IL-12, absence of T-cell response, less VEGF, lower level of monocyte chemotactic protein 1, the upregulation of immediate-early (IE) genes, such Nur77.
New perspectiver of diagnosis [82]	NGS is more sensitive than a conventional urine culture in the detection of uropathogens, highlighting an increased microbiome diversity in the recurrent cystitis group. Additional NGS tests can facilitate rapid decision-making and therapeutic advancement.
New perspectives of theraphy [8,32,38,55,140,144,145,152]	Following the understanding of the importance of lactobacilli and oestrogen in the pathophysiology of rUTIs, several studies demonstrated their benefits as therapies.
	The intravaginal administration of lactobacillus and/or oestrogens is associated with a significant reduction in rUTIs, especially if they are integrated with nonantibiotic therapeutical options as well as modification of behaviour, specific diet, integration with probiotics, and d-mannos, use of local oestrogens therapy, and systemic or local immunostimulants. The administration of one or more of these approaches provides the beneficial treatment to reduce rUTI risk.

Author Contributions: B.G. and M.D. designed the structure of the manuscript. M.L.V., C.M., A.G., M.F.P., S.B. and M.T. contributed to the literature search. A.L.S. and M.D. wrote the manuscript. M.D., B.G. and A.L.S. reviewed and revised the initial manuscript and approved the final manuscript as submitted. All authors approved the submitted version. All authors have read and agreed to the published version of the manuscript.

Funding: The study is supported by grants of the Italian ministry of health, "ricerca corrente" to the IRCCS Fondazione Policlinico San Matteo, Pavia, Italy.

Institutional Review Board Statement: Ethical review and approval were waived for this study because it is a systematic review of literature.

Informed Consent Statement: Patient consent was waived for this study because it is a systematic review of literature.

Data Availability Statement: The literature data analyzed during the current review are available from the corresponding author on reasonable request.

Conflicts of Interest: The authors declare no conflict of interest.

References

1. Stamm, W.E.; Norrby, S.R. Urinary Tract Infections: Disease Panorama and Challenges. *J. Infect. Dis.* **2001**, *183* (Suppl. 1), S1–S4. [CrossRef] [PubMed]
2. Cox, C.E.; Lacy, S.S.; Hinman, F., Jr. The Urethra and its Relationship to Urinary Tract Infection. II. The Urethral Flora of the Female with Recurrent Urinary Infection. *J. Urol.* **1968**, *99*, 632–638. [CrossRef]
3. Al-Badr, A.; Al-Shaikh, G. Recurrent Urinary Tract Infections Management in Women: A review. *Sultan Qaboos Univ. Med. J.* **2013**, *13*, 359–367. [CrossRef]
4. Renard, J.; Ballarini, S.; Mascarenhas, T.; Zahran, M.; Quimper, E.; Choucair, J.; Iselin, C.E. Recurrent Lower Urinary Tract Infections Have a Detrimental Effect on Patient Quality of Life: A Prospective, Observational Study. *Infect. Dis. Ther.* **2014**, *4*, 125–135. [CrossRef]
5. Dason, S.; Dason, J.T.; Kapoor, A. Guidelines for the diagnosis and management of recurrent urinary tract infection in women. *Can. Urol. Assoc. J.* **2013**, *5*, 316–322. [CrossRef]
6. Sabih, A.; Leslie, S.W. Complicated Urinary Tract Infections. In *StatPearls*; StatPearls Publishing: Treasure Island, FL, USA, 2022. Available online: https://www-ncbi-nlm-nih-gov.offcampus.lib.washington.edu/books/NBK436013/ (accessed on 12 August 2021).
7. Bonkat, G.; Pickard, R.; Bartoletti, R.; Bruyère, F.; Geerlings, S.; Wagenlehner, F.; Wullt, B.; Pradere, B.; Veeratterapillay, R. *EAU Guidelines on Urological Infections*; European Association of Urology: Arnhem, The Netherlands, 2018.
8. Sihra, N.; Goodman, A.; Zakri, R.; Sahai, A.; Malde, S. Nonantibiotic prevention and management of recurrent urinary tract infection. *Nat. Rev. Urol.* **2018**, *15*, 750–776. [CrossRef] [PubMed]
9. Boldogh, I.; Albrecht, T.; Porter, D.D. Persistent Viral Infections. In *Medical Microbiology*, 4th ed.; Baron, S., Ed.; University of Texas Medical Branch at Galveston: Galveston, TX, USA, 1996; Chapter 46. Available online: https://www.ncbi.nlm.nih.gov/books/NBK8538/ (accessed on 30 January 2023).
10. Foxman, B. Urinary Tract Infection Syndromes: Occurrence, recurrence, bacteriology, risk factors, and disease burden. *Infect. Dis. Clin. N. Am.* **2014**, *28*, 1–13. [CrossRef]
11. Foxman, B.; Gillespie, B.; Koopman, J.; Zhang, L.; Palin, K.; Tallman, P.; Marsh, J.V.; Spear, S.; Sobel, J.D.; Marty, M.J.; et al. Risk Factors for Second Urinary Tract Infection among College Women. *Am. J. Epidemiol.* **2000**, *151*, 1194–1205. [CrossRef] [PubMed]
12. Foxman, B.; Manning, S.; Tallman, P.; Bauer, R.; Zhang, L.; Koopman, J.S.; Gillespie, B.; Sobel, J.D.; Marrs, C.F. Uropathogenic *Escherichia coli* Are More Likely than Commensal E. coli to Be Shared between Heterosexual Sex Partners. *Am. J. Epidemiol.* **2002**, *156*, 1133–1140. [CrossRef]
13. Murray, B.E.; Rensimer, E.R.; DuPont, H.L. Emergence of high-level trimethoprim resistance in fecal *Escherichia coli* during oral ad-ministration of trimethoprim or trimethoprim—Sulfamethoxazole. *N. Engl. J. Med.* **1982**, *306*, 130–135. [CrossRef]
14. Wright, S.W.; Wrenn, K.D.; Haynes, M.L. Trimethoprim-sulfamethoxazole resistance among urinary coliform isolates. *J. Gen. Intern. Med.* **1999**, *14*, 606–609. [CrossRef] [PubMed]
15. Kristiansen, J.E. The antimicrobial activity of non-antibiotics. Report from a congress on the antimicrobial effect of drugs other than antibiotics on bacteria, viruses, protozoa, and other organisms. *APMIS. Suppl.* **1992**, *30*, 7–14. [PubMed]
16. Ulett, G.C.; Schembri, M.A. Bacterial pathogenesis: Remodelling recurrent infection. *Nat. Microbiol.* **2016**, *2*, 16256. [CrossRef]
17. Langford, B.J.; Brown, K.A.; Diong, C.; Marchand-Austin, A.; Adomako, K.; Saedi, A.; Schwartz, K.L.; Johnstone, J.; MacFadden, D.R.; Matukas, L.M.; et al. The Benefits and Harms of Antibiotic Prophylaxis for Urinary Tract Infection in Older Adults. *Clin. Infect. Dis.* **2021**, *73*, e782–e791. [CrossRef] [PubMed]
18. Gasiorek, M.; Hsieh, M.H.; Forster, C.S. Utility of DNA Next-Generation Sequencing and Expanded Quantitative Urine Culture in Diagnosis and Management of Chronic or Persistent Lower Urinary Tract Symptoms. *J. Clin. Microbiol.* **2019**, *58*, e00204-19. [CrossRef] [PubMed]
19. Thomas-White, K.; Brady, M.; Wolfe, A.J.; Mueller, E.R. The Bladder Is Not Sterile: History and Current Discoveries on the Urinary Microbiome. *Curr. Bladder Dysfunct. Rep.* **2016**, *11*, 18–24. [CrossRef]
20. Pohl, H.G.; Groah, S.L.; Pérez-Losada, M.; Ljungberg, I.; Sprague, B.M.; Chandal, N.; Caldovic, L.; Hsieh, M. The Urine Microbiome of Healthy Men and Women Differs by Urine Collection Method. *Int. Neurourol. J.* **2020**, *24*, 41–51. [CrossRef]
21. Ley, R.E.; Peterson, D.A.; Gordon, J.I. Ecological and Evolutionary Forces Shaping Microbial Diversity in the Human Intestine. *Cell* **2006**, *124*, 837–848. [CrossRef]

22. Higgins, J.; Altman, D.; Sterne, J. Chapter 8: Assessing risk of bias in included studies. In *Cochrane Handbook for Systematic Reviews of Interventions, Version 5.2.0*; Higgins, J.P.T., Churchill, R., Chandler, J., Cumpston, M.S., Eds.; John Wiley and Sons: Chichester, UK, 2017.
23. Schünemann, H.J.; Higgins, J.P.; Vist, G.E.; Glasziou, P.; Akl, E.A.; Skoetz, N.; Guyatt, G.H.; Cochrane GRADEing Methods Group; Cochrane Statistical Methods Group. Chapter 14: Completing 'Summary of findings' tables and grading the certainty of the evidence. In *Cochrane Handbook for Systematic Reviews of Interventions, Version 6.2*; Higgins, J.P., Thomas, J., Chandler, J., Cumpston, M., Li, T., Page, M.J., Welch, V.A., Eds.; John Wiley and Sons: Chichester, UK, 2021.
24. Czaja, C.A.; Stamm, W.E.; Stapleton, A.E.; Roberts, P.L.; Hawn, T.R.; Scholes, D.; Samadpour, M.; Hultgren, S.J.; Hooton, T.M. Prospective Cohort Study of Microbial and Inflammatory Events Immediately Preceding *Escherichia coli* Recurrent Urinary Tract Infection in Women. *J. Infect. Dis.* **2009**, *200*, 528–536. [CrossRef]
25. Ravel, J.; Gajer, P.; Abdo, Z.; Schneider, G.M.; Koenig, S.S.K.; McCulle, S.L.; Karlebach, S.; Gorle, R.; Russell, J.; Tacket, C.O.; et al. Vaginal microbiome of reproductive-age women. *Proc. Natl. Acad. Sci. USA* **2011**, *108* (Suppl. S1), 4680–4687. [CrossRef]
26. Romero, R.; Hassan, S.S.; Gajer, P.; Tarca, A.L.; Fadrosh, D.W.; Nikita, L.; Galuppi, M.; Lamont, R.F.; Chaemsaithong, P.; Miranda, J.; et al. The composition and stability of the vaginal microbiota of normal pregnant women is different from that of non-pregnant women. *Microbiome* **2014**, *2*, 4. [CrossRef]
27. Tamarelle, J.; Thiébaut, A.; de Barbeyrac, B.; Bébéar, C.; Ravel, J.; Delarocque-Astagneau, E. The vaginal microbiota and its association with human papillomavirus, Chlamydia trachomatis, Neisseria gonorrhoeae and Mycoplasma genitalium infections: A systematic review and meta-analysis. *Clin. Microbiol. Infect.* **2019**, *25*, 35–47. [CrossRef]
28. Borges, S.; Silva, J.; Teixeira, P. The role of lactobacilli and probiotics in maintaining vaginal health. *Arch. Gynecol. Obstet.* **2013**, *289*, 479–489. [CrossRef] [PubMed]
29. Tachedjian, G.; Aldunate, M.; Bradshaw, C.S.; Cone, R.A. The role of lactic acid production by probiotic Lactobacillus species in vaginal health. *Res. Microbiol.* **2017**, *168*, 782–792. [CrossRef] [PubMed]
30. Lewis, A.L.; Gilbert, N.M. Roles of the vagina and the vaginal microbiota in urinary tract infection: Evidence from clinical correlations and experimental models. *GMS Infect. Dis.* **2020**, *8*, DOC02. [CrossRef] [PubMed]
31. Hudson, P.L.; Hung, K.J.; Bergerat, A.; Mitchell, C. Effect of Vaginal Lactobacillus Species on *Escherichia coli* Growth. *Urogynecology* **2020**, *26*, 146–151. [CrossRef]
32. Vagios, S.; Hesham, H.; Mitchell, C. Understanding the potential of lactobacilli in recurrent UTI prevention. *Microb. Pathog.* **2020**, *148*, 104544. [CrossRef]
33. Pfau, A.; Sacks, T. The Bacterial Flora of the Vaginal Vestibule, Urethra and Vagina in Premenopausal Women with Recurrent Urinary Tract Infections. *J. Urol.* **1981**, *126*, 630–634. [CrossRef]
34. Gupta, K.; Stapleton, A.; Hooton, T.M.; Roberts, P.L.; Fennell, C.L.; Stamm, W.E. Inverse Association of H2O2-Producing Lactobacilli and Vaginal *Escherichia coli* Colonization in Women with Recurrent Urinary Tract Infections. *J. Infect. Dis.* **1998**, *178*, 446–450. [CrossRef]
35. Hooton, T.M.; Fihn, S.D.; Johnson, C.; Roberts, P.L.; Stamm, W.E. Association between bacterial vaginosis and acute cystitis in women using diaphragms. *Arch. Intern. Med.* **1989**, *149*, 1932–1936. [CrossRef]
36. Hooton, T.M.; Roberts, P.L.; Stamm, W.E. Effects of Recent Sexual Activity and Use of a Diaphragm on the Vaginal Microflora. *Clin. Infect. Dis.* **1994**, *19*, 274–278. [CrossRef]
37. Harmanli, O.H.; Cheng, G.Y.; Nyirjesy, P.; Chatwani, A.; Gaughan, J.P. Urinary Tract Infections in Women with Bacterial Vaginosis. *Obstet. Gynecol.* **2000**, *95*, 710–712. [CrossRef]
38. Stapleton, A.E.; Au-Yeung, M.; Hooton, T.M.; Fredricks, D.N.; Roberts, P.L.; Czaja, C.A.; Yarova-Yarovaya, Y.; Fiedler, T.; Cox, M.; Stamm, W.E. Randomized, Placebo-Controlled Phase 2 Trial of a Lactobacillus crispatus Probiotic Given Intravaginally for Prevention of Recurrent Urinary Tract Infection. *Clin. Infect. Dis.* **2011**, *52*, 1212–1217. [CrossRef] [PubMed]
39. Amatya, R.; Bhattarai, S.; Mandal, P.K.; Tuladhar, H.; Karki, B.M.S. Urinary tract infection in vaginitis: A condition often overlooked. *Nepal. Med. Coll. J.* **2013**, *15*, 65–67.
40. Navas-Nacher, E.L.; Dardick, F.; Venegas, M.F.; Anderson, B.E.; Schaeffer, A.J.; Duncan, J.L. Relatedness of *Escherichia coli* Colonizing Women Longitudinally. *Mol. Urol.* **2001**, *5*, 31–36. [CrossRef]
41. Muder, R.R.; Brennen, C.; Rihs, J.D.; Wagener, M.M.; Obman, A.; Stout, J.E.; Yu, V.L. Isolation of Staphylococcus aureus from the Urinary Tract: Association of Isolation with Symptomatic Urinary Tract Infection and Subsequent Staphylococcal Bacteremia. *Clin. Infect. Dis.* **2006**, *42*, 46–50. [CrossRef]
42. Baraboutis, I.G.; Tsagalou, E.P.; Lepinski, J.L.; Papakonstantinou, I.; Papastamopoulos, V.; Skoutelis, A.T.; Johnson, S. Primary Staphylococcus aureus urinary tract infection: The role of undetected hematogenous seeding of the urinary tract. *Eur. J. Clin. Microbiol. Infect. Dis.* **2010**, *29*, 1095–1101. [CrossRef]
43. Gilbert, N.M.; O'Brien, V.P.; Hultgren, S.; Macones, G.; Lewis, W.G.; Lewis, A.L. Urinary Tract Infection as a Preventable Cause of Pregnancy Complications: Opportunities, Challenges, and a Global Call to Action. *Glob. Adv. Health Med.* **2013**, *2*, 59–69. [CrossRef] [PubMed]
44. Kline, K.A.; Lewis, A.L. Gram-Positive Uropathogens, Polymicrobial Urinary Tract Infection, and the Emerging Microbiota of the Urinary Tract. *Microbiol. Spectr.* **2016**, *4*, UTI-0012-2012. [CrossRef] [PubMed]
45. Allsworth, J.E.; Lewis, V.A.; Peipert, J.F. Viral Sexually Transmitted Infections and Bacterial Vaginosis: 2001–2004 National Health and Nutrition Examination Survey Data. *Sex. Transm. Dis.* **2008**, *35*, 791–796. [CrossRef]

46. Klein, S.; Nurjadi, D.; Horner, S.; Heeg, K.; Zimmermann, S.; Burckhardt, I. Significant increase in cultivation of Gardnerella vaginalis, Alloscardovia omnicolens, Actinotignum schaalii, and Actinomyces spp. in urine samples with total laboratory automation. *Eur. J. Clin. Microbiol. Infect. Dis.* **2018**, *37*, 1305–1311. [CrossRef]
47. Sumati, A.; Saritha, N. Association of urinary tract infection in women with bacterial vaginosis. *J. Glob. Infect. Dis.* **2009**, *1*, 151–152. [CrossRef] [PubMed]
48. Gilbert, N.M.; O'Brien, V.P.; Lewis, A.L. Transient microbiota exposures activate dormant *Escherichia coli* infection in the bladder and drive severe outcomes of recurrent disease. *PLoS Pathog.* **2017**, *13*, e1006238. [CrossRef] [PubMed]
49. Donders, G.G.; Vereecken, A.; Bosmans, E.; Dekeersmaecker, A.; Salembier, G.; Spitz, B. Definition of a type of abnormal vaginal flora that is distinct from bacterial vaginosis: Aerobic vaginitis. *BJOG Int. J. Obstet. Gynaecol.* **2002**, *109*, 34–43. [CrossRef] [PubMed]
50. Tan, C.K.; Ulett, K.B.; Steele, M.; Benjamin, W.H., Jr.; Ulett, G.C. Prognostic value of semi-quantitative bacteriuria counts in the diagnosis of group B streptococcus urinary tract infection: A 4-year retrospective study in adult patients. *BMC Infect. Dis.* **2012**, *12*, 273. [CrossRef] [PubMed]
51. Gottschick, C.; Deng, Z.-L.; Vital, M.; Masur, C.; Abels, C.; Pieper, D.H.; Wagner-Döbler, I. The urinary microbiota of men and women and its changes in women during bacterial vaginosis and antibiotic treatment. *Microbiome* **2017**, *5*, 99. [CrossRef]
52. Groah, S.L.; Pérez-Losada, M.; Caldovic, L.; Ljungberg, I.H.; Sprague, B.M.; Castro-Nallar, E.; Chandel, N.J.; Hsieh, M.H.; Pohl, H. Redefining Healthy Urine: A Cross-Sectional Exploratory Metagenomic Study of People with and Without Bladder Dysfunction. *J. Urol.* **2016**, *196*, 579–587. [CrossRef]
53. Forster, C.S.; Pohl, H. Diagnosis of Urinary Tract Infection in the Neuropathic Bladder: Changing the Paradigm to Include the Microbiome. *Top. Spinal Cord Inj. Rehabil.* **2019**, *25*, 222–227. [CrossRef]
54. Whiteside, S.A.; Razvi, H.; Dave, S.; Reid, G.; Burton, J.P. The microbiome of the urinary tract—A role beyond infection. *Nat. Rev. Urol.* **2015**, *12*, 81–90. [CrossRef]
55. Atassi, F.; Ahn, D.L.P.V.; Moal, V.L.-L. Diverse Expression of Antimicrobial Activities Against Bacterial Vaginosis and Urinary Tract Infection Pathogens by Cervicovaginal Microbiota Strains of Lactobacillus gasseri and Lactobacillus crispatus. *Front. Microbiol.* **2019**, *10*, 2900. [CrossRef]
56. De Seta, F.; Lonnee-Hoffmann, R.M.; Campisciano, G.; Comar, M.; Verstraelen, H.M.; Vieira-Baptista, P.; Ventolini, G.M.; Lev-Sagie, A. The Vaginal Microbiome: III. The Vaginal Microbiome in Various Urogenital Disorders. *J. Low. Genit. Tract Dis.* **2022**, *26*, 85–92. [CrossRef]
57. Morand, A.; Cornu, F.; Dufour, J.-C.; Tsimaratos, M.; Lagier, J.-C.; Raoult, D. Human Bacterial Repertoire of the Urinary Tract: A Potential Paradigm Shift. *J. Clin. Microbiol.* **2019**, *57*, e00675-18. [CrossRef]
58. Dubourg, G.; Morand, A.; Mekhalif, F.; Godefroy, R.; Corthier, G.; Yacouba, A.; Diakite, A.; Cornu, F.; Cresci, M.; Brahimi, S.; et al. Deciphering the Urinary Microbiota Repertoire by Culturomics Reveals Mostly Anaerobic Bacteria from the Gut. *Front. Microbiol.* **2020**, *11*, 513305. [CrossRef]
59. Neugent, M.L.; Hulyalkar, N.V.; Nguyen, V.H.; Zimmern, P.E.; De Nisco, N.J. Advances in Understanding the Human Urinary Microbiome and Its Potential Role in Urinary Tract Infection. *Mbio* **2020**, *11*, e00218-20. [CrossRef]
60. Bossa, L.; Kline, K.; McDougald, D.; Lee, B.B.; Rice, S.A. Urinary catheter-associated microbiota change in accordance with treatment and infection status. *PLoS ONE* **2017**, *12*, e0177633. [CrossRef] [PubMed]
61. Burnett, L.A.; Hochstedler, B.R.; Weldon, K.; Wolfe, A.J.; Brubaker, L. Recurrent urinary tract infection: Association of clinical profiles with urobiome composition in women. *Neurourol. Urodyn.* **2021**, *40*, 1479–1489. [CrossRef] [PubMed]
62. Elliott, T.; Reed, L.; Slack, R.; Bishop, M. Bacteriology and ultrastructure of the bladder in patients with urinary tract infections. *J. Infect.* **1985**, *11*, 191–199. [CrossRef] [PubMed]
63. Robino, L.; Scavone, P.; Araujo, L.; Algorta, G.; Zunino, P.; Pírez, M.C.; Vignoli, R. Intracellular Bacteria in the Pathogenesis of *Escherichia coli* Urinary Tract Infection in Children. *Clin. Infect. Dis.* **2014**, *59*, e158–e164. [CrossRef]
64. Rosen, D.A.; Hooton, T.M.; Stamm, W.E.; Humphrey, P.A.; Hultgren, S.J. Detection of Intracellular Bacterial Communities in Human Urinary Tract Infection. *PLoS Med.* **2007**, *4*, e329. [CrossRef]
65. Liu, S.-C.; Han, X.-M.; Shi, M.; Pang, Z.-L. Persistence of uropathogenic Escherichia Coli in the bladders of female patients with sterile urine after antibiotic therapies. *J. Huazhong Univ. Sci. Technol.* **2016**, *36*, 710–715. [CrossRef]
66. De Nisco, N.J.; Neugent, M.; Mull, J.; Chen, L.; Kuprasertkul, A.; de Souza Santos, M.; Palmer, K.L.; Zimmern, P.; Orth, K. Direct detection of tissue-resident bacteria and chronic inflammation in the bladder wall of postmenopausal women with recurrent urinary tract infection. *J. Mol. Biol.* **2019**, *431*, 4368–4379. [CrossRef] [PubMed]
67. Ejrnaes, K.; Sandvang, D.; Lundgren, B.; Ferry, S.; Holm, S.; Monsen, T.; Lundholm, R.; Frimodt-Moller, N. Pulsed-Field Gel Electrophoresis Typing of *Escherichia coli* Strains from Samples Collected before and after Pivmecillinam or Placebo Treatment of Uncomplicated Community-Acquired Urinary Tract Infection in Women. *J. Clin. Microbiol.* **2006**, *44*, 1776–1781. [CrossRef] [PubMed]
68. Luo, Y.; Ma, Y.; Zhao, Q.; Wang, L.; Guo, L.; Ye, L.; Zhang, Y.; Yang, J. Similarity and Divergence of Phylogenies, Antimicrobial Susceptibilities, and Virulence Factor Profiles of *Escherichia coli* Isolates Causing Recurrent Urinary Tract Infections That Persist or Result from Reinfection. *J. Clin. Microbiol.* **2012**, *50*, 4002–4007. [CrossRef] [PubMed]
69. Skjøt-Rasmussen, L.; Olsen, S.; Jakobsen, L.; Ejrnæs, K.; Scheutz, F.; Lundgren, B.; Frimodt-Møller, N.; Hammerum, A. *Escherichia coli* clonal group A causing bacteraemia of urinary tract origin. *Clin. Microbiol. Infect.* **2013**, *19*, 656–661. [CrossRef] [PubMed]

70. Kõljalg, S.; Truusalu, K.; Stsepetova, J.; Pai, K.; Vainumäe, I.; Sepp, E.; Mikelsaar, M. The *Escherichia coli* phylogenetic group B2 with integrons prevails in childhood recurrent urinary tract infections. *Apmis* **2014**, *122*, 452–458. [CrossRef]
71. Yoo, J.-J.; Song, J.S.; Bin Kim, W.; Yun, J.; Shin, H.B.; Jang, M.-A.; Ryu, C.B.; Kim, S.S.; Chung, J.C.; Kuk, J.C.; et al. *Gardnerella vaginalis* in Recurrent Urinary Tract Infection Is Associated with Dysbiosis of the Bladder Microbiome. *J. Clin. Med.* **2022**, *11*, 2295. [CrossRef]
72. Stapleton, A.E. The Vaginal Microbiota and Urinary Tract Infection. *Microbiol. Spectr.* **2016**, *4*, 79–86. [CrossRef]
73. Raz, R. Urinary Tract Infection in Postmenopausal Women. *Korean J. Urol.* **2011**, *52*, 801–808. [CrossRef]
74. Muhleisen, A.L.; Herbst-Kralovetz, M.M. Menopause and the vaginal microbiome. *Maturitas* **2016**, *91*, 42–50. [CrossRef]
75. Mitchell, C.M.; Waetjen, L.E. Genitourinary changes with aging. *Obstet. Gynecol. Clin. N. Am.* **2018**, *45*, 737–750. [CrossRef]
76. Bhide, A.; Tailor, V.; Khullar, V. Interstitial cystitis/bladder pain syndrome and recurrent urinary tract infection and the potential role of the urinary microbiome. *Post Reprod. Health* **2020**, *26*, 87–90. [CrossRef] [PubMed]
77. Jung, C.; Brubaker, L. The etiology and management of recurrent urinary tract infections in postmenopausal women. *Climacteric* **2019**, *22*, 242–249. [CrossRef]
78. Hugenholtz, F.; van der Veer, C.; Terpstra, M.L.; Borgdorff, H.; van Houdt, R.; Bruisten, S.; Geerlings, S.E.; van de Wijgert, J.H.H.M. Urine and vaginal microbiota compositions of postmenopausal and premenopausal women differ regardless of recurrent urinary tract infection and renal transplant status. *Sci. Rep.* **2022**, *12*, 2698. [CrossRef]
79. Vaughan, M.H.; Mao, J.; Karstens, L.A.; Ma, L.; Amundsen, C.L.; Schmader, K.E.; Siddiqui, N.Y. The Urinary Microbiome in Postmenopausal Women with Recurrent Urinary Tract Infections. *J. Urol.* **2021**, *206*, 1222–1231. [CrossRef] [PubMed]
80. Curtiss, N.; Balachandran, A.; Krska, L.; Peppiatt-Wildman, C.; Wildman, S.; Duckett, J. Age, menopausal status and the bladder microbiome. *Eur. J. Obstet. Gynecol. Reprod. Biol.* **2018**, *228*, 126–129. [CrossRef]
81. Biagi, E.; Candela, M.; Fairweather-Tait, S.; Franceschi, C.; Brigidi, P. Ageing of the human metaorganism: The microbial counterpart. *Age* **2011**, *34*, 247–267. [CrossRef]
82. Yoo, J.-J.; Shin, H.B.; Song, J.S.; Kim, M.; Yun, J.; Kim, Z.; Lee, Y.M.; Lee, S.W.; Lee, K.W.; Kim, W.b.; et al. Urinary Microbiome Characteristics in Female Patients with Acute Uncomplicated Cystitis and Recurrent Cystitis. *J. Clin. Med.* **2021**, *10*, 1097. [CrossRef]
83. Ansaldi, Y.; Weber, B.M.d.T. Urinary tract infections in pregnancy. *Clin. Microbiol. Infect.* **2022**. [CrossRef] [PubMed]
84. DiGiulio, D.B.; Callahan, B.J.; McMurdie, P.J.; Costello, E.K.; Lyell, D.J.; Robaczewska, A.; Sun, C.L.; Goltsman, D.S.A.; Wong, R.J.; Shaw, G.; et al. Temporal and spatial variation of the human microbiota during pregnancy. *Proc. Natl. Acad. Sci. USA* **2015**, *112*, 11060–11065. [CrossRef]
85. Fettweis, J.M.; Serrano, M.G.; Brooks, J.P.; Edwards, D.J.; Girerd, P.H.; Parikh, H.I.; Huang, B.; Arodz, T.J.; Edupuganti, L.; Glascock, A.L.; et al. The vaginal microbiome and preterm birth. *Nat. Med.* **2019**, *25*, 1012–1021. [CrossRef]
86. Dominguez-Bello, M.G. Gestational shaping of the maternal vaginal microbiome. *Nat. Med.* **2019**, *25*, 882–883. [CrossRef] [PubMed]
87. Hooton, T.M.; Gupta, K. *Recurrent Urinary Tract Infection in Women*; UpToDate: Waltham, MA, USA, 2016.
88. Eschenbach, D.A.; Patton, D.L.; Meier, A.; Thwin, S.S.; Aura, J.; Stapleton, A.; Hooton, T.M. Effects of oral contraceptive pill use on vaginal flora and vaginal epithelium. *Contraception* **2000**, *62*, 107–112. [CrossRef] [PubMed]
89. Gupta, K.; Hillier, S.L.; Hooton, T.M.; Roberts, P.L.; Stamm, W.E. Effects of Contraceptive Method on the Vaginal Microbial Flora: A Prospective Evaluation. *J. Infect. Dis.* **2000**, *181*, 595–601. [CrossRef]
90. Hooton, T.M.; Hillier, S.; Johnson, C.; Roberts, P.L.; Stamm, W.E. *Escherichia coli* Bacteriuria and Contraceptive Method. *JAMA* **1991**, *265*, 64–69. [CrossRef]
91. Hooton, T.M.; Scholes, D.; Roberts, P.L.; Stapleton, A.; Stergachis, A.; Stamm, W.E. A prospective cohort study of the association between UTI and contraceptive method. *Abstr. Intersci. Conf. Antimicrob. Agents Chemother.* **1994**, *34*, 134.
92. Hooton, T.M.; Fennell, C.L.; Clark, A.M.; Stamm, W.E. Nonoxynol-9: Differential Antibacterial Activity and Enhancement of Bacterial Adherence to Vaginal Epithelial Cells. *J. Infect. Dis.* **1991**, *164*, 1216–1219. [CrossRef] [PubMed]
93. Achilles, S.L.; Hillier, S.L. The complexity of contraceptives: Understanding their impact on genital immune cells and vaginal microbiota. *AIDS* **2013**, *27* (Suppl 1), S5–S15. [CrossRef]
94. Raz, R.; Stamm, W.E. A Controlled Trial of Intravaginal Estriol in Postmenopausal Women with Recurrent Urinary Tract Infections. *N. Engl. J. Med.* **1993**, *329*, 753–756. [CrossRef]
95. Stapleton, A.; Latham, R.H.; Johnson, C.; Stamm, W.E. Postcoital antimicrobial prophylaxis for recurrent urinary tract infection. A randomized, double-blind, placebo-controlled trial. *JAMA* **1990**, *264*, 703–706. [CrossRef]
96. Stamatiou, C.; Bovis, C.; Panagopoulos, P.; Petrakos, G.; Economou, A.; Lycoudt, A. Sex-induced cystitis–patient burden and other epidemiological features. *Clin. Exp. Obstet. Gynecol.* **2005**, *32*, 180–182.
97. Hooton, T.M.; Scholes, D.; Hughes, J.P.; Winter, C.; Roberts, P.L.; Stapleton, A.E.; Stergachis, A.; Stamm, W.E. A Prospective Study of Risk Factors for Symptomatic Urinary Tract Infection in Young Women. *N. Engl. J. Med.* **1996**, *335*, 468–474. [CrossRef] [PubMed]
98. Scholes, D.; Hooton, T.M.; Roberts, P.L.; Stapleton, A.; Gupta, K.; Stamm, W.E. Risk Factors for Recurrent Urinary Tract Infection in Young Women. *J. Infect. Dis.* **2000**, *182*, 1177–1182. [CrossRef]
99. Shreiner, A.B.; Kao, J.Y.; Young, V.B. The gut microbiome in health and in disease. *Curr. Opin. Gastroenterol.* **2015**, *31*, 69–75. [CrossRef]

100. Cumpanas, A.A.; Bratu, O.G.; Bardan, R.; Ferician, O.C.; Cumpanas, A.D.; Horhat, F.G.; Licker, M.; Pricop, C.; Cretu, O.M. Urinary Microbiota—Are We Ready for Prime Time? A Literature Review of Study Methods' Critical Steps in Avoiding Contamination and Minimizing Biased Results. *Diagnostics* **2020**, *10*, 343. [CrossRef] [PubMed]
101. Meštrović, T.; Matijašić, M.; Perić, M.; Čipčić Paljetak, H.; Barešić, A.; Verbanac, D. The Role of Gut, Vaginal, and Urinary Microbiome in Urinary Tract Infections: From Bench to Bedside. *Diagnostics* **2021**, *11*, 7. [CrossRef] [PubMed]
102. Wolfe, A.J.; Brubaker, L. Urobiome updates: Advances in urinary microbiome research. *Nat. Rev. Urol.* **2019**, *16*, 73–74. [CrossRef]
103. Lewis, D.A.; Brown, R.; Williams, J.; White, P.; Jacobson, S.K.; Marchesi, J.R.; Drake, M.J. The human urinary microbiome; bacterial DNA in voided urine of asymptomatic adults. *Front. Cell. Infect. Microbiol.* **2013**, *3*, 41. [CrossRef]
104. Finucane, T.E. 'Urinary tract infection' and the microbiome. *Am. J. Med.* **2017**, *130*, e97–e98. [CrossRef]
105. Ackerman, A.L.; Chai, T.C. The Bladder is Not Sterile: An Update on the Urinary Microbiome. *Curr. Bladder Dysfunct. Rep.* **2019**, *14*, 331–341. [CrossRef]
106. Amabebe, E.; Anumba, D.O.C. Female Gut and Genital Tract Microbiota-Induced Crosstalk and Differential Effects of Short-Chain Fatty Acids on Immune Sequelae. *Front. Immunol.* **2020**, *11*, 2184. [CrossRef]
107. Brubaker, L.; Wolfe, A.J. The new world of the urinary microbiota in women. *Am. J. Obstet. Gynecol.* **2015**, *213*, 644–649. [CrossRef]
108. Wolfe, A.J.; Toh, E.; Shibata, N.; Rong, R.; Kenton, K.; FitzGerald, M.; Mueller, E.R.; Schreckenberger, P.; Dong, Q.; Nelson, D.E.; et al. Evidence of Uncultivated Bacteria in the Adult Female Bladder. *J. Clin. Microbiol.* **2012**, *50*, 1376–1383. [CrossRef]
109. Hilt, E.E.; McKinley, K.; Pearce, M.M.; Rosenfeld, A.B.; Zilliox, M.J.; Mueller, E.R.; Brubaker, L.; Gai, X.; Wolfe, A.J.; Schreckenberger, P.C. Urine Is Not Sterile: Use of Enhanced Urine Culture Techniques to Detect Resident Bacterial Flora in the Adult Female Bladder. *J. Clin. Microbiol.* **2014**, *52*, 871–876. [CrossRef]
110. Price, T.K.; Dune, T.; Hilt, E.E.; Thomas-White, K.J.; Kliethermes, S.; Brincat, C.; Brubaker, L.; Wolfe, A.J.; Mueller, E.R.; Schreckenberger, P.C. The Clinical Urine Culture: Enhanced Techniques Improve Detection of Clinically Relevant Microorganisms. *J. Clin. Microbiol.* **2016**, *54*, 1216–1222. [CrossRef]
111. Pearce, M.M.; Hilt, E.E.; Rosenfeld, A.B.; Zilliox, M.J.; Thomas-White, K.; Fok, C.; Kliethermes, S.; Schreckenberger, P.C.; Brubaker, L.; Gai, X.; et al. The Female Urinary Microbiome: A Comparison of Women with and without Urgency Urinary Incontinence. *Mbio* **2014**, *5*, e01283-14. [CrossRef] [PubMed]
112. Khasriya, R.; Sathiananthamoorthy, S.; Ismail, S.; Kelsey, M.; Wilson, M.; Rohn, J.L.; Malone-Lee, J. Spectrum of Bacterial Colonization Associated with Urothelial Cells from Patients with Chronic Lower Urinary Tract Symptoms. *J. Clin. Microbiol.* **2013**, *51*, 2054–2062. [CrossRef] [PubMed]
113. McDonald, M.; Kameh, D.; Johnson, M.E.; Johansen, T.E.B.; Albala, D.; Mouraviev, V. A Head-to-Head Comparative Phase II Study of Standard Urine Culture and Sensitivity Versus DNA Next-generation Sequencing Testing for Urinary Tract Infections. *Rev. Urol.* **2017**, *19*, 213–220. [CrossRef] [PubMed]
114. Ishihara, T.; Watanabe, N.; Inoue, S.; Aoki, H.; Tsuji, T.; Yamamoto, B.; Yanagi, H.; Oki, M.; Kryukov, K.; Nakagawa, S.; et al. Usefulness of next-generation DNA sequencing for the diagnosis of urinary tract infection. *Drug Discov. Ther.* **2020**, *14*, 42–49. [CrossRef]
115. Bennett, J.E.; Dolin, R.; Blaser, M.J. *Mandell, Douglas, and Bennett's Principles and Practice of Infectious Diseases*; Elsevier Health Sciences: Philadelphia, PA, USA, 2014; Volume 2.
116. Hooton, T.M. Recurrent urinary tract infection in women. *Int. J. Antimicrob. Agents* **2001**, *17*, 259–268. [CrossRef] [PubMed]
117. Brannon, J.R.; Dunigan, T.L.; Beebout, C.J.; Ross, T.; Wiebe, M.A.; Reynolds, W.S.; Hadjifrangiskou, M. Invasion of vaginal epithelial cells by uropathogenic Escherichia coli. *Nat. Commun.* **2020**, *11*, 2803. [CrossRef]
118. Rosen, D.A.; Pinkner, J.S.; Jones, J.M.; Walker, J.N.; Clegg, S.; Hultgren, S.J. Utilization of an Intracellular Bacterial Community Pathway in *Klebsiella pneumoniae* Urinary Tract Infection and the Effects of FimK on Type 1 Pilus Expression. *Infect. Immun.* **2008**, *76*, 3337–3345. [CrossRef] [PubMed]
119. Robino, L.; Scavone, P.; Araujo, L.; Algorta, G.; Zunino, P.; Vignoli, R. Detection of intracellular bacterial communities in a child with *Escherichia coli* recurrent urinary tract infections. *Pathog. Dis.* **2013**, *68*, 78–81. [CrossRef]
120. Schilling, J.D.; Lorenz, R.G.; Hultgren, S.J. Effect of Trimethoprim-Sulfamethoxazole on Recurrent Bacteriuria and Bacterial Persistence in Mice Infected with Uropathogenic *Escherichia coli*. *Infect. Immun.* **2002**, *70*, 7042–7049. [CrossRef]
121. Mysorekar, I.U.; Hultgren, S.J. Mechanisms of uropathogenic *Escherichia coli* persistence and eradication from the urinary tract. *Proc. Natl. Acad. Sci. USA* **2006**, *103*, 14170–14175. [CrossRef] [PubMed]
122. Kim, A.; Ahn, J.H.; Choi, W.S.; Park, H.K.; Kim, S.; Paick, S.H.; Kim, H.G. What is the Cause of Recurrent Urinary Tract Infection? Contemporary Microscopic Concepts of Pathophysiology. *Int. Neurourol. J.* **2021**, *25*, 192–201. [CrossRef]
123. Simpson, B.W.; May, J.M.; Sherman, D.J.; Kahne, D.; Ruiz, N. Lipopolysaccharide transport to the cell surface: Biosynthesis and extraction from the inner membrane. *Philos. Trans. R. Soc. Lond. B Biol. Sci.* **2015**, *370*, 20150029. [CrossRef]
124. Zhang, G.; Meredith, T.C.; Kahne, D. On the essentiality of lipopolysaccharide to Gram-negative bacteria. *Curr. Opin. Microbiol.* **2013**, *16*, 779–785. [CrossRef] [PubMed]
125. Hunstad, D.A.; Justice, S.S.; Hung, C.S.; Lauer, S.R.; Hultgren, S.J. Suppression of Bladder Epithelial Cytokine Responses by Uropathogenic *Escherichia coli*. *Infect. Immun.* **2005**, *73*, 3999–4006. [CrossRef] [PubMed]
126. Yang, Y.; Wang, H.; Kouadir, M.; Song, H.; Shi, F. Recent advances in the mechanisms of NLRP3 inflammasome activation and its inhibitors. *Cell Death Dis.* **2019**, *10*, 128. [CrossRef]

127. Hughes, F.M., Jr.; Vivar, N.P.; Kennis, J.G.; Pratt-Thomas, J.D.; Lowe, D.W.; Shaner, B.E.; Nietert, P.J.; Spruill, L.S.; Purves, J.T. Inflammasomes are important mediators of cyclo¬phosphamide-induced bladder inflammation. *Am. J. Physiol. Ren. Physiol.* **2014**, *306*, F299–F308. [CrossRef]
128. Jaillon, S.; Moalli, F.; Ragnarsdottir, B.; Bonavita, E.; Puthia, M.; Riva, F.; Barbati, E.; Nebuloni, M.; Krajinovic, L.C.; Markotic, A.; et al. The Humoral Pattern Recognition Molecule PTX3 Is a Key Component of Innate Immunity against Urinary Tract Infection. *Immunity* **2014**, *40*, 621–632. [CrossRef]
129. Bishop, B.L.; Duncan, M.J.; Song, J.; Li, G.; Zaas, D.; Abraham, S.N. Cyclic AMP–regulated exocytosis of *Escherichia coli* from infected bladder epithelial cells. *Nat. Med.* **2007**, *13*, 625–630. [CrossRef] [PubMed]
130. O'Brien, V.P.; Lewis, A.L.; Gilbert, N.M. Bladder Exposure to Gardnerella Activates Host Pathways Necessary for *Escherichia coli* Recurrent UTI. *Front. Cell. Infect. Microbiol.* **2021**, *11*, 788229. [CrossRef]
131. Yoon, K.; Lee, S.-O.; Cho, S.-D.; Kim, K.; Khan, S.; Safe, S. Activation of nuclear TR3 (NR4A1) by a diindolylmethane analog induces apoptosis and proapoptotic genes in pancreatic cancer cells and tumors. *Carcinog.* **2011**, *32*, 836–842. [CrossRef]
132. Gao, H.; Chen, Z.; Fu, Y.; Yang, X.; Weng, R.; Wang, R.; Lu, J.; Pan, M.; Jin, K.; McElroy, C.; et al. Nur77 exacerbates PC12 cellular injury in vitro by aggravating mitochondrial impairment and endoplasmic reticulum stress. *Sci. Rep.* **2016**, *6*, 34403. [CrossRef] [PubMed]
133. Rajpal, A.; Cho, Y.A.; Yelent, B.; Koza-Taylor, P.H.; Li, D.; Chen, E.; Whang, M.; Kang, C.; Turi, T.G.; Winoto, A. Transcriptional activation of known and novel apoptotic pathways by Nur77 orphan steroid receptor. *EMBO J.* **2003**, *22*, 6526–6536. [CrossRef] [PubMed]
134. Herring, J.A.; Elison, W.S.; Tessem, J.S. Function of Nr4a Orphan Nuclear Receptors in Proliferation, Apoptosis and Fuel Utilization Across Tissues. *Cells* **2019**, *8*, 1373. [CrossRef]
135. Rodríguez-Calvo, R.; Tajes, M.; Vázquez-Carrera, M. The NR4A subfamily of nuclear receptors: Potential new therapeutic targets for the treatment of inflammatory diseases. *Expert Opin. Ther. Targets* **2017**, *21*, 291–304. [CrossRef]
136. Liebmann, M.; Hucke, S.; Koch, K.; Eschborn, M.; Ghelman, J.; Chasan, A.I.; Glander, S.; Schädlich, M.; Kuhlencord, M.; Daber, N.M.; et al. Nur77 serves as a molecular brake of the metabolic switch during T cell activation to restrict autoimmunity. *Proc. Natl. Acad. Sci. USA* **2018**, *115*, E8017–E8026. [CrossRef]
137. Hanna, R.N.; Carlin, L.M.; Hubbeling, H.G.; Nackiewicz, D.; Green, A.M.; Punt, J.A.; Geissmann, F.; Hedrick, C.C. The transcription factor NR4A1 (Nur77) controls bone marrow differentiation and the survival of Ly6C− monocytes. *Nat. Immunol.* **2011**, *12*, 778–785. [CrossRef]
138. O'Brien, V.P.; Joens, M.S.; Lewis, A.L.; Gilbert, N.M. Recurrent *Escherichia coli* Urinary Tract Infection Triggered by Gardnerella vaginalis Bladder Exposure in Mice. *J. Vis. Exp.* **2020**, *166*, e61967. [CrossRef]
139. Kirjavainen, P.V.; Pautler, S.; Baroja, M.L.; Anukam, K.; Crowley, K.; Carter, K.; Reid, G. Abnormal Immunological Profile and Vaginal Microbiota in Women Prone to Urinary Tract Infections. *Clin. Vaccine Immunol.* **2009**, *16*, 29–36. [CrossRef]
140. Neugent, M.L.; Kumar, A.; Hulyalkar, N.V.; Lutz, K.C.; Nguyen, V.H.; Fuentes, J.L.; Zhang, C.; Nguyen, A.; Sharon, B.M.; Kuprasertkul, A.; et al. Recurrent urinary tract infection and estrogen shape the taxonomic ecology and function of the postmenopausal urogenital microbiome. *Cell Rep. Med.* **2022**, *3*, 100753. [CrossRef]
141. Akgul, T.; Karakan, T. The role of probiotics in women with recurrent urinary tract infections. *Turk. J. Urol.* **2018**, *44*, 377–383. [CrossRef] [PubMed]
142. Boswell-Ruys, C.L.; Toh, S.-L.; Lee, B.S.B.; Simpson, J.M.; Clezy, K.R. Probiotics for preventing urinary tract infection in people with neuropathic bladder. *Cochrane Database Syst. Rev.* **2017**, *9*, 010723. [CrossRef]
143. Goneau, L.W.; Yeoh, N.S.; MacDonald, K.W.; Cadieux, P.A.; Burton, J.P.; Razvi, H.; Reid, G. Selective Target Inactivation Rather than Global Metabolic Dormancy Causes Antibiotic Tolerance in Uropathogens. *Antimicrob. Agents Chemother.* **2014**, *58*, 2089–2097. [CrossRef]
144. Uehara, S.; Monden, K.; Nomoto, K.; Seno, Y.; Kariyama, R.; Kumon, H. A pilot study evaluating the safety and effectiveness of Lactobacillus vaginal suppositories in patients with recurrent urinary tract infection. *Int. J. Antimicrob. Agents* **2006**, *28* (Suppl. 1), 30–34. [CrossRef]
145. Sadahira, T.; Wada, K.; Araki, M.; Mitsuhata, R.; Yamamoto, M.; Maruyama, Y.; Iwata, T.; Watanabe, M.; Watanabe, T.; Kariyama, R.; et al. Efficacy of *Lactobacillus* vaginal suppositories for the prevention of recurrent cystitis: A phase II clinical trial. *Int. J. Urol.* **2021**, *28*, 1026–1031. [CrossRef]
146. Reid, G.; Charbonneau, D.; Erb, J.; Kochanowski, B.; Beuerman, D.; Poehner, R.; Bruce, A.W. Oral use of Lactobacillus rhamnosus GR-1 and L. fermentum RC-14 significantly alters vaginal flora: Randomized, placebo-controlled trial in 64 healthy women. *FEMS Immunol. Med. Microbiol.* **2003**, *35*, 131–134. [CrossRef]
147. Garofalo, L.; Nakama, C.; Hanes, D.; Zwickey, H. Whole-Person, Urobiome-Centric Therapy for Uncomplicated Urinary Tract Infection. *Antibiotics* **2022**, *11*, 218. [CrossRef]
148. Heinemann, C.; Reid, G. Vaginal microbial diversity among postmenopausal women with and without hormone replacement therapy. *Can. J. Microbiol.* **2005**, *51*, 777–781. [CrossRef]
149. Raz, R. Hormone Replacement Therapy or Prophylaxis in Postmenopausal Women with Recurrent Urinary Tract Infection. *J. Infect. Dis.* **2001**, *183*, S74–S76. [CrossRef] [PubMed]

150. Cauci, S.; Driussi, S.; De Santo, D.; Penacchioni, P.; Iannicelli, T.; Lanzafame, P.; De Seta, F.; Quadrifoglio, F.; de Aloysio, D.; Guaschino, S. Prevalence of Bacterial Vaginosis and Vaginal Flora Changes in Peri- and Postmenopausal Women. *J. Clin. Microbiol.* **2002**, *40*, 2147–2152. [CrossRef] [PubMed]
151. Eriksen, B.C. A randomized, open, parallel-group study on the preventive effect of an estradiol-releasing vaginal ring (Estring) on recurrent urinary tract infections in postmenopausal women. *Am. J. Obstet. Gynecol.* **1999**, *180*, 1072–1079. [CrossRef] [PubMed]
152. Krause, M.; Wheeler, T.L., 2nd; Snyder, T.E.; Richter, H.E. Local Effects of Vaginally Administered Estrogen Therapy: A Review. *J. Pelvic Med. Surg.* **2009**, *15*, 105–114. [CrossRef]
153. Mehta, J.; Utkarsh, K.; Fuloria, S.; Singh, T.; Sekar, M.; Salaria, D.; Rolta, R.; Begum, M.Y.; Gan, S.H.; Rani, N.N.I.M.; et al. Antibacterial Potential of *Bacopa monnieri* (L.) Wettst. and Its Bioactive Molecules against Uropathogens—An In Silico Study to Identify Potential Lead Molecule(s) for the Development of New Drugs to Treat Urinary Tract Infections. *Molecules* **2022**, *27*, 4971. [CrossRef] [PubMed]

Disclaimer/Publisher's Note: The statements, opinions and data contained in all publications are solely those of the individual author(s) and contributor(s) and not of MDPI and/or the editor(s). MDPI and/or the editor(s) disclaim responsibility for any injury to people or property resulting from any ideas, methods, instructions or products referred to in the content.

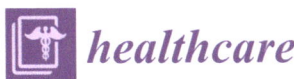

Article

Pelvic Floor Muscle Exercises as a Treatment for Urinary Incontinence in Postmenopausal Women: A Systematic Review of Randomized Controlled Trials

María Paz López-Pérez [1], Diego Fernando Afanador-Restrepo [2], Yulieth Rivas-Campo [3], Fidel Hita-Contreras [1], María del Carmen Carcelén-Fraile [1], Yolanda Castellote-Caballero [1,*], Carlos Rodríguez-López [4] and Agustín Aibar-Almazán [1]

1 Department of Health Sciences, Faculty of Health Sciences, University of Jaén, 23071 Jaen, Spain
2 Faculty of Health Sciences and Sport, University Foundation of the Área Andina-Pereira, Pereira 660004, Colombia
3 Faculty of Human and Social Sciences, University of San Buenaventura-Cali, Santiago de Cali 760016, Colombia
4 Gimbernat-Cantabria School of Physiotherapy, University of Cantabria, 39005 Santander, Spain
* Correspondence: mycastel@ujaen.es

Abstract: Women frequently suffer from urinary incontinence due to atrophic changes in the urogenital tract. Recommended conservative treatment includes evaluation of pelvic-floor strength and the functional use of pelvic-floor-muscle (PFM) training. Following the PRISMA 2020 guidelines, a search was conducted in the electronic databases PubMed, Web of Science, and Scopus for articles with at least one group performing PFM exercises in post-menopausal women with urinary incontinence. Eight articles were included, and each study had at least one group of PFM exercise-based intervention alone or combined. The volume or duration, frequency, and number of sessions were heterogeneous. All the studies reported significant differences in favor of PFM exercise in strength, quality of life, and/or severity of urinary incontinence. PFM exercise is a highly recommended intervention to treat urinary incontinence in postmenopausal women. However, more research is needed to establish specific factors such as dose–response relationships and to standardize methods for measuring effects.

Keywords: urinary incontinence; pelvic-floor-muscle exercises; postmenopausal women; systematic review

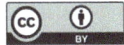

1. Introduction

Urinary incontinence was defined in 2003 as the complaint of any involuntary leakage of urine [1]. This condition is associated with risk factors such as pelvic-floor-muscle (PFM) deficits, pelvic surgery, prolapse, urinary-tract infections, obesity, smoking, constipation, diabetes mellitus, high-impact physical exercise, being female, increasing age, parity, and menopause [2,3].

Postmenopausal women frequently suffer from urinary incontinence as a result of increased intra-abdominal pressure, such as sneezing, coughing, jumping, laughing, or sexual relations [4]. Estrogen deficiency at this stage of the life cycle generates atrophic changes in the urogenital tract and vaginal and periurethral tissues [5], and has been associated with involuntary urine loss due to stress and increased urinary urgency and frequency [6]. Despite this association, there has been no evidence of improvement with hormonal management [7].

Among the options based on non-invasive and non-pharmacological intervention are therapeutic targeted exercise such as PFM training, which focuses on improving the function, muscle tone, strength, coordination, and endurance of the pelvic-floor musculature [8]. Other active treatment techniques are Kegel exercises, which focus on enhancing the strength and improving the function of the PFM [9], or pelvic-floor contraction exercises coupled with coactivation of the trunk-stabilizing muscles [10].

Conservative treatment, recommended as first line by the International Continence Society, includes assessment of pelvic-floor strength and functional use of PFM training [11]. The success of this intervention lies in the achievement of increased contraction and holding strength, coordination, speed, and endurance of the pelvic-floor musculature to keep the bladder elevated during demanding activities. Likewise, PFM training allows adequate urethral closure pressure to be maintained and supports and stabilizes the pelvic organs [12]. For postmenopausal women who receive regular supervision, it has been observed that they are more likely to comply and report a decrease in urinary incontinence than women who perform PFM training with little or no supervision [13].

Other systematic reviews related to exercise in this population can be found in the literature; however, they focused on determining the effects of exercise on quality of life or on comparing different interventions with this type of training on multiple variables associated with the pathology [14,15]. Therefore, the aim of the present review was to perform a systematic review of randomized controlled clinical trials that evaluated the effect of targeted PFM exercise in postmenopausal women for the treatment of urinary incontinence.

2. Materials and Methods

This systematic review was performed following the guidelines of the PRISMA statement (Preferred Reporting Items for Systematic reviews and Meta-Analysis) [16]. The pre-specified protocol was registered in PROSPERO under the code CRD42022373488.

2.1. Eligibility Criteria

Articles were selected according to the following criteria: clinical trial, randomized control trial with objective measures of urinary incontinence before and after an exercise-based intervention in postmenopausal women. Regarding the intervention, articles in which the PFM training method was used for the treatment of urinary incontinence during the postmenopausal period were included.

2.2. Information Sources

Data collection took place from October to November 2022 by consulting the following databases: Pubmed (MEDLINE), Scopus, and Web of Science.

2.3. Search Strategy

The keywords used were ("postmenopausal period" OR "postmenopausal" OR "postmenopausal women") AND ("diurnal enuresis" OR "enuresis" OR "daytime wetting" OR "daytime urinary incontinence" OR "urinary incontinence") AND ("pelvic floor muscle training" OR "pelvic floor exercises" OR "pelvic floor muscle exercise" OR "pelvic floor muscles") AND ("severity" OR "frequency of urination" OR "urinary frequency" OR "urination behaviors" OR "frequency of micturition" OR "micturition" OR "quality of life" OR "mental health" OR "depression" OR "sexual activity").

2.4. Selection Process

The search results were exported to the Rayyan QCRI application (https://rayyan.qcri.org/welcome accessed on 15 November 2021) [17]. Two blinded independent researchers conducted the literature review and decided on the inclusion of the articles separately. The pre-selection of the studies was performed based on reading of the title and abstract. Subsequently, the pre-selected articles were read in full text and the articles that met the criteria were included. In case of discrepancies, a third author resolved them.

2.5. Data-Collection Process

The main variable of this review was the objective measurement of urinary incontinence, mainly in terms of strength, quality of life, and severity of the incontinence. We included information on the authors, the year of publication, the country of publication, and the country in which the study was conducted; likewise, we collected the type, duration or volume, frequency, number of sessions, and number of weeks of the interventions performed, as well as the follow-up time and the results obtained in each measurement.

2.6. Assessment of Methodological Quality

The methodological quality of the articles included in this review was assessed using the PEDro scale [18], with a maximum score of 10 points, as the first item ("eligibility criteria") is not used in the final score calculation. Each item can be answered as either "Yes" (1 point) or "No" (0 points) [19]. A score between 0 and 3 was considered "Poor" quality, 4–5 "Fair," 6–8 "Good," and >9 "Excellent" [20]. The scores were consulted in the PEDro database; when scores were not found, two authors evaluated the methodological quality of articles, and in situations where a discrepancy was generated, it was resolved by a third author.

3. Results

3.1. Selection of the Studies

The database search resulted in a total of 91 articles, which were revised to identify duplicates, discarding 35 and leaving 56 unique articles. After a title-and-abstract screen, 11 potentially eligible articles remained. Finally, only eight articles [21–28] met the eligibility criteria established for this review (Figure 1).

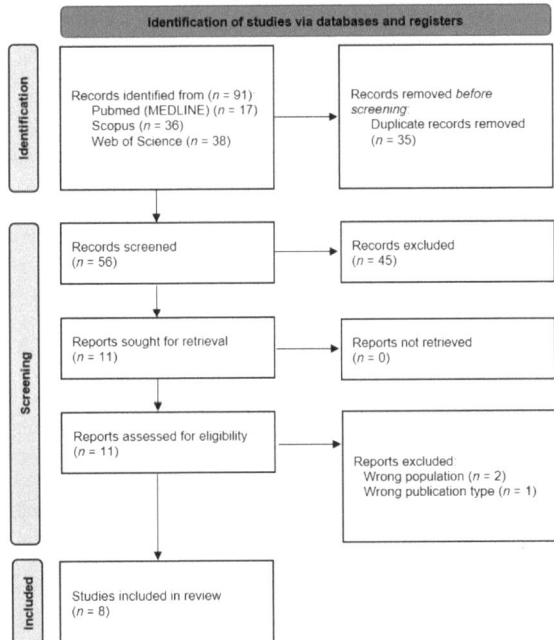

Figure 1. Flow diagram of the study-selection process.

3.2. Methodological Quality

Methodological quality was assessed using the PEDro scale. The scores of seven of the articles [21–27] were obtained from the PEDro website, whereas the remaining article [28] was calculated manually. Seven of the articles [22–28] included in this review presented "Good" methodological quality, and only one [21] had "Fair" methodological quality (Table 1).

Table 1. Methodological quality of the articles included.

Article	1	2	3	4	5	6	7	8	9	10	11	Total
Aksac et al., 2003 [21]	Y	Y	Y	Y	N	N	N	N	N	Y	Y	5
Sherburn et al., 2011 [22]	Y	Y	Y	Y	N	N	Y	Y	Y	Y	Y	8
Pereira et al., 2012 [23]	Y	Y	Y	N	N	N	N	Y	Y	Y	Y	6
Pereira et al., 2013 [24]	Y	Y	Y	Y	N	N	N	Y	N	Y	Y	6
Flávia et al., 2015 [25]	Y	Y	Y	Y	N	N	Y	Y	Y	Y	Y	8
Sran et al., 2016 [26]	Y	Y	Y	Y	N	N	Y	Y	Y	Y	Y	8
Bertotto et al., 2016 [27]	Y	Y	Y	Y	N	N	N	Y	N	Y	Y	6
Ghoniem et al., 2022 [28]	Y	Y	Y	Y	N	N	N	Y	N	Y	Y	6

Items: 1 = eligibility criteria; 2 = random allocation; 3 = concealed allocation; 4 = baseline comparability; 5 = blind subjects; 6 = blind therapists; 7 = blind assessors; 8 = adequate follow-up; 9 = intention-to-treat analysis; 10 = between-group comparisons; 11 = point estimates and variability; Y = Yes; N = No.

3.3. Characteristics of the Studies

The articles included in this systematic review were all randomized controlled clinical trials published in Switzerland [21,25], the United Kingdom [22–24], the United States [26,27], and Poland [28]; however, the studies were conducted in countries other than those in which they were published, such as Turkey [21], Australia [22], Brazil [23–25,27], Canada [26], and Egypt [28].

A total of 376 postmenopausal women aged 60.31 ± 6.73 years participated in the included studies. Out of the overall population, 196 postmenopausal women were part of the groups that received PFM exercise-based treatments (Table 2).

3.4. Study Intervention

Every study [21–28] included at least one group with a PFM exercise-based intervention. Six studies [21–25,27] performed PFM exercise-based interventions only, whereas Sran et al. [26] combined it with physiotherapy and Ghoniem et al. [28] with Pilates.

Although all the interventions included PFM exercises, the prescription of the volume or duration, frequency, and number of sessions was heterogeneous. Regarding frequency, one study proposed an intervention program with only one intervention per week [26], five studies proposed two sessions per week [23–25,27,28], one study maintained three sessions per day but did not specify the number of days per week [21], and one study did not specify either sessions per day or per week. The number of sessions ranged from 8 [27] to 12 [23,24,26] to 24 [25,28]; however, two studies did not specify the number of sessions [21,22].

Concerning the volume or duration of the exercises, four of the studies [23,24,26,27] dosed the exercises based on time, with sessions lasting from 20 min to 60 min. On the other hand, three studies [21,25,28] dosed the exercise based on the number of contractions and positions used, ranging from 10 contractions and one single position [21], to four positions and 10 contractions in each [25], and to positions with up to 52 contractions after the adaptation period [28].

3.5. Study Results

All the articles found a significant difference in favor of the PFM-exercise intervention in at least one variable related to the strength of this musculature, severity of incontinence, and/or quality of life [21–28]. In addition, when PFM exercises were applied in combination with other interventions, no significant differences were observed with the groups that did PFM exercises alone [28].

Table 2. Characteristics of the included studies.

Author and Year	Control Group	Sample CG/IG	Type of Urinary Incontinence	Population Characteristics	Intervention Group			
					Intervention Type	Variable Observed-Initial Measure	Modifications over Time	
Aksac et al., 2003 [21]	No treatment	10/20	Stress urinary incontinence	Age: 52.5 ± 7.9 Body weight: 59.4 ± 6.1 Parity: 2.8 ± 0.5	T: PFM exercises V: 10 contractions/session F: 3 sessions/day S: Not specified	1 h pad test, g 9.9 (SD = 2.5) Perineometry, cmH₂O 20.3 (SD = 6.2) PFM strength with digital palpation 3.5 (SD = 0.5) Incontinence frequency 2.3 (SD = 0.7) SAI 4.5 (SD = 0.3)	8 weeks 1 h pad test, g 2.1 (SD = 0.4) * Perineometry, cmH₂O 37.5 (SD = 8.7) * PFM strength with digital palpation 4.8 (SD = 0.4) * Incontinence frequency 3.5 (SD = 0.5) * SAI 7.5 (SD = 1.2) *	—
Sherburn et al., 2011 [22]	Bladder training	41/43	Stress urinary incontinence	Age: 71.6 ± 4.73 BMI: 27.6 ± 3.88 Parity: 3.2 ± 1.6	T: PFM exercises V: Not specified F: Not specified S: Not specified	Stress test—cough (g) 0.8 (IQR = 4.9) Stress test—brace/cough (g) 0.2 (IQR = 2.2)	1 month Stress test—cough 0.9 (IQR = 2.0) Stress test—brace/cough 0.2 (IQR = 0.5)	3 months Stress test—cough 0.6 (IQR = 2.8) Stress test—brace/cough 0 (IQR = 0.5) *	5 months Stress test—cough 0.1 (IRQ = 1.5) * Stress test—brace/cough 0 (IRQ = 0.3) *
Pereira et al., 2012 [23]	No treatment	14/15	Stress urinary incontinence	Age 63 ± 10.73 BMI: 25.65 ± 2.79 Parity: 2.26 ± 1.09	T: PFM exercises D: 40 min F: 2 times/week S: 12 sessions	Urinary leakage (g) 3.70 (SD = 4.35) PFM pressure 12.55 (SD = 9.20). General health 33.34 (SD = 18.09) Incontinence impact 55.82 (SD = 39.32) Gravity measures 41.33 (SD = 25.47)	6 weeks Urinary leakage (g) 0.19 (SD = 0.27) * PFM pressure 37.38 (SD = 18.18) * General health 23.33 (SD = 6.45) Incontinence impact 7.69 (SD = 14.6) * Gravity measures 5.91 (SD = 6.26) *	12 weeks Urinary leakage (g) 0.29 (SD = 0.31) * PFM pressure 35.22 (SD = 18.96) * General health 30.01 (SD = 16.90) Incontinence impact 17.76 (SD = 24.7) * Gravity measures 15.11 (SD = 23.0) *	—
Pereira et al., 2013 [24]	No treatment	13/13	Stress or urgency urinary incontinence	Age 62 (51–85) BMI: 25.7 (24.3–31.8) Parity: 2.0 (0–4)	T: PFM exercises D: 40 min F: 2 times/week S: 12 sessions	Urinary leakage (g) 1.9 (1.0–15.2) * PFM pressure (cmH₂O) 0.7 (2.7–43.3) General health 33.3 (0–100) Incontinence impact 46.7 (6–73.3) *	3 months Urinary leakage (g) 0.1 (0–0.9) * PFM pressure (cmH₂O) 37.3 (15.3–60) General health 25.0 (0–25) Incontinence impact 0.0 (0–33) * Gravity measures 0.0 (0–7) *	6 months Urinary leakage (g) 0.1 (0–1.2) * PFM pressure (cmH₂O) 15.3 (7.3–60) * General health 25.0 (0–25) Incontinence impact 0.0 (0–0) * Gravity measures 0.0 (0–20) *	—
Flavia et al., 2015 [25]	No treatment	41/47	Stress or urgency urinary incontinence	Age 52.9 ± 4.1 BMI: 28.5 ± 5.4 Vaginal births: 1.1 ± 1.4	T: PFM exercises V: 4 positions with 10 voluntary maximal contractions each F: 2 times/week S: 24 sessions	PFM strength (cmH₂O) 38.5 (SD = 23.6) Prevalence of UI, n/N (%) 21/47 (44.7%) UI severity (0 to 21) 3.8 (SD = 5.0) *	12 weeks PFM strength (cmH₂O) 44.7 (SD = 24.0) * Prevalence of UI, n/N (%) 17/47 (36.2%) * UI severity (0 to 21) 1.9 (SD = 2.9)	—	

Table 2. Cont.

Author and Year	Sample CG/IG	Control Group	Type of Urinary Incontinence	Population Characteristics	Intervention Type	Intervention Group Variable Observed-Initial Measure	Intervention Group Modifications over Time
Sran et al., 2016 [26]	24/24	Osteoporosis education	Stress, urgency, or mixed urinary incontinence	Age 66.17 ± 6.66 BMI: 24.69 ± 3.93 Parity: 1.35 ± 1.15	T: Physical therapy + PFM training D: 30–60 min F: 1 time/week S: 12 sessions	3 months # of leakage episodes 8.00 (4.00–10.50) Pad test (weight, g) 6.50 (3.00–25.50) UDI total score 113.07 (75.85–137.41) IIQ total score 53.06 (22.33–88.13) Self-perceived efficacy 0.51 (0.38–0.68)	12 months # of leakage episodes 2.00 (0.00–5.75) * Pad test (weight, g) 2.50 (1.00–3.75) * UDI total score 66.29 (20.54–90.91) * IIQ total score 6.95 (0.00–26.39) Self-perceived efficacy 0.64 (0.51–0.76)
Bertotto et al., 2016 [27]	15/15	No treatment	Stress urinary incontinence	Age 59.3 ± 4.9 BMI: 27.7 ± 3.6 Number of pregnancies: 2.3 ± 1.3	T: PFM exercises D: 20 min F: 2 times/week S: 8 sessions	Precontraction 0.13 (SD = 0.9) Initial EMG baseline (µv) 14.7 (SD = 4.4) Final EMG baseline (µv) 15.5 (SD = 3.3) DEC (s) 1.66 (SD = 2.55) MVC (µv) 10.3 (SD = 2.11) ICIQ-SF quality-of-life score 11.1 (SD = 2.9)	6 weeks Precontraction 0.67 (SD = 0.12) * Initial EMG baseline (µv) 16.3 (SD = 2.9) * Final EMG baseline (µv) 15.9 (SD = 2.4) DEC (s) 6.8 (SD = 2.01) * MVC (µv) 20 (SD = 5.21) * ICIQ-SF quality-of-life score 4.3 (SD = 3.2) *	—
Ghoniem et al., 2022 [28]	15/15	Same program without Pilates	Stress urinary incontinence	Age 55.13 ± 4.48 BMI: 26.86 ± 1.92 Parity: not reported	T: PFM exercises + Pilates D: 3 positions with up to 52 contractions F: 2 times/week S: 24 sessions	Squeeze vaginal pressure CG: 18.1 (SD = 6.25) IG: 18.33 (SD = 6.45) Urinary-incontinence scale CG: 11.46 (SD = 1.95) IG: 10.93 (SD = 2.08)	12 weeks Squeeze vaginal pressure CG: 23.33 (SD = 9.29) * IG: 26.66 (SD = 9.29) * Urinary-incontinence scale CG: 10.33(SD = 2.19) * IG: 9.06 (SD = 1.62) * No significant difference between groups	—

CG: control group; IG: intervention group; T: type; D: duration; F: frequency; I: intensity; PFM: pelvic-floor muscles; SAI: social activity index; IQR: interquartile range; SD: standard deviation; UI: urinary incontinence; #: number; DEC: duration of endurance contraction; MVC: maximum voluntary contraction; ICIQ-SF: International Consultation Incontinence Questionnaire—Short Form; UDI: Urogenital Distress Inventory; IIQ: Incontinence Impact Questionnaire; EMG: electromyographic; *: statistically significant.

Similarly, to the interventions, the outcomes measured remained heterogeneous. Statistically significant changes ($p < 0.05$) were observed in the 1 h pad test [21,26], perineometry [21], PFM strength with digital palpation [21], incontinence frequency [21], stress test [22], urinary leakage [23,24], PFM pressure [23,24], incontinence impact [23,24], gravity measures [23,24], urinary-incontinence severity [25], number of leakage episodes [26], Urogenital Distress Inventory total score [26], precontraction [27], initial electromyographic baseline [27], duration of endurance contraction [27], maximum voluntary contraction [27], International Consultation Incontinence Questionnaire—Short Form [27], squeeze vaginal pressure [28], and the Urinary Incontinence Scale [28].

4. Discussion

The present systematic review aimed to determine the effects of PFM exercises in the treatment of urinary incontinence in postmenopausal women. The review included eight randomized controlled trials that met the selection criteria [21–28]. After analysis of the studies, scientific evidence was found to support the use of PFM training as an effective intervention for incontinence in the studied population.

Several risk factors predispose to the development of urinary incontinence in women, such as high parity, history of vaginal deliveries, and menopause [29–31]. In addition, obesity and aging are also important variables for the development of urinary incontinence independent of sex [32]. Within the eight articles included in this review, six studied overweight postmenopausal women (BMI > 25 Kg/m^2–<30 Kg/m^2) [22–25,27,28], one included postmenopausal women with normal weight [26], and finally, one article did not report BMI [21]. However, regardless of the BMI of the participants, the effects were statistically significant in all studies, which is in agreement with the systematic review made by Woodley et al. [33], who also conducted studies with varied BMI populations and observed favorable effects in all articles.

From the eight articles included in this review, 5 = five [21–23,27,28] focused on stress urinary incontinence only, two [24,25] included patients with stress or urgency urinary incontinence, and just one [26] of the articles included patients with stress, urgency, or mixed urinary incontinence; however, the effects of PFM training were statistically significant irrespective of this factor.

All studies used different measurement techniques to assess strength, quality of life, and the severity and prevalence of the urinary incontinence. Regarding strength, six articles [21,23–25,27] found statistically significant favorable changes in all of them. This is congruent with the findings of Alouini et al. [34], who reported similar results regarding the improvement of strength through PFM exercises in women. Strength production is mainly due to two factors: muscle-fiber trophism and motor-unit recruitment capacity. Current evidence suggests that changes in strength, at least during the first 8 weeks of a training protocol, are mainly caused by an increase in motor-unit recruitment capacity [35,36]. The protocols included in this review that found favorable results in terms of strength ranged from 6 to 12 weeks, finding in neural adaptations an explanation for their results. Additionally, one study evaluated the long-term effects [24], reporting that after 6 months, the strength gain decreased, however the change was not large enough to reach baseline.

The prevalence and severity of urinary incontinence was evaluated in seven of the studies [21–26,28], with statistically significant changes observed, both acutely and chronically, in favor of the groups that performed PFM exercise. The most prevalent ways to measure this variable were the pad test [21,26] and the amount or number of urinary leakages [23,24,26]. These results are similar to those obtained by other authors who determined the effects of PFM training in other population groups [33,37–39].

Quality of life was assessed in six [21,23–27] out of the eight studies included in this review, using different instruments such as the Social Activity Index [21], the International Consultation Incontinence Questionnaire—Short Form [25,27], the Incontinence Impact Questionnaire [26], and three domains (general health, incontinence impact, and gravity) of the King's Health Questionnaire [23,24]. Only one of the studies [25] did not show statistically significant changes in this variable, mainly because the population of the intervention and control groups were not balanced from baseline (intergroup difference at baseline $p = 0.03$). Usually, patients with urinary incontinence present discomfort, low self-esteem, mood deterioration, and a feeling of helplessness, which generates an important psychological impact that ends up affecting the quality of life of the patient [37,40–42]. This is why interventions that generate a decrease in urinary incontinence are associated with an improvement in quality of life [43].

This systematic review is the first to evaluate the effects of PFM exercises in postmenopausal women with urinary incontinence; however, it has several limitations, and the results should be interpreted with discretion. The great heterogeneity in the exercise prescription does not allow an optimal prescription of the intervention to be established. In addition, no study was carried out in a European population; hence, a geographic bias was observed. Finally, it was not possible to calculate the size of the effects through a meta-analysis due to the great variety in the variables and the instruments and measurement techniques used by the different authors.

5. Conclusions

PFM exercise is a highly recommended intervention for treating urinary incontinence in postmenopausal women, whether it is applied alone or in combination with other interventions. Although the studies included in this review suggest that PFM training is effective regardless of the type of urinary incontinence, the current evidence is insufficient to be certain. Additionally, it is necessary to establish specific criteria for prescribing PFM exercises and measuring their results. More research in this field is needed, focused mainly on establishing the dose–response relationship of this intervention and on standardizing the methods of measuring the effects.

Author Contributions: Conceptualization, M.P.L.-P., C.R.-L. and Y.R.-C.; methodology, A.A.-A., F.H.-C. and M.d.C.C.-F.; writing—original draft preparation, M.P.L.-P, D.F.A.-R. and Y.C.-C.; writing—review and editing, Y.R.-C., M.d.C.C.-F., A.A.-A. and C.R.-L.; supervision, D.F.A.-R., Y.C.-C. and F.H.-C. All authors have read and agreed to the published version of the manuscript.

Funding: This research received no external funding.

Institutional Review Board Statement: Not applicable.

Informed Consent Statement: Not applicable.

Data Availability Statement: Not applicable.

Conflicts of Interest: The authors declare no conflict of interest.

References

1. Abrams, P.; Cardozo, L.; Fall, M.; Griffiths, D.; Rosier, P.; Ulmsten, U.; Van Kerrebroeck, P.; Victor, A.; Wein, A. The standardisation of terminology in lower urinary tract function: Report from the standardisation sub-committee of the international continence society. *Urology* **2003**, *61*, 37–49. [CrossRef] [PubMed]
2. National Institute for Health and Care. *Risk Factors for Pelvic Floor Dysfunction*; National Institute for Health and Care: London, UK, 2021.
3. Robles, J.E. La incontinencia urinaria %j anales del sistema sanitario de navarra. *An. Sis San Navar.* **2006**, *29*, 219–231. Available online: http://scielo.isciii.es/scielo.php?script=sci_arttext&pid=S1137-66272006000300006&nrm=iso (accessed on 8 October 2022).
4. Tubaro, A. Defining overactive bladder: Epidemiology and burden of disease. *Urology* **2004**, *64*, 2–6. [CrossRef] [PubMed]
5. Robinson, D.; Cardozo, L.D. The role of estrogens in female lower urinary tract dysfunction. *Urology* **2003**, *62*, 45–51. [CrossRef] [PubMed]
6. Seyyedi, F. Comparison of the effects of vaginal royal jelly and vaginal estrogen on quality of life, sexual and urinary function in postmenopausal women. *J. Clin. Diagn. Res.* **2016**, *10*, Qc01-5. [CrossRef]
7. Ces, J.; Lago, I.; Liceras, J. Menopausia e incontinencia urinaria femenina: Acerca del posible efecto de la terapia hormonal sustitutiva. *Clínica E Investig. En Ginecol. Y Obstet.* **2007**, *34*, 224–229. [CrossRef]
8. Dumoulin, C.; Cacciari, L.P.; Hay-Smith, E.J.C. Pelvic Floor Muscle Training Versus no Treatment, or Inactive Control Treatments, for Urinary Incontinence in Women. Available online: https://pubmed.ncbi.nlm.nih.gov/30288727/ (accessed on 8 October 2022).

9. Arañó, P.; Rebollo, P.; Alsina, D.G.-S. Afectación de la calidad de vida relacionada con la salud en mujeres con incontinencia urinaria mixta. *Actas Urológicas Españolas* **2009**, *33*, 410–415. [CrossRef] [PubMed]
10. Hay-Smith, E.J.C.; Herderschee, R.; Dumoulin, C.; Herbison, G.P. Comparisons of approaches to pelvic floor muscle training for urinary incontinence in women. *Cochrane Database Syst. Rev.* **2011**, *2011*, CD009508. [CrossRef] [PubMed]
11. Chamochumbi, C.C.M.; Nunes, F.R.; Guirro, R.R.D.J.; Guirro, E.C.D.O. Comparison of active and passive forces of the pelvic floor muscles in women with and without stress urinary incontinence. *Rev. Bras Fisioter.* **2012**, *16*, 314–319. [CrossRef] [PubMed]
12. Berghmans; Hendriks; Bø; Smith, H.; Bie, D.; Van Doorn, V.W. Conservative treatment of stress urinary incontinence in women: A systematic review of randomized clinical trials. *Br. J. Urol.* **1998**, *82*, 181–191. [CrossRef]
13. Wu, C.; Newman, D.; Schwartz, T.A.; Zou, B.; Miller, J.; Palmer, M.H. Effects of unsupervised behavioral and pelvic floor muscle training programs on nocturia, urinary urgency, and urinary frequency in postmenopausal women: Secondary analysis of a randomized, two-arm, parallel design, superiority trial (tulip study). *Maturitas* **2021**, *146*, 42–48. [CrossRef] [PubMed]
14. Malinauskas, A.P.; Bressan, E.F.M.; de Melo, A.M.Z.R.P.; Brasil, C.A.; Lordêlo, P.; Torelli, L. Efficacy of pelvic floor physiotherapy intervention for stress urinary incontinence in postmenopausal women: Systematic review. *Arch. Gynecol. Obstet.* **2022**. [CrossRef] [PubMed]
15. Nguyen, T.M.; Do, T.T.T.; Tran, T.N.; Kim, J.H. Exercise and quality of life in women with menopausal symptoms: A systematic review and meta-analysis of randomized controlled trials. *Int. J. Environ. Res. Public Health* **2020**, *17*, 7049. [CrossRef] [PubMed]
16. Page, M.J.; McKenzie, J.E.; Bossuyt, P.M.; Boutron, I.; Hoffmann, T.C.; Mulrow, C.D.; Shamseer, L.; Tetzlaff, J.M.; Akl, E.A.; Brennan, S.E.; et al. The prisma 2020 statement: An updated guideline for reporting systematic reviews. *Syst. Rev.* **2021**, *10*, 105906. [CrossRef] [PubMed]
17. Ouzzani, M.; Hammady, H.; Fedorowicz, Z.; Elmagarmid, A. Rayyan—A web and mobile app for systematic reviews. *Syst. Rev.* **2016**, *5*, 210. [CrossRef]
18. Macedo, L.G.; Elkins, M.R.; Maher, C.G.; Moseley, A.M.; Herbert, R.D.; Sherrington, C. There was evidence of convergent and construct validity of physiotherapy evidence database quality scale for physiotherapy trials. *J. Clin. Epidemiol.* **2010**, *63*, 920–925. [CrossRef]
19. Armijo-Olivo, S.; Pitance, L.; Singh, V.; Neto, F.; Thie, N.; Michelotti, A. Effectiveness of manual therapy and therapeutic exercise for temporomandibular disorders: Systematic review and meta-analysis. *Phys. Ther.* **2016**, *96*, 9–25. [CrossRef]
20. Rivas-Campo, Y.; García-Garro, P.A.; Aibar-Almazán, A.; Martínez-Amat, A.; Vega-Ávila, G.C.; Afanador-Restrepo, D.F.; León-Morillas, F.; Hita-Contreras, F. The effects of high-intensity functional training on cognition in older adults with cognitive impairment: A systematic review. *Healthcare* **2022**, *10*, 670. [CrossRef]
21. Aksac, B.; Aki, S.; Karan, A.; Yalcin, O.; Isikoglu, M.; Eskiyurt, N. Biofeedback and pelvic floor exercises for the rehabilitation of urinary stress incontinence. *Gynecol. Obs. Investig.* **2003**, *56*, 23–27. [CrossRef]
22. Sherburn, M.; Bird, M.; Carey, M.; Bø, K.; Galea, M.P. Incontinence improves in older women after intensive pelvic floor muscle training: An assessor-blinded randomized controlled trial. *Neurourol. Urodyn.* **2011**, *30*, 317–324. [CrossRef]
23. Pereira, V.S.; De Melo, M.V.; Correia, G.N.; Driusso, P. Vaginal cone for postmenopausal women with stress urinary incontinence: Randomized, controlled trial. *Climacteric* **2012**, *15*, 45–51. [CrossRef] [PubMed]
24. Pereira, V.S.; de Melo, M.V.; Correia, G.N.; Driusso, P. Long-term effects of pelvic floor muscle training with vaginal cone in post-menopausal women with urinary incontinence: A randomized controlled trial. *Neurourol. Urodyn.* **2013**, *32*, 48–52. [CrossRef] [PubMed]
25. Antônio, F.I.; Herbert, R.D.; Bø, K.; Rosa-E-Silva, A.C.J.S.; Lara, L.A.S.; Franco, M.D.M.; Ferreira, C.H.J. Pelvic floor muscle training increases pelvic floor muscle strength more in post-menopausal women who are not using hormone therapy than in women who are using hormone therapy: A randomised trial. *J. Physiother.* **2018**, *64*, 166–171. [CrossRef] [PubMed]
26. Sran, M.; Mercier, J.; Wilson, P.; Lieblich, P.; Dumoulin, C. Physical therapy for urinary incontinence in postmenopausal women with osteoporosis or low bone density: A randomized controlled trial. *Menopause* **2016**, *23*, 286–293. [CrossRef] [PubMed]
27. Bertotto, A.; Schvartzman, R.; Uchôa, S.; Wender, M. Effect of electromyographic biofeedback as an add-on to pelvic floor muscle exercises on neuromuscular outcomes and quality of life in postmenopausal women with stress urinary incontinence: A randomized controlled trial. *Neurourol. Urodyn.* **2017**, *36*, 2142–2147. [CrossRef]
28. Ghoniem, W.M.; Youssef, A.M.; Mohamed, S.A.; Elinin, M.F.A.; Hasanin, M.E. Effect of pilates exercises on stress urinary incontinence in post menopausal women: A randomized control trial. *Fizjoterapia Pol.* **2022**, *22*, 82–87. Available online: https://www.scopus.com/inward/record.uri?eid=2-s2.0-85133327931&partnerID=40&md5=4d91ebea1b9969fe4f72be6c7407f97f (accessed on 28 October 2022).
29. MacArthur, C.; Lewis, M.; Bick, D. Stress incontinence after childbirth. *Br. J. Midwifery* **1993**, *1*, 207–215. [CrossRef]
30. Wilson, P.D.; Herbison, R.M.; Herbison, G.P. Obstetric practice and the prevalence of urinary incontinence three months after delivery. *BJOG Int. J. Obstet. Gynaecol.* **1996**, *103*, 154–161. [CrossRef]
31. Thom, D.H.; Eeden, S.K.V.D.; Brown, J.S. Evaluation of parturition and other reproductive variables as risk factors for urinary incontinence in later life. *Obstet. Gynecol.* **1997**, *90*, 983–989. [CrossRef]
32. Irwin, G.M. Urinary incontinence. *Prim Care* **2019**, *46*, 233–242. [CrossRef]
33. Woodley, S.J.; Boyle, R.; Cody, J.D.; Mørkved, S.; Hay-Smith, E.J.C. Pelvic floor muscle training for prevention and treatment of urinary and faecal incontinence in antenatal and postnatal women. *Cochrane Database Syst. Rev.* **2017**, *12*, Cd007471. [CrossRef] [PubMed]

34. Alouini, S.; Memic, S.; Couillandre, A. Pelvic floor muscle training for urinary incontinence with or without biofeedback or electrostimulation in women: A systematic review. *Int. J. Environ. Res. Public Health* **2022**, *19*, 2789. [CrossRef]
35. Škarabot, J.; Brownstein, C.G.; Casolo, A.; Del Vecchio, A.; Ansdell, P. The knowns and unknowns of neural adaptations to resistance training. *Eur. J. Appl. Physiol.* **2021**, *121*, 675–685. [CrossRef] [PubMed]
36. Gabriel, D.A.; Kamen, G.; Frost, G. Neural adaptations to resistive exercise: Mechanisms and recommendations for training practices. *Sport. Med.* **2006**, *36*, 133–149. [CrossRef] [PubMed]
37. Radzimińska, A.; Strączyńska, A.; Weber-Rajek, M.; Styczyńska, H.; Strojek, K.; Piekorz, Z. The impact of pelvic floor muscle training on the quality of life of women with urinary incontinence: A systematic literature review. *Clin. Interv. Aging.* **2018**, *13*, 957–965. [CrossRef] [PubMed]
38. Hagen, S.; Elders, A.; Stratton, S.; Sergenson, N.; Bugge, C.; Dean, S.; Hay-Smith, J.; Kilonzo, M.; Dimitrova, M.; Abdel-Fattah, M.; et al. Effectiveness of pelvic floor muscle training with and without electromyographic biofeedback for urinary incontinence in women: Multicentre randomised controlled trial. *BMJ* **2020**, *371*, m3719. [CrossRef]
39. Sayılan, A.A.; Özbaş, A. The effect of pelvic floor muscle training on incontinence problems after radical prostatectomy. *Am. J. Mens Health* **2018**, *12*, 1007–1015. [CrossRef] [PubMed]
40. Melville, J.L.; Fan, M.-Y.; Rau, H.; Nygaard, I.E.; Katon, W.J. Major depression and urinary incontinence in women: Temporal associations in an epidemiologic sample. *Am. J. Obs. Gynecol.* **2009**, *201*, 490.e1–490.e7. [CrossRef]
41. Felde, G.; Bjelland, I.; Hunskaar, S. Anxiety and depression associated with incontinence in middle-aged women: A large norwegian cross-sectional study. *Int. Urogynecol. J.* **2012**, *23*, 299–306. [CrossRef]
42. Tettamanti, G.; Altman, D.; Iliadou, A.N.; Bellocco, R.; Pedersen, N.L. Depression, neuroticism, and urinary incontinence in premenopausal women: A nationwide twin study. *Twin Res. Hum. Genet.* **2013**, *16*, 977–984. [CrossRef]
43. Gordon, S.; Ruivo, D.B.; Viscardi, L.G.A.; de Oliveira, A.S. Effects of the pilates method isolated and associated with manual therapy in women with urinary incontinence. *Man. Ther. Posturol. Rehabil. J.* **2020**, *18*, 1–6. [CrossRef]

Disclaimer/Publisher's Note: The statements, opinions and data contained in all publications are solely those of the individual author(s) and contributor(s) and not of MDPI and/or the editor(s). MDPI and/or the editor(s) disclaim responsibility for any injury to people or property resulting from any ideas, methods, instructions or products referred to in the content.

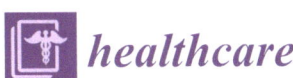

Article

Coexistent Detrusor Overactivity-Underactivity in Patients with Pelvic Floor Disorders

Matteo Frigerio [1,2,*], Marta Barba [2], Giuseppe Marino [2], Silvia Volontè [2], Tomaso Melocchi [2], Desirèe De Vicari [2], Marco Torella [3], Stefano Salvatore [4], Andrea Braga [5], Maurizio Serati [6], Stefano Manodoro [7] and Alice Cola [1,2]

1. San Gerardo Hospital, ASST Monza, 20900 Monza, Italy
2. Department of Obstetrics and Gynecology, Milano-Bicocca University, 20900 Monza, Italy
3. Department of Woman, Luigi Vanvitelli University of Campania, 80138 Naples, Italy
4. Obstetrics and Gynaecology Department, Vita-Salute University and IRCCS San Raffaele Hospital, 20133 Milan, Italy
5. EOC-Beata Vergine Hospital, 6850 Mendrisio, Switzerland
6. Del Ponte Hospital, University of Insubria, 21100 Varese, Italy
7. ASST Santi Paolo e Carlo, San Paolo Hospital, 20132 Milano, Italy
* Correspondence: frigerio86@gmail.com; Tel.: +39-2339434; Fax: +39-2339433

Abstract: Introduction and Hypothesis: Pelvic floor disorders represent a series of conditions that share, in part, the same etiological mechanisms, so they tend to be concomitant. Recently, awareness of a new lower urinary tract clinical syndrome has risen, namely the coexisting overactive–underactive bladder (COUB). The etiopathogenetic process, prevalence, and related instrumental findings of COUB are not well-established. We aimed to evaluate the prevalence, clinical features, and urodynamic findings of patients with COUB in a large cohort of patients with pelvic floor disorders. *Methods:* A cohort of 2092 women was retrospectively analyzed. A clinical interview, urogenital examination, and urodynamic assessment were performed by a trained urogynecologist. Based on baseline symptoms, patients were divided into COUB and non-COUB groups, and the degree of concordance between COUB and urodynamic findings, and other parameters related to the clinical aspects of these patients were measured and analyzed. *Results:* 18.8% of patients were classified as COUB. The association between COUB and patients with coexisting detrusor overactivity–underactivity (DOU) was statistically significant and there were substantial similarities in terms of population characteristics, symptoms, and urodynamic findings. *Conclusions:* Our study showed a high prevalence of COUB, and a link between this clinical syndrome and DOU was demonstrated. They showed substantial similarities in terms of clinical and urodynamics correlates. Based on these findings, we do think that urodynamic tests can be useful to improve knowledge on COUB and may be of help in the management of this condition.

Keywords: coexistent detrusor overactivity-underactivity; pelvic organ prolapse; underactive bladder; urodynamics; surgery; coexistent overactive-underactive bladder

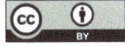

1. Introduction

Pelvic floor disorders (PFDs) represent a series of conditions—including prolapse, lower urinary tract, bowel, and sexual disorders—usually related to pelvic floor obstetric trauma and quality-of-life impairment [1,2]. Since all these conditions share—at least in part—the same etiological mechanisms, they tend to be concomitant. For instance, patients with pelvic organ prolapse (POP) often complain about lower urinary tract symptoms (LUTS), who tend to recover after prolapse surgery [3,4]. Specifically, LUTS are traditionally divided into storage and voiding symptoms [4,5].

Recently, a new lower urinary tract clinical syndrome, named the coexisting overactive–underactive bladder (COUB), has been identified. This is defined as a syndrome "characterized by coexisting storage and emptying symptoms in the same patient, without implying any specific urodynamic/functional findings or causative physiology; and that these symptoms are suggestive of urodynamically demonstrable coexistent detrusor overactivity/underactivity, but can be caused by other forms of urethro-vesical dysfunctions" [6]. COUB is thought to be multifactorial and involves neurogenic and non-neurogenic factors. Specifically, aging is believed to play a major role due to degeneration and biochemical changes due to cellular damage and apoptosis [6]. However, the etiopathogenetic process is yet to be fully understood, and different hypotheses have been proposed [6–10], including:

(1) Afferent dysfunctions leading to a decrease or an early start and end of the micturition reflex.

(2) Detrusor rest impairment during the filling phase due to abnormal activation, leading to muscle inefficiency and exhaustion in the voiding phase.

(3) Chronic ischemic-reperfusion injury due to blood supply impairment, involving patchy denervation and substitution of the detrusor muscle with fibrous connective.

(4) Autonomous contraction of small areas of the detrusor ("micromotions") during the voiding phase due to sparse denervation, inducing detrusor contractions during storage and inefficient activation during the voiding phase.

(5) Bladder outlet obstruction-induced remodeling of the detrusor, involving initial compensatory hypertrophy and later impairment and decompensation [10].

To date, the prevalence of COUB and related instrumental findings are not well-established. Specifically, urodynamic tests are not routinely recommended and reserved in the presence of unclear cases or in cases not responding to initial treatment [4]. However, the urodynamic correlates of this syndrome are poorly known, and detrusor overactivity (DO) and/or detrusor underactivity (DU) may or may not be recorded. The definition of clinical and urodynamic patterns of patients with DU and coexisting DO (DOU) may help in the future to establish reliable diagnostic criteria for COUB. This uncertainty led the International Consultation on Incontinence Research Society in 2019 to identify the definition of urodynamic findings of COUB as a research priority. This would be of the utmost importance to better understand the clinical characteristics, natural evolution, and adequate management of COUB syndrome.

However, to date, there is a paucity of urodynamic studies on the relationship between COUB, and urodynamics diagnoses such as DO and DU. As a consequence, we aimed to evaluate the prevalence, association, clinical features, and urodynamic findings of patients with COUB and/or DOU in a large cohort of patients with pelvic floor disorders.

2. Material and Methods

Women who underwent outpatient urodynamics evaluation for PFDs between 2008 and 2016 were retrospectively analyzed. A clinical interview was performed to investigate the presence of LUTS, including overactive bladder syndrome (OAB), urge urinary incontinence (UUI), stress urinary incontinence (SUI), voiding symptoms (VS), and bulging symptoms. All definitions conformed to IUGA/ICS terminology [11]. A gynecological examination was carried out and prolapse-staged according to the POP-Q system. We considered a significant prolapse as any compartment descensus staged $\geq$ II. The urodynamic assessment was performed including filling cystometry, pressure/flow study, and post-void residual volume (PVR) by a trained clinician, as previously described [12]. All procedures and definitions conformed to the Good Urodynamic Practice Guidelines of the International Continence Society [13]. The following parameters were evaluated during the storage phase: Bladder volume at first desire to void, maximum bladder capacity, presence or absence of leakage with intra-abdominal pressure increasing maneuvers, presence or absence of urgency, presence or absence of leakage with urgency, and maximum filling pressure (PdetMax). The urodynamic observation of involuntary detrusor contractions during the filling phase (spontaneous or provoked) was defined as detrusor overactivity. Urinary leakage during the Valsalva maneuver in the absence of a detrusor contraction was considered urodynamic stress urinary incontinence (USUI), while any leakage associated with detrusor overactivity (DO) was recorded as urge urinary incontinence. During the voiding phase, the following parameters were noted: Maximum flow (Qmax), detrusor pressure at opening (Pdet@op), detrusor pressure at maximal flow(pDet@Qmax), detrusor pressure at closure (Pdet@clo), and postvoid residual (PVR). Voiding dysfunction was defined—according to ICS—as "abnormally slow and/or incomplete micturition, based on abnormally slow urine flow rates and or abnormally high post-void residuals". Positive PVR (PPVR) volume was defined as a post-micturition residual >100 mL. Detrusor underactivity was evaluated through the Bladder Contractility Index (BCI) (pDet@Qmax + Qmax × 5) proposed by Abrams [14] A BCI < 100 was considered indicative of DU. Based on baseline symptoms, patients were divided into COUB and non-COUB groups. Specifically, in the case of coexisting storage and emptying symptoms in the same patient, she was diagnosed as COUB, otherwise as non-COUB. According to urodynamic findings, the population was divided into DOU and non-DOU. Specifically, in the case of coexisting detrusor overactivity and detrusor underactivity in the same patient, she was diagnosed as DOU, otherwise as non-DOU.

The study obtained local ethics committee approval. Statistical analysis was performed using JMP software version 9.0 (SAS, Cary, NC, USA). Continuous data are reported as mean ± standard deviation, while non-continuous data are shown as the absolute (relative) frequency. The degree of concordance/agreement between COUB and DOU was measured with Cohen's Kappa [10]. Differences were tested using Student's t-test for continuous parametric data, the Wilcoxon test for continuous nonparametric data, and Pearson's Chi-squared test for noncontinuous data. A p-value < 0.05 was considered statistically significant.

3. Results

This study represents a secondary analysis of a previous paper focusing on the agreement of lower urinary tract symptoms and corresponding urodynamic diagnosis [15]. In total, 2092 women with PFDs underwent outpatient urodynamic evaluation in the study period. Full records were available for 1972 of them (5.7% exclusion rate due to partial data). The population characteristics are reported in Table 1. The mean age of the patients was 61.0 ± 12.8 years. Lower urinary tract symptoms and anterior pelvic supports are shown in Table 2. The reasons for performing urodynamic evaluation were stress urinary incontinence in 61.6%, overactive bladder syndrome in 57.5%, and voiding in 35.6% of patients. Bulging symptoms were reported by 42.1% of women, and a significant anterior prolapse (≥2 stage) was found in 43.4% of patients. According to baseline symptoms, 371 (18.8%) patients were classified as having COUB, while the remaining 1601 (81.2%) were classified as non-COUB. Urodynamic findings are reported in Table 3. The most frequent urodynamic findings were voiding dysfunction (50.8%), urodynamic stress urinary incontinence (47.6%), and detrusor overactivity (33.5%). Based on preoperative urodynamic findings, the population was divided into 243 (12.3%) women with DOU and 1729 (87.7%) patients without DOU. The association between COUB and DOU was statistically significant (p < 0.001), and the observed proportionate agreement was 75.8%, but agreement according to Cohen κ coefficient (κ = 0.09) resulted in only being slight. The two conditions (COUB and DOU) showed substantial similarities in terms of population characteristics, symptoms, and urodynamic findings, compared to the corresponding controls (non-COUB and non-DOUS). Specifically, age (p < 0.001) and menopausal status (p < 0.001) were associated with both COUB and DOU (Table 4). Both conditions were related to OAB syndrome, urge incontinence, and voiding symptoms, but inversely related to the presence of SUI (Table 5). Moreover, on a urodynamic basis, both COUB and DOU demonstrated a reproducible footprint, characterized by lower volumes and flow, but higher pressures and postvoid residuals (Table 6). Urodynamic diagnoses demonstrated a higher prevalence of detrusor overactivity, voiding dysfunction, positive postvoid residuals, and a lower bladder contractility index for both conditions. However, while COUB was found to be related to bulging symptoms and significant anterior compartment prolapse, this association was not demonstrated for DOU.

Table 1. Population characteristics. Continuous data shown as mean ± standard deviation. Non-continuous data shown as absolute frequency (relative frequency).

Age (years)	61.0 ± 12.8
Body Mass Index (kg/m^2)	26.5 ± 4.7
Parity (n)	1.9 ± 1.2
Instrumental delivery	183 (9.3%)
Maximal birth-weight (g)	3479 ± 702
Menopausal status	1580 (80.1%)

Table 2. Lower urinary tract symptoms and pelvic supports. Data shown as absolute frequency (relative frequency).

Overactive bladder syndrome	1134 (57.5%)
Urge urinary incontinence	790 (40.1%)
Stress urinary incontinence	1215 (61.6%)
Voiding symptoms	703 (35.6%)
Bulging symptoms	817 (42.1%)
Anterior prolapse stage ≥ 2	855 (43.4%)

Table 3. Urodynamic findings. Continuous data shown as mean ± standard deviation. Non-continuous data shown as absolute frequency (relative frequency).

First desire to void (mL)	155 ± 81
Maximum cystometric capacity (mL)	396 ± 99
Opening detrusor pressure (cmH$_2$O)	21 ± 14
Maximum flow (mL/s)	19 ± 10
Detrusor pressure at maximum flow (cmH$_2$O)	25 ± 18
Closure detrusor pressure (cmH$_2$O)	22 ± 16
Urodynamic stress urinary incontinence	939 (47.6%)
Detrusor overactivity	660 (33.5%)
Voiding dysfunction	1002 (50.8%)
Positive post-void residual	280 (14.2%)

Table 4. Population characteristics: COUB versus non-COUB; DOU versus non-DOU. Continuous data shown as mean ± standard deviation. Non-continuous data shown as absolute frequency (relative frequency). Abbreviations: COUB, coexisting overactive–underactive bladder; DOU, detrusor overactivity–underactivity. Statistically significant associations shown in bold.

	COUB			DOU		
	Yes	No	*p* Value	Yes	No	*p* Value
Age (years)	63.4 ± 12.4	60.5 ± 10.8	**<0.001**	66.5 ± 10.8	60.3 ± 12.9	**<0.001**
Body Mass Index (kg/m^2)	26.3 ± 4.8	26.6 ± 4.7	0.397	27.5 ± 4.7	26.4 ± 4.7	**0.026**
Parity (n)	1.9 ± 1.1	1.9 ± 1.2	0.322	2.1 ± 1.5	1.9 ± 1.1	0.142
Instrumental delivery	35 (9.4%)	148 (9.2%)	0.921	15 (6.2%)	168 (9.7%)	0.096
Maximal birth-weight (g)	3502 ± 692	3477 ± 715	0.831	3493 ± 750	3480 ± 706	0.181
Menopausal status	321 (86.5%)	1259 (78.6%)	**<0.001**	222 (91.4%)	1358 (78.5%)	**<0.001**

Table 5. Lower urinary tract symptoms and pelvic supports: COUB versus non-COUB; DOU versus non-DOU. Continuous data shown as mean ± standard deviation. Non-continuous data shown as absolute frequency (relative frequency). Abbreviations: COUB, coexisting overactive–underactive bladder; DOU, detrusor overactivity–underactivity. Statistically significant associations shown in bold.

	COUB			DOU		
	Yes	No	p Value	Yes	No	p Value
Overactive bladder syndrome	371 (100%)	763 (47.7%)	**<0.001**	186 (76.5%)	948 (54.8%)	**<0.001**
Urge urinary incontinence	235 (63.3%)	555 (34.7%)	**<0.001**	129 (53.1%)	661 (33.2%)	**<0.001**
Stress urinary incontinence	212 (57.2%)	1003 (62.7%)	**0.049**	128 (52.7%)	1087 (62.9%)	**0.002**
Voiding symptoms	371 (100%)	332 (20.7%)	**<0.001**	103 (42.4%)	600 (34.7%)	**0.019**
Bulging symptoms	199 (53.8%)	618 (39.3%)	**<0.001**	113 (47.5%)	704 (41.3%)	0.071
Anterior prolapse stage ≥ 2	185 (49.9%)	644 (40.2%)	**<0.001**	99 (40.7%)	730 (42.2%)	0.662

Table 6. Urodynamic findings: COUB versus non-COUB; DOU versus non-DOU. Continuous data shown as mean ± standard deviation. Non-continuous data shown as absolute frequency (relative frequency). Abbreviations: COUB, coexisting overactive–underactive bladder; DOU, detrusor overactivity–underactivity. BCI = Bladder Contractility Index; MCC = Maximum Cystometric Capacity; pDet@MCC = Detrusor Pressure at Maximum Cystometric Capacity; pDet@Qmax = Detrusor Pressure at Maximum Flow; Qmax = Maximum Flow; PVR = PostVoid Residual; PVR% = PVR/MCC × 100; USUI = Urodynamic Stress Urinary Incontinence. Statistically significant associations shown in bold.

	COUB			DOU		
	Yes	No	p Value	Yes	No	p Value
First desire volume (mL)	150 ± 78	156 ± 82	0.168	133 ± 70	158 ± 82	**<0.001**
MCC (mL)	384 ± 94	398 ± 100	**0.005**	352 ± 101	402 ± 98	**<0.001**
pDet@MCC (cmH$_2$O)	10 ± 8	9 ± 9	**0.011**	16 ± 12	9 ± 8	**<0.001**
pDet@op (cmH$_2$O)	23 ± 13	20 ± 14	**<0.001**	25 ± 14	20 ± 14	**<0.001**
Qmax (mL/s)	16 ± 9	19 ± 10	**<0.001**	10 ± 4	20 ± 10	**<0.001**
pDet@Qmax (cmH$_2$O)	26 ± 15	25 ± 18	**0.009**	26 ± 12	25 ± 18	**0.016**
pDet@clo (cmH$_2$O)	24 ± 17	22 ± 16	**0.022**	24 ± 15	22 ± 16	**0.002**
PVR (%)	16 ± 26	10 ± 23	**<0.001**	26 ± 30	10 ± 23	**<0.001**
BCI	109 ± 48	121 ± 52	**<0.001**	74 ± 21	125 ± 51	**<0.001**
USUI	161 (43.4%)	778 (48.6%)	0.071	107 (44.0%)	832 (48.1%)	0.232
DO	152 (41.0%)	508 (31.7%)	**<0.001**	243 (100%)	417 (24.1%)	**<0.001**
VD	237 (63.9%)	765 (48.8%)	**<0.001**	181 (74.5%)	821 (47.5%)	**<0.001**
PPVR	74 (20.0%)	206 (12.9%)	**<0.001**	72 (29.6%)	208 (12.0%)	**<0.001**

4. Discussion

Up-to-date COUB diagnostic criteria have not yet been established, and the urodynamic correlates of this syndrome are poorly understood. Although the definition of COUB suggests a correlation with coexistent DOU, it does not rely on urodynamics tests, which are thus not considered mandatory in the diagnostic workup. This uncertainty is exacerbated by incomplete knowledge about COUB development and the paucity of etiopathogenetic models. Our study showed a high prevalence of both conditions, with 18.8% and 12.3% of women having COUB and DOU, respectively. However, these results were comparable to those previously reported in other populations, such as in women scheduled for prolapse repair [16]. A significant link between the two conditions was demonstrated, with a 75.8% proportion of agreement between COUB and DOU. Moreover, they showed substantial similarities in terms of clinical and urodynamics correlates.

Specifically, we confirmed the central role of aging in COUB/DOU development, since, in both conditions, age was significantly higher than in respective controls. This is thought to be related to progressive degeneration and biochemical changes caused by cellular damage and apoptosis, thus impairing both neural and/or nonneural functions [6]. This is consistent with previous studies reporting that both male and female patients with DO and concomitant impaired contractility were significantly older than controls [17–19]. Estrogen deprivation may also play a role, as suggested by the higher prevalence of menopausal women in both COUB and DOU patients.

Moreover, as expected, both conditions were associated with a higher prevalence of OAB, urge incontinence, and voiding dysfunction. On the contrary, both COUB and DOU were associated with lower SUI. A possible explanation is that one of the most frequent mechanisms of SUI is found in the decrease in urethral resistance, while one of the proposed mechanisms of COUB and DOU is, on the contrary, represented by bladder outlet obstruction [19,20]. The increase in urethral resistance may induce compensatory hypertrophy of the detrusor at the beginning, which may subsequently evolve into decompensation with progressive deterioration of bladder function. The relationship with bladder outlet obstruction was particularly evident in patients with COUB, in which a significant association was found with both bulging symptoms and anterior compartment prolapse. On the contrary, this was not found in patients with DOU. A possible explanation of this difference is that in patients with neglected prolapse, progressive cumulative detrusor damage is more likely to evolve in isolated DU than coexistent DU and DO. This is consistent with previous papers, reporting up to 40% DU in women with severe prolapse scheduled for surgical repair, but only 6% DOU [16,19].

In our study, urodynamic tests demonstrated substantial similarities in terms of urodynamic findings between the two conditions. In particular, both COUB and DOU showed lower maximum cystometric capacity (MCC) and maximum flow (Qmax), and higher detrusor pressures, including pressure at MCC, opening, Qmax, and closure. Moreover, we recorded a higher prevalence of detrusor overactivity, voiding dysfunction, positive postvoid residuals, and a lower bladder contractility index for both conditions. These findings indicate that COUB and DOU incorporate urodynamic characteristics of both bladder overactivity—such as lower MCC and higher detrusor pressures—and bladder underactivity—such as lower Qmax and higher residuals in the same patient [4,19,21]. In addition to this common urodynamic profile, DOU patients also demonstrated a lower first-desire volume. A possible explanation for the consistent agreement between the two conditions and the substantial similarities in urodynamics findings is that they represent a continuum, with DOU likely representing the most severe form of detrusor abnormalities. This hypothesis is consistent with the fact that patients with DOU presented with additional urodynamic alterations, such as low first-desire volume. This has already been reported by previous studies in which patients with concomitant DU and DO demonstrated lower bladder volumes at first desire to void compared to controls [16,17]. Based on these findings, we do think that urodynamic tests can be useful to improve knowledge about COUB and may be of great help in the management of patients with this condition.

To the best of our knowledge, this is the largest work to evaluate the prevalence, association, and clinical and urodynamic features of COAB and DOU in a cohort of patients with pelvic floor disorders. This may be of great help to better understand this condition. A limitation is the retrospective study design. Future efforts should be addressed to standardize the COUB definition including urodynamic parameters.

5. Conclusions

Our study showed a high prevalence of COUB and DOU in women with PFDs, and a significant association between the two conditions was demonstrated. COUB and DOU showed substantial similarities in terms of clinical and urodynamics correlates.

Regarding preoperative urodynamics, continuous data are shown as mean ± standard deviation and non-continuous data are shown as absolute (relative) frequency. BCI = Bladder Contractility Index; MCC = Maximum Cystometric Capacity; pDet@MCC = Detrusor Pressure at Maximum Cystometric Capacity; pDet@Qmax = Detrusor Pressure at Maximum Flow; Qmax = Maximum Flow; PVR = PostVoid Residual; PVR% = PVR/MCC × 100; USUI = Urodynamic Stress Urinary Incontinence.

Author Contributions: M.F., M.B., G.M., S.V., T.M., D.D.V. and A.C.: Project development, data collection and analysis, manuscript writing and revision. M.T., S.S., A.B., M.S. and S.M.: Project development, manuscript writing and revision. All authors have read and agreed to the published version of the manuscript.

Funding: This research received no external funding.

Institutional Review Board Statement: The study was conducted in accordance with the Declaration of Helsinki, and approved by the Institutional Review Board ASST Monza Ethical committee. Approval Code: RE-PFDs. Approval Date: 11 February 2022.

Informed Consent Statement: Not applicable.

Conflicts of Interest: The authors declare no conflict of interest.

References

1. Rørtveit, G.; Hannestad, Y.S. Association between mode of delivery and pelvic floor dysfunction. *Tidsskr. Nor. Laegeforen.* **2014**, *134*, 1848–1852. (In English and Norwegian) [CrossRef] [PubMed]
2. Mota, R.L. Female urinary incontinence and sexuality. *Int. Braz. J. Urol.* **2017**, *43*, 20–28. [CrossRef] [PubMed]
3. Lowder, J.L.; Frankman, E.A.; Chetti, C.; Burrows, L.J.; Krohn, M.A.; Moalli, P.; Zyczynski, H. Lower urinary tract symptoms in women with pelvic organ prolapse. *Int. Urogynecol. J.* **2010**, *21*, 665–672. [CrossRef] [PubMed]
4. Frigerio, M.; Manodoro, S.; Cola, A.; Palmieri, S.; Spelzini, F.; Milani, R. Risk factors for persistent, de novo and overall overactive bladder syndrome after surgical prolapse repair. *Eur. J. Obstet. Gynecol. Reprod. Biol.* **2019**, *233*, 141–145. [CrossRef]
5. Palmieri, S.; Manodoro, S.; Cola, A.; Spelzini, F.; Milani, R.; Frigerio, M. Pelvic organ prolapse and voiding function before and after surgery. *Minerva Ginecol.* **2019**, *71*, 253–256. [CrossRef]
6. Mancini, V.; Tarcan, T.; Serati, M.; Wyndaele, M.; Carrieri, G.; Abrams, P. Is coexistent overactive-underactive bladder (with or without detrusor overactivity and underactivity) a real clinical syndrome? ICI-RS 2019. *Neurourol. Urodyn.* **2020**, *39* (Suppl. 3), S50–S59. [CrossRef] [PubMed]
7. Aldamanhori, R.; Osman, N.I.; Chapple, C.R. Underactive bladder: Pathophysiology and clinical significance. *Asian J. Urol.* **2018**, *5*, 17–21. [CrossRef] [PubMed]
8. Nordling, J. The aging bladder—A significant but underestimated role in the development of lower urinary tract symptoms. *Exp. Gerontol.* **2002**, *37*, 991–999. [CrossRef]
9. Drake, M.J.; Kanai, A.; Bijos, D.A.; Ikeda, Y.; Zabbarova, I.; Vahabi, B.; Fry, C.H. The potential role of unregulated autonomous bladder micromotions in urinary storage and voiding dysfunction; overactive bladder and detrusor underactivity. *BJU Int.* **2017**, *119*, 22–29. [CrossRef] [PubMed]
10. Fusco, F.; Creta, M.; De Nunzio, C.; Iacovelli, V.; Mangiapia, F.; Li Marzi, V.; Finazzi Agrò, E. Progressive bladder remodeling due to bladder outlet obstruction: A systematic review of morphological and molecular evidences in humans. *BMC Urol.* **2018**, *18*, 15. [CrossRef] [PubMed]
11. Haylen, B.T.; de Ridder, D.; Freeman, R.M.; Swift, S.E.; Berghmans, B.; Lee, J.; Monga, A.; Petri, E.; Rizk, D.E.; Sand, P.K.; et al. An International Urogynecological Association (IUGA)/International Continence Society (ICS) joint report on the terminology for female pelvic floor dysfunction. *Neurourol. Urodyn.* **2010**, *29*, 4–20. [CrossRef] [PubMed]
12. Manodoro, S.; Spelzini, F.; Frigerio, M.; Nicoli, E.; Verri, D.; Milani, R. Is Occult Stress Urinary Incontinence a Reliable Predictive Marker? *Female Pelvic Med. Reconstr. Surg.* **2016**, *22*, 280–282. [CrossRef] [PubMed]
13. Abrams, P.; Cardozo, L.; Wagg, A.; Wein, A. (Eds.) *Incontinence*, 6th ed.; International Continence Society (ICI-ICS): Bristol, UK, 2017; ISBN 978-0956960733.
14. Abrams, P. Bladder outlet obstruction index, bladder contractility index and bladder voiding efficiency: Three simple indices to define bladder voiding function. *BJU Int.* **1999**, *84*, 14–15. [CrossRef] [PubMed]

15. D'Alessandro, G.; Palmieri, S.; Cola, A.; Barba, M.; Manodoro, S.; Frigerio, M. Correlation between urinary symptoms and urodynamic findings: Is the bladder an unreliable witness? *Eur. J. Obstet. Gynecol. Reprod. Biol.* **2022**, *272*, 130–133. [CrossRef] [PubMed]
16. Frigerio, M.; Barba, M.; Cola, A.; Spelzini, F.; Milani, R.; Manodoro, S. Coexisting overactive-underactive bladder and detrusor overactivity-underactivity in pelvic organ prolapse. *Int. J. Gynaecol. Obstet.* **2022**, *in press*. [CrossRef]
17. Gammie, A.; Kaper, M.; Steup, A.; Yoshida, S.; Dorrepaal, C.; Kos, T.; Abrams, P. What are the additional signs and symptoms in patients with detrusor underactivity and coexisting detrusor overactivity? *Neurourol. Urodyn.* **2018**, *37*, 2220–2225. [CrossRef] [PubMed]
18. Stav, K.; Shilo, Y.; Zisman, A.; Lindner, A.; Leibovici, D. Comparison of lower urinary tract symptoms between women with detrusor overactivity and impaired contractility, and detrusor overactivity and preserved contractility. *J. Urol.* **2013**, *189*, 2175–2178. [CrossRef] [PubMed]
19. Frigerio, M.; Manodoro, S.; Cola, A.; Palmieri, S.; Spelzini, F.; Milani, R. Detrusor underactivity in pelvic organ prolapse. *Int. Urogynecol. J.* **2018**, *29*, 1111–1116. [CrossRef] [PubMed]
20. D'Alessandro, G.; Palmieri, S.; Cola, A.; Barba, M.; Manodoro, S.; Frigerio, M. Detrusor underactivity prevalence and risk factors according to different definitions in women attending urogynecology clinic. *Int. Urogynecol. J.* **2022**, *33*, 835–840. [CrossRef] [PubMed]
21. Araki, I.; Haneda, Y.; Mikami, Y.; Takeda, M. Incontinence and detrusor dysfunction associated with pelvic organ prolapse: Clinical value of preoperative urodynamic evaluation. *Int. Urogynecol. J. Pelvic Floor Dysfunct.* **2009**, *20*, 1301–1306. [CrossRef] [PubMed]

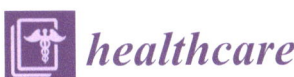

Article

Effect of Immersive Virtual Reality on Post-Baccalaureate Nursing Students' In-Dwelling Urinary Catheter Skill and Learning Satisfaction

Chu-Ling Chang

Nursing Department, HungKuang University, No. 1018, Sec. 6, Taiwan Boulevard, Shalu District, Taichung City 43304, Taiwan; sxc46851@sunrise.hk.edu.tw; Tel.: +886-4-26318652 (ext. 3151)

Abstract: A fundamental skill required from nursing students is how to manage the insertion of in-dwelling urinary catheters, and this skill is a core competency for nurses. However, practice with conventional test models is insufficient for learning this skill and leads to inadequate proficiency among students. To address this problem, this study created an immersive virtual reality (IVR) scheme, based on the theory of situated learning, to simulate clinical situations. Innovative approaches were adopted to design clinical cases, construct three-dimensional environments, design character dialogs, and integrate artificial intelligence voice recognition. The effect of these design elements on students' in-dwelling urinary catheter skills and learning satisfaction was explored. First, nursing experts assessed the quality of the IVR scheme. Over a 4-week period, 43 students in a post-baccalaureate nursing program used conventional test models to practice the management of in-dwelling urinary catheters in female patients, and their learning was supplemented by at least two practice sessions with IVR. Data were collected from in-class observation records, a questionnaire survey on student satisfaction, and focused group interviews. The results showed that the participating students were highly satisfied with the IVR scheme and stated that it provided a pleasurable learning experience and exerted a positive impact on them. The IVR scheme provided situations closely resembling real clinical environments, helping the students to memorize the steps for catheter management. The students also noted that the IVR scheme should incorporate other nursing skills, such as empathetical and solicitous care and patient companionship. This enables nursing students to fulfill their role and care for patients in clinical settings.

Keywords: immersive virtual reality; post-baccalaureate nursing students; skill for managing female in-dwelling urinary catheters

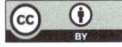

Citation: Chang, C.-L. Effect of Immersive Virtual Reality on Post-Baccalaureate Nursing Students' In-Dwelling Urinary Catheter Skill and Learning Satisfaction. *Healthcare* **2022**, *10*, 1473. https://doi.org/10.3390/healthcare10081473

Academic Editors: Matteo Frigerio and Stefano Manodoro

Received: 7 July 2022
Accepted: 3 August 2022
Published: 5 August 2022

Publisher's Note: MDPI stays neutral with regard to jurisdictional claims in published maps and institutional affiliations.

Copyright: © 2022 by the author. Licensee MDPI, Basel, Switzerland. This article is an open access article distributed under the terms and conditions of the Creative Commons Attribution (CC BY) license (https://creativecommons.org/licenses/by/4.0/).

1. Introduction

When using immersive virtual reality (IVR), users can see, hear, and interact with virtual environments, enabling them to completely immerse themselves in simulated scenarios [1]. New IVR technologies offer unprecedentedly vivid environments and realistic and immersive experiences [2]. The phrase "immersive experience" refers to an experience in which users fully immerse themselves in a simulated situation. That is, digital technology or an environment that employs augmented reality (AR), virtual reality (VR), mixed reality (MR), or projection technology is employed to create a near-realistic situation and the users become fully immersed in the situation, connecting and resonating with it. Immersive learning involves guiding learners into a fully immersive environment, reducing external interferences. In this immersive experience, learners' brains actively grasp and memorize information. Gamifying neonatal resuscitation training using immersive VR has effectively enhanced nursing students' neonatal resuscitation knowledge, problem-solving skills, self-confidence, and learning motivations [3]. Interactive media have been widely studied and applied abroad. For example, one study investigated the use of interactive media for entertainment, specifically for providing theater audiences with a sense of realism [4].

Several studies evaluating the applications of IVR in medical care have yielded favorable results. For example, in one pediatric care study, researchers compared the use of IVR and kaleidoscopes in helping child patients to understand the treatment process before undergoing venipuncture, thus minimizing the patients' pain and anxiety. The results indicated that compared with kaleidoscopes, IVR could more effectively minimize the patients' pain and anxiety [5]. In another study, scholars used IVR to prepare child patients with cancer and their families for regular pediatric radiation therapy. The results of the study provided preliminary support for the use of IVR to achieve favorable clinical and surgical outcomes in pediatric populations [6]. Another study revealed that interactive media–based interventions are effective in treating depression [7]. Regarding medical or nurse education, IVR improved skills focusing on cooperative learning and reinforcement [8]. In one study, game-based VR was applied in tracheostomy care education for nursing students, to help the students hone their psychomotor skills [9]. Another study applied IVR in an interprofessional round training program for healthcare students. By participating in an IVR simulation program, the students gained a profound understanding of the distinct roles of the different members of interprofessional teams and how to interact with their team members. The IVR simulation program thus reduced the gap between nursing school and clinical settings [10]. IVR simulations designed to simulate teamwork enabled users to cooperate and interact with one another within the system [1]. According to one study, VR is an effective assistive tool that students can use to learn specific clinical skills, such as inserting urinary catheters [11]. In another study, IVR was used to teach undergraduate nursing students how to care for a patient with a foreign body in their right lung. The results revealed that the students proactively participated in the IVR simulation and expressed the opinion that the IVR-based teaching method was beneficial to their learning [12]. Another study used IVR to educate nursing students on simple triage in a simulated mass casualty incident, and the results revealed that the IVR training program was as effective as a clinical simulation [13]. In another study in which IVR was used to simulate a mass casualty incident, the sense of presence in an immersive scenario was determined to be correlated with immersion propensity [14]. Another study on health education focused on participants' feelings when they used gamified two-dimensional, three-dimensional, and IVA-based educational tools to study clinical cases. The participants perceived the IVR-based tool to be the most conducive to improving their learning performance [15]. In a recent study evaluating VR simulation training for adult students, the students had high expectations regarding the VR simulation training and offered suggestions for improvement after completing the VR simulation training; these suggestions may serve as a reference for nursing educators in developing more effective VR-based training programs [16].

In Taiwan, the applications of interactive media have proliferated in recent years. One such application is in entertainment devices at theme parks, which enable visitors to immerse themselves in simulated environments [17]. One Taiwanese pilot study evaluated the use of interactive media in ecotourism for older adults, which yielded favorable results [18]. However, most applications of IVR in Taiwan have been limited to the fields of art, culture, and recreation. To create new experiences for users, IVR simulations should emphasize pleasure, inspiration, and creativity [19]. According to a survey of university-education personnel, antidrug teaching materials integrated with IVR technology exerted substantial effects on the behavior of high-school students and were more effective than conventional teaching methods [20]. In medical education in Taiwan, VR has been applied in pre-internship pharmaceutical education at teaching hospitals, specifically for the purposes of training new pharmacists in dispensing medicine. Participating in a VR-simulation training program enhanced participants' motivation and learning performance and helped them to accumulate hands-on experience [21]. Clinical nursing supervisors in Taiwan have suggested that because VR is interactive and provides a sense of touch and movement when simulating the human body or sensory organs, it effectively piques the learners' interest, thereby improving their learning performance and comprehension. IVR is suitable for helping nurse practitioners to hone their critical thinking skills, including those related to speculation, reasoning, and differentiation [22]. One medical center in Taiwan offered a flipped training course in which a VR-based lesson plan was used to help nurses practice placing peripherally inserted central catheters. The nurses were interested in the course and, using VR, were able to effectively learn and retain knowledge regarding the correct way to perform the procedure [23]. Nevertheless, there have been no previous studies conducted in Taiwan that explored the applications of IVR in university nursing programs. However, most university nursing students are not in-service students, and universities often experience difficulties in providing opportunities for nursing students to practice clinical skills in actual clinical settings. Researchers and practitioners must consider how to overcome this problem to help students hone their hands-on abilities.

The technique regarding how to place Foley catheters ins female patients is one of the most common and basic clinical nursing skills that every nursing student must have mastered before commencing clinical work. Moreover, according to the worksheet used in the present study, we discovered that the post-baccalaureate nursing students who participated in this study faced difficulties learning such skills, including "having to memorize the operational steps without a clinical scenario," being "unable to memorize the steps," and "having difficulty memorizing all the items involved in the technical operation". One approach to helping students gain clinical experience, memorize operational steps, and overcome other difficulties in learning these skills involves the use of IVR. The research participants were students in a post-baccalaureate nursing program. Their difficulties lay in the students' inability to install an in-dwelling urinary catheter completely and correctly, which necessitates numerous complicated steps. The research question of this study was whether employing IVR teaching could resolve their learning issues. The research objective was to explore the effect (i.e., solving the students' problem and offering learning satisfaction) of IVR teaching on learning performance regarding in-dwelling urinary catheter skills.

2. Materials and Methods

2.1. Materials

The development of IVR teaching materials consists of writing simulation scenarios and dialogs, constructing three-dimensional scenes, and designing characters, as well as integrating artificial intelligence voice recognition capabilities and coordinating with media engineers to convert the developed content into engineering documents. Certain pieces of hardware, such as headgear and computers, were required to use the IVR platform.

2.2. Research Design

This study adopted a quasi-experimental design. The independent variable of this study was IVR teaching, while the dependent variable was learning performance. Learning performance consisted of solving students' learning problems, providing learning satisfaction, and discerning their learning experiences and feelings toward their in-dwelling urinary catheter skills. We designed a clinical scenario and collaborated with an information technology engineering team to produce an IVR-based lesson plan on how to place Foley catheters in female patients (Figures 1 and 2). We used a model to demonstrate how to place Foley catheters in female patients and used the IVR platform for additional demonstrations and explanations. The participants of this study were 43 freshman students of a postbaccalaureate nursing department, all of whom had earned bachelor's degrees in non-nursing majors and were aged 23–38 years. All the participants were first-time learners of the technique for inserting in-dwelling urinary catheters. This study was approved by the Institutional Review Board, and all the participants were full-time students. The students were instructed on the goals of the VR teaching and research procedure and had signed informed consents before this study commenced. Students who were unable or unwilling to use the VR technology were excluded from this study, without repercussions on their grades. Over a 4-week period, each student used the model to study how to place

Foley catheters in female patients and used the IVR platform to practice performing the procedure at least twice. We collected and statistically analyzed class observation records, satisfaction questionnaires, and focus group interviews. The measurement tool of this study was a learning satisfaction and learning impact questionnaire that was produced for this study. The questionnaire employed a 5-point Likert scale design and the questionnaire comprised 10 items. The questionnaire was administered after its reliability and validity were tested. The items were as follows:

1. Using VR can partially resolve the difficulties in learning in-dwelling urinary catheter skills.
2. Using VR helps me memorize the steps.
3. Using VR makes me feel as if I were in a clinical setting.
4. Using VR solves my learning issues.
5. Using VR improves my learning performance.
6. After using VR, I feel the VR is of good quality.
7. Using VR to practice is convenient.
8. I think that VR is a suitable assistive learning device for learning nursing skills.
9. Using VR to practice skills makes me uncomfortable.
10. In the future, I would like to use VR again to help my learning.

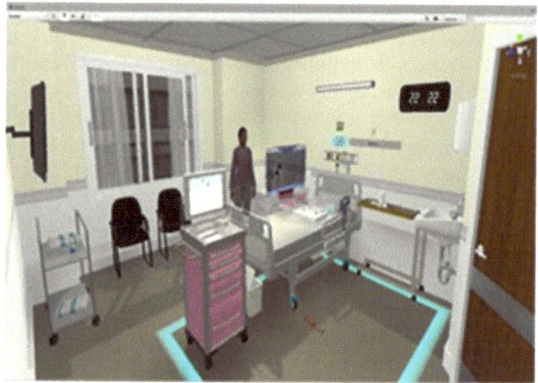

Figure 1. IVR simulation regarding how to place Foley catheters in female patients.

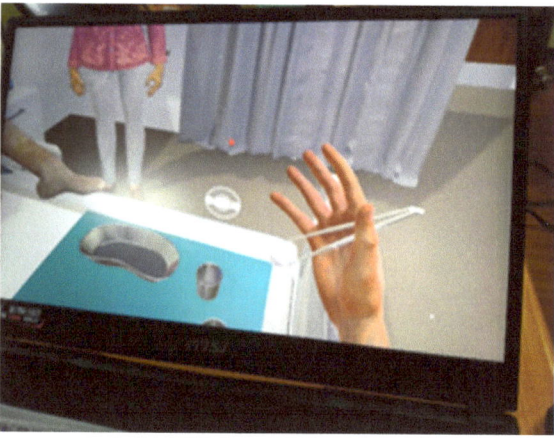

Figure 2. The participant's viewpoint.

This study held focus-group interviews to understand students' learning experiences and feelings. The interview was conducted 3 days after the students engaged in VR training. The interview outline consisted of the following examples: "Have you ever used VR?", "How do you feel about using VR this time?", "How does the VR application help or influence your skills in handling in-dwelling urinary catheters in female patients?" and "What are some suggestions you have for using VR?" The interview guidelines were inspected by teacher experts in the same department as the author. The focus group interview was hosted by the author. At the beginning of the interview, the interview rules were explained to the interviewees: "Each participant is allowed to express their opinions and must raise their hand to speak. Do not interrupt others when they are speaking and do not speak in an interrogating tone".

2.3. Procedure

The study process comprised three stages, namely, the pre-teaching, teaching, and post-teaching stages (Table 1). In the teaching stage, we demonstrated how to place Foley catheters in female patients in real life and by using the IVR platform (Figure 3). During the VR demonstration process, the view from the operator was projected onto a screen to enable the whole class to observe the VR operation process. Each student practiced the technique, using the VR system, at least twice (Figure 4).

Table 1. Research process.

Stage		Content
Pre-teaching	1.	Key points about how to place Foley catheters in female patients (5-min digital teaching materials).
	2.	VR instructions (5-min digital teaching materials).
Teaching	1.	In class, the teacher demonstrated how to place Foley catheters in female patients by using VR.
	2.	The students were divided into seven groups of 5–6 students to practice the technique by using VR. The researchers and teaching assistants moved among the groups to observe and guide the students when practicing. When a group member was practicing using VR, the other group members observed the projected screen simultaneously.
	3.	The VR case scenario was used in class for the teacher and students to discuss.
Post-teaching	1.	Each student was required to practice the technique with the VR system at least twice.
	2.	After the VR practice, the students completed the learning satisfaction questionnaires.
	3.	After all the group members finished practicing, focus group discussions were conducted to gather the students' feedback on how to modify the VR training in the future.

2.4. Data Analysis

The analytical approach of this study involved a combination of qualitative and quantitative methods. We analyzed the qualitative and quantitative data collected via a learning satisfaction questionnaire survey and a focus group interview. Each item on the learning satisfaction questionnaire was scored on a 5-point Likert scale. We used Microsoft Excel to calculate the frequency of each score (as a percentage) and the mean score for each item. We recruited 11 of the students as voluntary participants for the focus-group interview. The interview outline includes the questions "Have you ever heard of or used VR?" and "How did you feel when you first used VR?" The interviewees were also asked about the effects of using the IVR system to practice how to place Foley catheters in female patients and their suggestions on how to improve the process. All the interviewees agreed to be voice recorded. The recording of each interview was transcribed for inductive content analysis. After the focus group interview, the recordings of the interview were transcribed. The author compiled and coded the transcripts and the transcripts were inspected by a teacher from the same department as the author. The students' experiences and feelings about practicing using VR were discussed in terms of three topics and five categories.

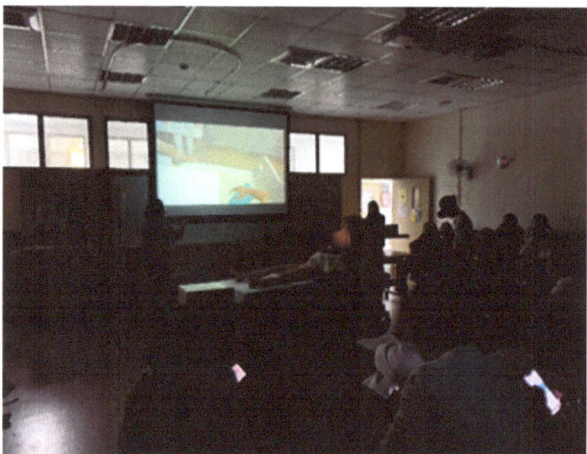

Figure 3. The researcher explaining IVR to the students.

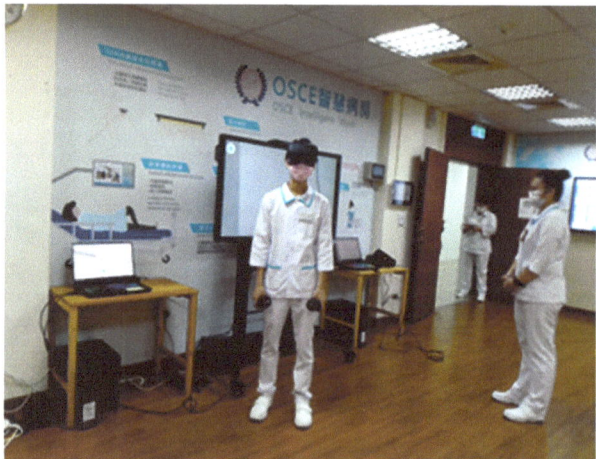

Figure 4. A student practicing using the IVR system.

3. Results

A total of 43 first-year students in a post-baccalaureate nursing program participated in the study. All the participants had a bachelor's degree (100%), and their ages ranged from 23 to 40 years old (mean: 25 years). Nine (21%) of the participants were men, and 34 (79%) were women.

3.1. Learning Satisfaction

We evaluated the students' satisfaction and experiences with using VR to learn how to place Foley catheters in female patients. The participants' mean score on the learning satisfaction questionnaire was 4.37. Their mean scores on the VR scenario and content, the innovative teaching method, and the VR operation procedure were components of the satisfaction questionnaire and were 4.42, 4.40, and 4.42, respectively, indicating that most of the students were highly satisfied with the IVR-based lesson on how to position Foley catheters in female patients.

3.2. Effects of Using VR to Learn and Practice How to Insert Foley Catheters in Female Patients

Regarding the effects of using VR to learn how to position Foley catheters inside female patients, 25 (58.6%) of the students reported that the IVR platform helped them overcome the difficulties that they had experienced in learning the technique; the remaining 18 (41.4%) students' responses were neutral. Regarding the statement, "Using VR can help me memorize the operation procedure," six (13.8%) of the students strongly agreed, 21 (48.3%) agreed, 15 (34.5%) were neutral, and one disagreed. Regarding the statement "Using VR to practice makes me feel as though I were in a clinical setting," two (4.6%) of the students strongly agreed, 20 (44.8%) agreed, 18 (41.4%) were neutral, 3 (6.9%) disagreed, and 3 (6.9%) strongly disagreed. A total of 39 (90.7%) of the students reported that they thought using VR to practice the technique was convenient; the remaining 4 (9.3%) reported that it was inconvenient. Regarding the suitability of using VR to learn how to position Foley catheters inside female patients, 30 (69.8%) of the students reported that it was suitable or extremely suitable, one (2.3%) reported that it was unsuitable, and 12 (27.9%) were neutral. Regarding whether the students would like to continue using VR to learn, 36 (82.8%) of the students said they would, and the remaining 7 (17.2%) said they would not. Overall, most of the students expressed a positive attitude toward using VR to learn.

3.3. Learning Experience and Feelings about the IVR Training

We divided the students' experiences with and feelings toward using VR to learn how to place Foley catheters in female patients, as described in the focus group interview, into three themes and five categories (Table 2).

Table 2. Learning experience summary table.

Themes	Categories
1. Pleasurable experience	1. Fun
2. Effective learning	2. Experiencing clinical scenarios
	3. Memorizing steps of the technique
	4. Understanding clinical situations before working at the hospital
3. Critical thinking	5. Inability to reflect the role of nurses as care providers

3.4. Pleasurable Experience

Most of the participants had not previously used VR. When they first used it, they felt a sense of novelty. They stated that during the IVR practice, they could see different scenarios; for example, one student said, "I was shocked because there were such scenes. I thought, wow, this world turned out to be fun" (Student 8). The students' interest in using VR to practice was stimulated during the training, and some of the students even directly expressed the opinion that using VR to learn was fun ("It was kind of fun" (Student 5); "It was super fun" (Student 9)). While observing the students who were practicing using the IVR platform, we noted that most of the students were interested in VR and actively engaged in the IVR training.

3.5. Effective Learning

Some of the students reported that using VR to practice effectively helped them to learn how to place Foley catheters in female patients. Exposure to a simulated clinical scenario helped them memorize the steps involved in the procedure regarding the placement of

Foley catheters in female patients. They were given a sense of the clinical and practical aspects of the procedure before starting a hospital internship, and they acquired a new understanding of the applications of technology in medicine.

3.5.1. Being in a Clinical Scenario

Some of the students stated that using VR to practice was like being in an actual clinical setting. For example, students made the following statements: "I could feel a sense of presence, and the visual effect" (Student 1); "Back then, it was a more fragmented concept. Now, it's real. It has the actual sense of clinic-ness" (Student 4); "It has a sense of body" (Student 9); "It has a sense of touch" (Student 2); and "It provides a sense of interaction" (Student 7).

3.5.2. Memorizing the Steps of the Procedure Regarding the Placement of Foley Catheters in Female Patients

Many of the students maintained that using VR to practice how to place Foley catheters in female patients helped them to memorize the steps involved in the procedure. For example, students made the following statements: "It has the advantage of enabling me to memorize all the steps" (Student 7); "It involves a step to memorize the procedure" (Student 12); "It enables a student to become familiar with a technique. I feel it consists of steps to help students familiarize themselves with the technique" (Student 5); "So far, it is for practice" (Student 10). "I use it to memorize the steps" (Student 11); "Using VR in our study prevents us from making numerous mistakes when we enter a clinical setting. I'm grateful for this learning opportunity" (Student 6); "The greatest help VR provides is the procedure" (Student 2); and "It enabled me to become familiar with the procedure. By continually operating the system, I came to see what I was doing" (Student 3). The technique of placing Foley catheters in female patients involves many operational steps, and the entire procedure must be performed in a sterile environment with sterile equipment, to prevent contamination and avoid subsequent infection. Therefore, the ability of the IVR practice to help the students to familiarize themselves with the steps involved in the procedure regarding the placement of Foley catheters in female patients is one of its most important benefits.

3.5.3. Understanding Clinical Situations before Internship

Some of the students also mentioned that using VR to practice helped them attain a more thorough understanding of actual clinical situations. Students made the following statements: "It has greater influence before our internship. We get to know about clinical situations ahead of time" (Student 4); "It was like seeing what we will see in a clinical setting, so we won't be shocked when seeing the real thing when we enter an actual clinical setting" (Student 8); and "I think we can practice what we will encounter in a clinical setting in the VR world ahead of time. I think it's not bad" (Student 9). Many of the students believed that experiencing the clinical scenarios before starting their internships would help them to succeed during their internships.

3.5.4. Understanding the Applications of IVR Technology in Medicine

Some of the students also mentioned that IVR-based practice made them more aware of the applications of technology in medicine. For example, students made the following statements: "(The school) prepared ahead of time and let us know that VR and many other artificial intelligence–related things will come" (Student 1); "(VR) broadened my vision!" (Student 5); and "VR is able to connect things that are related. Through it, I can see a lot of things. Now, it is applied in many areas" (Student 4). Some of the students felt that through the IVR practice, the school intended to make the students aware of the diverse applications of technology. They felt that the nursing education curriculum had been planned ahead of time to help students understand the various applications of VR and artificial intelligence.

3.6. Critical Thinking

Some of the students reported that using IVR to practice how to place Foley catheters in female patients was surprising, fun, and effective in helping them learn. Moreover, the experience inspired them to reflect on the use of VR in nursing education. For example, students made the following statements: "Regarding the technical aspect, machines can replace practice. However, I feel that the other role of nurses is to provide care and companionship" (Student 8); "(VR) is cold. For example, in our basic nursing theory course, we were taught to pay attention to the patients' reactions and use communication skills such as repeating (what the patients said). These were not applied [in the VR practice]" (Student 12); "During the IVR practice, we should care about the patients. I feel I couldn't engage in much communication" (Student 5); "I feel we, as nurses, sometimes should provide patients with strength" (Student 8); and "In principle, (VR) will not make you feel warmth, and it will not make the patient feel empathy" (Student 3). As reflected in these comments, the students thought critically about the IVR practice and were concerned about its ability to help them practice providing patient-centered care.

4. Discussion

According to the questionnaire survey and the focus group interview, over half of the students believed that the IVR training helped them overcome the difficulties they encountered in learning how to insert Foley catheters inside female patients (58.6%) and memorize the operational steps involved in the procedure regarding the placement of Foley catheters in female patients (62.8%). Furthermore, over half (52%) of the students agreed with the statement, "Using VR to practice makes me feel as though I were in a clinical setting." Some of the students mentioned that although they used VR to practice only the technique regarding how to place Foley catheters in female patients in the present study, in the future, VR could be used to help nursing students to practice providing care to patients with acute and severe symptoms, thereby helping students to feel less overwhelmed when starting a clinical internship or subsequent work. Student 6 said, "I wonder if VR can be integrated with lessons on addressing acute and severe symptoms or navigating the operating room. If I can experience the image of the trauma ahead of time, when I work in a clinical setting, I will not be too scared to know what to do." Our course observations revealed that the students were diligent in using VR to practice the technique. Their reflections on the IVR practice, therefore, provide valuable insights into the use of VR in nursing education. According to one study, using VR to practice a technique positively affects the nursing students' critical thinking abilities [24]. Another study revealed that by enabling students to undergo innovative simulations and training, VR can increase students' confidence [25]. Moreover, in the present study, over 90% (39) of the students maintained that using VR to practice how to place Foley catheters in female patients was convenient. Practicing the technique using the model involved many physical objects, such as sterilized cotton balls, urinary catheters, urine bags, and catheterization kits, which must be disposed of after the actual procedure, resulting in medical waste. Most of the students exhibited a positive attitude toward using VR to learn additional techniques in the future. According to the focus group interview, the IVR practice was a pleasant learning experience. Most of the students reported that IVR was novel and interesting. In another study in which nursing students were interviewed on the use of VR in nursing education, the researchers determined that VR effectively helped the students to learn skills by complementing conventional teaching methods with novel and intriguing content [26]. In the present study, students mentioned that using VR to practice how to place Foley catheters in female patients had a substantial impact on them because it helped them to gain a more thorough understanding of the technique before they started interning or working at the hospital. Student 4 said, "If I can learn the concept ahead of time, in the future, I will be more willing to use VR," and Student 7 said, "The school gave me the feeling that it had been preparing ahead of time to let us know about VR. In the future, many other artificial intelligence products may be involved." VR helped the students to effectively familiarize themselves with the operational steps involved in the procedure regarding the placement of Foley catheters in female patients and enabled the students to explore a clinical setting within the virtual environment. According to another study, the use of VR has become increasingly common in various fields. In addition to its applications in education, VR is helpful in the cognitive assessment of mental disorders and mood disorders [27] and in helping people recover from motion sickness [28]. In another study evaluating the use of mobile VR in operating-room nursing education, the nursing students who had completed a mobile VR–based course outperformed those who had not [29]. The results of the aforementioned study and of the present study may serve as a reference for the application of VR in nurse-training courses, especially those focused on specific clinical skills.

In addition to feeling that the IVR practice was effective in helping them learn, the students also reflected critically on the IVR practice. Although the students felt that using VR made them feel as though they were in an actual clinical setting, which helped them understand the operational steps involved in the procedure regarding the placement of Foley catheters in female patients, as well as the applications of technology in medical education, they also felt that clinical care should involve communication with patients, empathy, and compassion. They thought that the IVR training should have reflected the role of nurses as care providers. In the questionnaire, 18 of the participants (41.4%) indicated that their experience in learning how to insert in-dwelling urinary catheters through VR training was a mediocre experience. In the focus group interview, the participants expressed their feeling that the capacity for expressing empathy, concerns, and companionship was lacking in VR interactions. This demonstrates the participants' ability to express their opinions on VR and describe its pros and cons. One study of the effects of VR on the knowledge, attitudes, and behaviors of healthcare workers revealed that VR had considerable benefits related to the "affective domain of learning," especially in promoting empathy. Increased empathy helped improve the attitudes and behaviors of the participants in caring for patients, thereby helping them to provide a better quality of care [30]. The results of this study demonstrated the participants' ability to think critically about using VR. "We should learn to express empathy to patients in immersive VR training, but I do not feel we can communicate further in it" (Participant 5). The participants expressed concerns regarding learning how to provide empathic care. However, in the present study, many of the students reported that the simulated interaction in the VR practice did not require them to express empathy, compassion, or other principles of patient-centered care. In the future, principles of patient-centered care should be integrated into VR-based courses on clinical skills. In terms of equality of education, although only one participant expressed discomfort in using VR, this problem must be addressed in future studies. This study conducted focus-group interviews to collect students' VR usage experiences, and the responses provided by the students were analyzed. Some of the students had previous VR usage experiences, and their satisfaction with VR varied. This signified that the students' responses may have been biased, which was a limitation of this study.

5. Conclusions

The participants in this study, who were students in a postbaccalaureate nursing program, were satisfied with the experience of using IVR to learn how to place Foley catheters in female patients. They considered the IVR training to be convenient and reported that they would like to continue using IVR to practice clinical skills in the future. The IVR practice had multiple positive effects on the students, which are summarized as follows. (1) The students had a pleasurable learning experience. Most of the students who had not used VR in the past did not reject the IVR training; rather, they felt that it was surprising and interesting. (2) Using VR to practice made the students feel as though they were actually in a clinical setting. They felt a sense of presence and could interact with the patient in the simulation. (3) Using VR to practice effectively helped the students overcome their difficulties in learning the procedure, specifically by helping them to memorize the operational steps involved in learning how to place Foley catheters in female patients. (4) The students reported that the IVR practice made them feel more prepared for clinical practice and that they expected to feel shocked by actual clinical scenarios upon entering a hospital setting. (5) In addition, by helping the students to learn how to place Foley catheters in female patients, the IVR training encouraged the students to reflect critically on the use of technology in nursing education and provided them with a new perspective on the role of nurses as care providers. The students argued that VR-based training courses should integrate features that require students to express empathy, compassion, and other principles of patient-centered care.

Funding: This study was funded by Hungkuang University's Award for Teacher Improvement and Innovation (HKU-109-C14).

Institutional Review Board Statement: The study was conducted in accordance with the Declaration of Helsinki and was approved by the Institutional Review Board (KTGH 11026).

Informed Consent Statement: Not applicable.

Data Availability Statement: Not applicable.

Acknowledgments: The authors of this study are grateful to all the students from the postbaccalaureate nursing program who participated in this study.

Conflicts of Interest: The authors declare no conflict of interest.

References

1. D'Errico, M. Immersive Virtual Reality as an International Collaborative Space for Innovative Simulation Design. *Clin. Simul. Nurs.* **2021**, *54*, 30–34. [CrossRef]
2. Aebersold, M.; Rasmussen, J.; Mulrenin, T. Virtual Everest: Immersive Virtual Reality Can Improve the Simulation Experience. *Clin. Simul. Nurs.* **2020**, *38*, 1–4. [CrossRef]
3. Yang, S.-Y.; Oh, Y.-H. The effects of neonatal resuscitation gamification program using immersive virtual reality: A quasi-experimental study. *Nurse Educ. Today* **2022**, *117*, 105464. [CrossRef] [PubMed]
4. Sharma, R.S.; Yang, Y. A Hybrid Scenario Planning Methodology for Interactive Digital Media. *Long Range Plan.* **2015**, *48*, 412–429. [CrossRef]
5. Özkan, T.K.; Polat, F. The Effect of Virtual Reality and Kaleidoscope on Pain and Anxiety Levels during Venipuncture in Children. *J. PeriAnesthesia Nurs.* **2020**, *35*, 206–211. [CrossRef]
6. Tennant, M.; Anderson, N.; Youssef, G.J.; McMillan, L.; Thorson, R.; Wheeler, G.; McCarthy, M.C. Effects of immersive virtual reality exposure in preparing pediatric oncology patients for radiation therapy. *Tech. Innov. Patient Support Radiat. Oncol.* **2021**, *19*, 18–25. [CrossRef]
7. Sandoval, L.R.; Buckey, J.C.; Ainslie, R.; Tombari, M.; Stone, W.; Hegel, M.T. Randomized Controlled Trial of a Computerized Interactive Media-Based Problem Solving Treatment for Depression. *Behav. Ther.* **2017**, *48*, 413–425. [CrossRef]
8. Gan, B.; Menkhoff, T.; Smith, R. Enhancing students' learning process through interactive digital media: New opportunities for collaborative learning. *Comput. Hum. Behav.* **2015**, *51*, 652–663. [CrossRef]
9. Bayram, S.B.; Caliskan, N. Effect of a game-based virtual reality phone application on tracheostomy care education for nursing students: A randomized controlled trial. *Nurse Educ. Today* **2019**, *79*, 25–31. [CrossRef]
10. Liaw, S.Y.; Wu, L.T.; Soh, S.L.H.; Ringsted, C.; Lau, T.C.; Lim, W.S. Virtual Reality Simulation in Interprofessional Round Training for Health Care Students: A Qualitative Evaluation Study. *Clin. Simul. Nurs.* **2020**, *45*, 42–46. [CrossRef]
11. Smith, P.C.; Hamilton, B.K. The Effects of Virtual Reality Simulation as a Teaching Strategy for Skills Preparation in Nursing Students. *Clin. Simul. Nurs.* **2015**, *11*, 52–58. [CrossRef]
12. Botha, B.S.; de Wet, L.; Botma, Y. Undergraduate Nursing Student Experiences in Using Immersive Virtual Reality to Manage a Patient with a Foreign Object in the Right Lung. *Clin. Simul. Nurs.* **2021**, *56*, 76–83. [CrossRef]
13. Ferrandini Price, M.; Escribano Tortosa, D.; Nieto Fernandez-Pacheco, A.; Perez Alonso, N.; Cerón Madrigal, J.J.; Melendreras-Ruiz, R.; García-Collado, Á.J.; Pardo Rios, M.; Juguera Rodriguez, L. Comparative study of a simulated incident with multiple victims and immersive virtual reality. *Nurse Educ. Today* **2018**, *71*, 48–53. [CrossRef] [PubMed]
14. Servotte, J.-C.; Goosse, M.; Campbell, S.H.; Dardenne, N.; Pilote, B.; Simoneau, I.L.; Guillaume, M.; Bragard, I.; Ghuysen, A. Virtual Reality Experience: Immersion, Sense of Presence, and Cybersickness. *Clin. Simul. Nurs.* **2020**, *38*, 35–43. [CrossRef]
15. Chávez, O.L.; Rodríguez, L.-F.; Gutierrez-Garcia, J.O. A comparative case study of 2D, 3D and immersive-virtual-reality applications for healthcare education. *Int. J. Med. Inform.* **2020**, *141*, 104226. [CrossRef]
16. Jeon, J.; Kim, J.H.; Choi, E.H. Needs Assessment for a VR-Based Adult Nursing Simulation Training Program for Korean Nursing Students: A Qualitative Study Using Focus Group Interviews. *Int. J. Environ. Res. Public Health* **2020**, *17*, 8880. [CrossRef]

17. Wang, C.-M.; Tsai, T.-C.; Peng, C.-H. The research of applying interactive technology and multi-interactive interface of smartphone into theme park applications. *Int. J. Digit. Media Des.* **2016**, *8*, 12–24.
18. Lu, L.S.; Ho, Y.F. A study on the behavior and emotion of the active aging groups' ecotourism travel experience: Needs survey on the use of interactive technology. *J. Gerontechnol. Serv. Manag.* **2015**, *3*, 223–234. [CrossRef]
19. Hsieh, Y.-L.; Chen, C.-H.; Lai, Y.-H. Inspiration and creativity: Visitor study of virtual reality-based museum exhibition. *Museol. Q.* **2019**, *33*, 49–73. [CrossRef]
20. Wang, S.-W.; Xu, Q.; Lin, M.-L.; Wang, M.-C.; Guo, J.-L. Evaluation of University educators on the promotion of innovative anti-drug textbooks. *J. Healthy Life Success. Aging* **2019**, *11*, 56–73.
21. Cheng, S.W.; Chang, K.C.; Chen, J.T. Analyzing the effectiveness of using virtual reality in pharmacy education. *Cheng Ching Med. J.* **2021**, *18*, 22–27.
22. Lin, S.-C. Applying virtual reality assisted critical thinking training programs among nurse practitioners. *J. Nurs.* **2021**, *68*, 18–23. [CrossRef]
23. Jiang, R.P.; Chou, Y.F. Tutoring nursing via VR. *Tzu Chi Nurs. J.* **2021**, *21*, 32–33.
24. Wells-Beede, E.; Garcia, B.; Chun, S.W.; Kicklighter, C.; Seo, J.H. Creative Solutions for Complex Circumstances: The Utilization of Virtual Reality in a Specialty Course. *Clin. Simul. Nurs.* **2022**, *65*, 82–85. [CrossRef]
25. Wood, J.; Ebert, L.; Duff, J. Implementation Methods of Virtual Reality Simulation and the Impact on Confidence and Stress When Learning Patient Resuscitation: An Integrative Review. *Clin. Simul. Nurs.* **2022**, *66*, 5–17. [CrossRef]
26. Saab, M.M.; Hegarty, J.; Murphy, D.; Landers, M. Incorporating virtual reality in nurse education: A qualitative study of nursing students' perspectives. *Nurse Educ. Today* **2021**, *105*, 105045. [CrossRef]
27. Miskowiak, K.W.; Jespersen, A.E.; Kessing, L.V.; Aggestrup, A.S.; Glenthøj, L.B.; Nordentoft, M.; Ott, C.V.; Lumbye, A. Cognition Assessment in Virtual Reality: Validity and feasibility of a novel virtual reality test for real-life cognitive functions in mood disorders and psychosis spectrum disorders. *J. Psychiatr. Res.* **2022**, *145*, 182–189. [CrossRef] [PubMed]
28. Ugur, E.; Konukseven, B.O. The potential use of virtual reality in vestibular rehabilitation of motion sickness. *Auris Nasus Larynx* **2022**, *49*, 768–781. [CrossRef]
29. Sen, S.; Usta, E.; Bozdemir, H. The effect of mobile virtual reality on operating room nursing education. *Teach. Learn. Nurs.* **2022**, *17*, 199–202. [CrossRef]
30. Gillespie, G.L.; Farra, S.; Regan, S.L.; Brammer, S.V. Impact of Immersive Virtual Reality Simulations for Changing Knowledge, Attitudes, and Behaviors. *Nurse Educ. Today* **2021**, *105*, 105025. [CrossRef]

MDPI AG
Grosspeteranlage 5
4052 Basel
Switzerland
Tel.: +41 61 683 77 34

Healthcare Editorial Office
E-mail: healthcare@mdpi.com
www.mdpi.com/journal/healthcare

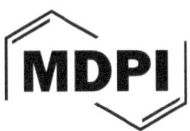

Disclaimer/Publisher's Note: The title and front matter of this reprint are at the discretion of the Guest Editors. The publisher is not responsible for their content or any associated concerns. The statements, opinions and data contained in all individual articles are solely those of the individual Editors and contributors and not of MDPI. MDPI disclaims responsibility for any injury to people or property resulting from any ideas, methods, instructions or products referred to in the content.

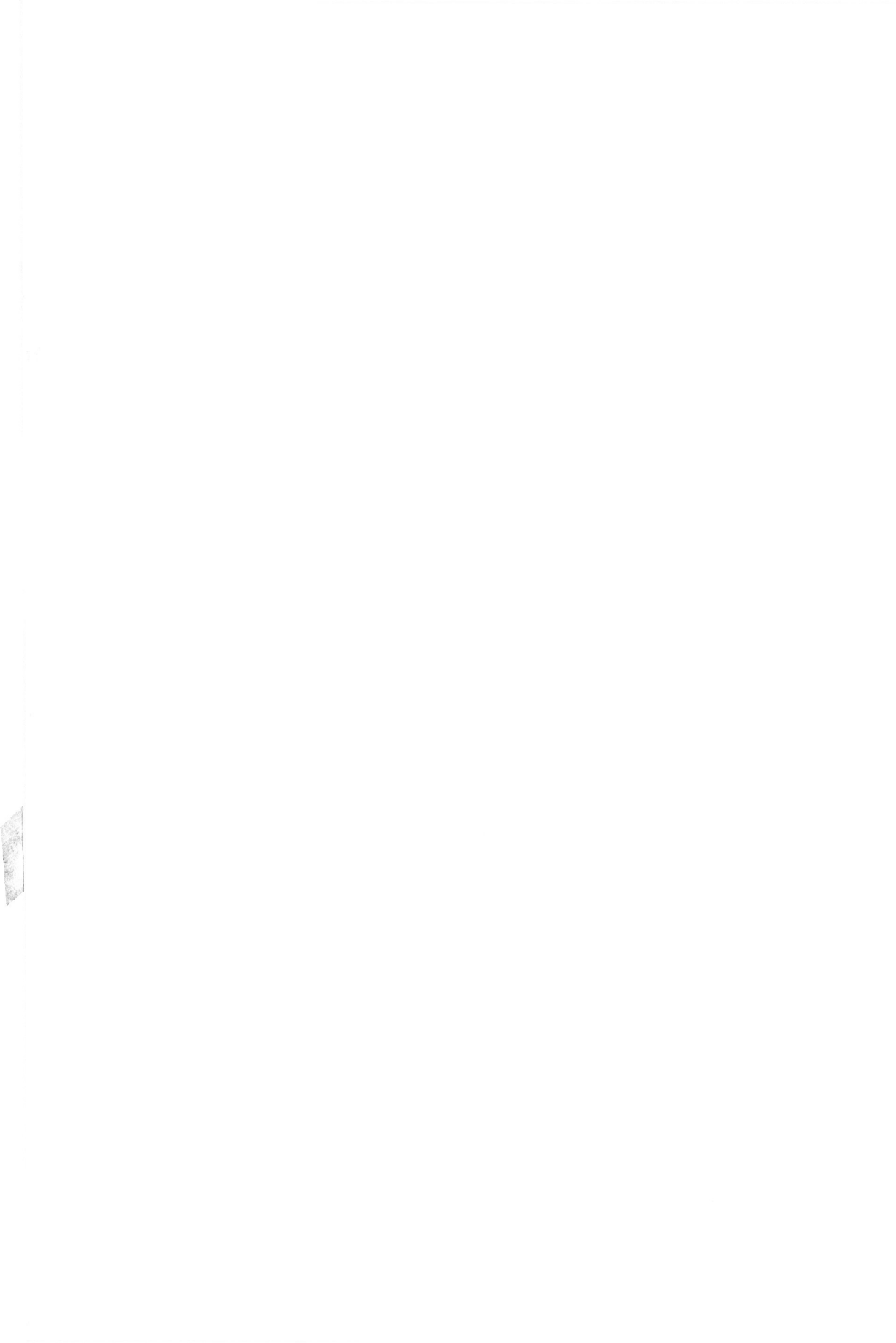

www.ingramcontent.com/pod-product-compliance
Lightning Source LLC
LaVergne TN
LVHW072357090526
838202LV00019B/2564